PROGRESS IN CLINICAL AND BIOLOGICAL RESEARCH

RECENT TITLES

Vol 50: **Rights and Responsibilities in Modern Medicine: The Second Volume in a Series on Ethics, Humanism, and Medicine**, Marc D. Basson, *Editor*

Vol 51: **The Function of Red Blood Cells: Erythrocyte Pathobiology**, Donald F. H. Wallach, *Editor*

Vol 52: **Conduction Velocity Distributions: A Population Approach to Electrophysiology of Nerve**, Leslie J. Dorfman, Kenneth L. Cummins, and Larry J. Leifer, *Editors*

Vol 53: **Cancer Among Black Populations**, Curtis Mettlin and Gerald P. Murphy, *Editors*

Vol 54: **Connective Tissue Research: Chemistry, Biology, and Physiology**, Zdenek Deyl and Milan Adam, *Editors*

Vol 55: **The Red Cell: Fifth Ann Arbor Conference**, George J. Brewer, *Editor*

Vol 56: **Erythrocyte Membranes 2: Recent Clinical and Experimental Advances**, Walter C. Kruckeberg, John W. Eaton, and George J. Brewer, *Editors*

Vol 57: **Progress in Cancer Control**, Curtis Mettlin and Gerald P. Murphy, *Editors*

Vol 58: **The Lymphocyte**, Kenneth W. Sell and William V. Miller, *Editors*

Vol 59: **Eleventh International Congress of Anatomy**, Enrique Acosta Vidrio, *Editor-in-Chief*. Published in 3 volumes:
Part A: **Glial and Neuronal Cell Biology**, Sergey Fedoroff, *Editor*
Part B: **Advances in the Morphology of Cells and Tissues**, Miguel A. Galina, *Editor*
Part C: **Biological Rhythms in Structure and Function**, Heinz von Mayersbach, Lawrence E. Scheving, and John E. Pauly, *Editors*

Vol 60: **Advances in Hemoglobin Analysis**, Samir M. Hanash and George J. Brewer, *Editors*

Vol 61: **Nutrition and Child Health: Perspectives for the 1980s**, Reginald C. Tsang and Buford Lee Nichols, Jr., *Editors*

Vol 62: **Pathophysiological Effects of Endotoxins at the Cellular Level**, Jeannine A. Majde and Robert J. Person, *Editors*

Vol 63: **Membrane Transport and Neuroreceptors**, Dale Oxender, Arthur Blume, Ivan Diamond, and C. Fred Fox, *Editors*

Vol 64: **Bacteriophage Assembly**, Michael S. DuBow, *Editor*

Vol 65: **Apheresis: Development, Applications, and Collection Procedures**, C. Harold Mielke, Jr., *Editor*

Vol 66: **Control of Cellular Division and Development**, Dennis Cunningham, Eugene Goldwasser, James Watson, and C. Fred Fox, *Editors*. Published in 2 Volumes.

Vol 67: **Nutrition in the 1980s: Constraints on Our Knowledge**, Nancy Selvey and Philip L. White, *Editors*

Vol 68: **The Role of Peptides and Amino Acids as Neurotransmitters**, J. Barry Lombardini and Alexander D. Kenny, *Editors*

Vol 69: **Twin Research 3, Proceedings of the Third International Congress on Twin Studies,** Luigi Gedda, Paolo Parisi, and Walter E. Nance, *Editors*. Published in 3 volumes:
Part A: **Twin Biology and Multiple Pregnancy**
Part B: **Intelligence, Personality, and Development**
Part C: **Epidemiological and Clinical Studies**

Vol 70: **Reproductive Immunology,** Norbert Gleicher, *Editor*

Vol 71: **Psychopharmacology of Clonidine,** Harbans Lal and Stuart Fielding, *Editors*

Vol 72: **Hemophilia and Hemostasis,** Doris Ménaché, D. MacN. Surgenor, and Harlan D. Anderson, *Editors*

Vol 73: **Membrane Biophysics: Structure and Function in Epithelia,** Mumtaz A. Dinno and Arthur B. Callahan, *Editors*

Vol 74: **Physiopathology of Endocrine Diseases and Mechanisms of Hormone Action,** Roberto J. Soto, Alejandro De Nicola, and Jorge Blaquier, *Editors*

Vol 75: **The Prostatic Cell: Structure and Function,** Gerald P. Murphy, Avery A. Sandberg, and James P. Karr, *Editors*. Published in 2 volumes:
Part A: **Morphologic, Secretory, and Biochemical Aspects**
Part B: **Prolactin, Carcinogenesis, and Clinical Aspects**

Vol 76: **Troubling Problems in Medical Ethics: The Third Volume in a Series on Ethics, Humanism, and Medicine,** Marc D. Basson, Rachel E. Lipson, and Doreen L. Ganos, *Editors*

Vol 77: **Nutrition in Health and Disease and International Development: Symposia From the XII International Congress of Nutrition,** Alfred E. Harper and George K. Davis, *Editors*

Vol 78: **Female Incontinence,** Norman R. Zinner and Arthur M. Sterling, *Editors*

Vol 79: **Proteins in the Nervous System: Structure and Function,** Bernard Haber, Joe Dan Coulter, and Jose Regino Perez-Polo, *Editors*

Vol 80: **Mechanism and Control of Ciliary Movement,** Charles J. Brokaw and Pedro Verdugo, *Editors*

Vol 81: **Physiology and Biology of Horseshoe Crabs: Studies on Normal and Environmentally Stressed Animals,** Joseph Bonaventura and Celia Bonaventura, *Editors*

Vol 82: **Clinical, Structural, and Biochemical Advances in Hereditary Eye Disorders,** Donna L. Daentl, *Editor*

Vol 83: **Issues in Cancer Screening and Communications,** Curtis Mettlin and Gerald P. Murphy, *Editors*

Vol 84: **Progress in Dermatoglyphic Research,** Christos S. Bartsocas, *Editor*

See pages 473-474 for previous titles in this series

PROGRESS IN DERMATOGLYPHIC RESEARCH

PROGRESS IN DERMATOGLYPHIC RESEARCH

Based on the Proceedings of an International Conference on Dermatoglyphics, Athens, Greece September 20–23, 1981

Editor

Christos S. Bartsocas
Second Department of Pediatrics
University of Athens
Athens, Greece

ALAN R. LISS, INC., NEW YORK

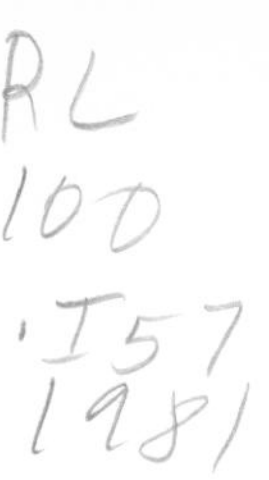

Address all Inquiries to the Publisher
Alan R. Liss, Inc., 150 Fifth Avenue, New York, NY 10011

Printed in the United States of America.

Library of Congress Cataloging in Publication Data

International Conference on Dermatoglyphics (1981:
Athens, Greece)
Progress in dermatoglyphic research.

(Progress in clinical and biological research;
v. 84)
Includes index.
1. Dermatoglyphics—Congresses. I. Bartsocas
Christos S. II. Title. III. Series
RL100.I57 1981 573′.677 82-215
ISBN 0-8451-0084-X AACR2

Contents

SESSION III

EMBRYOGENESIS

SESSION IV

NONHUMAN PRIMATE DERMATOGLYPHICS

SESSION V

POPULATION DERMATOGLYPHICS

SESSION VI

MEDICAL APPLICATIONS

Contributors

Nasr F. Abdullah [269]
Department of Biology, College of Education, Baghdad University, Baghdad, Iraq

Harmien W.M. Amesz-Voorhoeve [93]
State University Groningen, The Netherlands

Monika Bär [371]
Institute of Human Genetics, University of the Saar, Homburg, Federal Republic of Germany

Christos S. Bartsocas [xv, 139, 247]
Second Department of Pediatrics, University of Athens, Athens, Greece

Abdülbari Bener [145]
Istanbul Technical University, Department of Environmental Engineering, Taksim, Taskisla, Istanbul, Turkey

A.M. Budy [285, 295]
Department of Genetics and Cancer Center of Hawaii, University of Hawaii, Honolulu, Hawaii

M. Castello [385]
Department of Pediatrics II, State University of Rome, Rome, Italy

V. Curró [385]
Department of Pediatrics, Catholic University of Rome, Rome, Italy

Karen Davis [353]
Division of Medical Genetics, Department of Pediatrics, Meharry Medical College, Nashville, Tennessee

André G. de Wilde [93]
State University Groningen, The Netherlands

Awatif El-Mazni [393]
Department of Pediatrics, Children's Hospital, Cairo University, Cairo, Egypt

Lilly K. El Meniawi [393]
Human Genetics Department, National Research Center, Dokki, Cairo, Egypt

Carol E. Fahrenbruch [189]
Departments of Anthropology and Orthodontics and Regional Primate Research Center, University of Washington, Seattle, Washington

The bold face number in brackets following each contributor's name indicates the opening page of that author's paper.

Virginia Inés Fortich Baca [157]
Facultad de Filosofía y Letras, Departamento de Ciencias Antropológicas, Universidad de Buenos Aires, Buenos Aires, Argentina

Fawzia H. Hussien [393]
Human Genetics Department, National Research Center, Dokki, Cairo, Egypt

R.L. Jantz [325]
Veterans Administration Medical Center, Minneapolis, Minnesota and University of Tennessee, Knoxville, Tennessee

Sue Barden Johnson [33,325]
Veterans Administration Medical Center, Minneapolis, Minnesota and University of Tennessee, Knoxville, Tennessee

M. Shariff Kamali [317]
Center for Iranian Anthropology, Markaz Mardom Shenasi Iran, Ministry of Culture and Higher Education, Baharestan Tehran, Iran

B. Karmakar [111]
Anthropometry and Human Genetics Unit, Indian Statistical Institute, Calcutta, India

M. Bat-Miriam Katznelson [335, 435]
Department of Human Genetics, Tel-Aviv University Medical School, Institute of Human Genetics, The Sheba Medical Center, Tel-Hashomer, Israel

H. Warner Kloepfer [105]
Department of Anatomy, Tulane University, New Orleans, Louisiana

R. Kolski [427]
Department Genética, Facultad de Humanidades y Ciencias, Montevideo, Uruguay

S. Kritsikis [247]
Department of Cardiology, University of Athens, Athens, Greece

Danuta Z. Loesch [45]
Department of Genetics, Psychoneurological Institute, Warsaw, Poland

K.C. Malhotra [111, 203]
Anthropometry and Human Genetics Unit, Indian Statistical Institute, Calcutta, India

R. Mastrangelo [385]
Department of Pediatrics, Catholic University of Rome, Rome, Italy

P.P. Mastroiacovo [385]
Department of Pediatrics, Catholic University of Rome, Rome, Italy

Ichiro Matsui [129]
Divisions of Research Promotion and Medical Genetics, Kanagawa Children's Medical Center, Yokohama, Japan

Jamshed Mavalwala [13]
Department of Anthropology, University of Toronto, Toronto, Canada

Florence C.C. Mi [421]
Department of Genetics, University of Hawaii, Honolulu, Hawaii

M.P. Mi [285, 295, 421]
Department of Genetics and Cancer Center of Hawaii, University of Hawaii, Honolulu, Hawaii

Amal A. Moussa [393]
Pediatrics Department, Children's Hospital, Cairo University, Cairo, Egypt

Laura Newell-Morris [189]
Departments of Anthropology and Orthodontics and Regional Primate Research Center, University of Washington, Seattle, Washington

Michio Okajima [175]
Department of Forensic Medicine, Tokyo Medical and Dental University, Yushima, Bunkyo-ku, Tokyo, Japan

M. Oyhenart-Perera [427]
Department Genética, Facultad de Humanidades y Ciencias, Montevideo, Uruguay

Th. Panayotou [247]
Department of Cardiology, University of Athens, Athens, Greece

C.J. Papadatos [247]
Second Department of Pediatrics, University of Athens, P. and A. Kyriakou Children's Hospital, Athens, Greece

Chris C. Plato [1, 25, 247]
Gerontology Research Center NIA, NIH, Baltimore City Hospitals, Baltimore, Maryland

M.N. Rashad [285, 295]
Department of Genetics and Cancer Center of Hawaii, University of Hawaii, Honolulu, Hawaii

Sigrid Reicke [371]
Institute of Human Genetics, Univeristy of the Saar, Homburg, Federal Republic of Germany

D.F. Roberts [79]
Department of Human Genetics, University of Newcastle upon Tyne, England

Alexander Rodewald [371, 451]
Institute of Human Genetics, University of the Saar, Homburg, Federal Republic of Germany

C. Romagnoli [385]
Department of Pediatrics, Catholic University of Rome, Rome, Italy

Mouchira Abdel Salam [393]
Human Genetics Department, National Research Center, Dokki, Cairo, Egypt

G. Salvat [427]
Department Genética, Facultad de Humanidades y Ciencias, Montevideo, Uruguay

Blanka Schaumann [33, 325]
Veterans Administration Medical Center, Minneapolis, Minnesota

G. Segni [385]
Department of Pediatrics, Catholic University of Rome, Rome, Italy

Dharmdeo N. Singh [353]
Division of Medical Genetics, Department of Pediatrics, Meharry Medical College, Nashville, Tennessee

R.D. Singh [303]
Department of Sociology and Anthropology, University of Windsor, Windsor, Ontario, Canada

Samia A. Temtamy [393]
Human Genetics Department, National Research Center, Dokki, Cairo, Egypt

S. Varonos [247]
Athens Naval Hospital, Athens, Greece

M. Vijayakumar [111]
Anthropometry and Human Genetics Unit, Indian Statistical Institute, Calcutta, India

Wladimir Wertelecki [1,25]
Department of Medical Genetics, University of South Alabama Medical School, Mobile, Alabama

Cynthia Yost [189]
Departments of Anthropology and Orthodontics and Regional Primate Research Center, University of Washington, Seattle, Washington

Karen Zahn-Messow [451]
Department of Pediatrics, University of Munich, Federal Republic of Germany

Mouchira E. Zaki [393]
Human Genetics Department, National Research Center, Dokki, Cairo, Egypt

Klaus D. Zang [371]
Institute of Human Genetics, University of the Saar, Homburg, Federal Republic of Germany

Heinrich Zankl [371]
Division of Human Biology and Human Genetics, University of Kaiserlautern, Federal Republic of Germany

Merve Zankl [371]
Institute of Human Genetics, University of the Saar, Federal Republic of Germany

PREFACE

Dermatoglyphics as a tool in human or medical genetics and in physical anthropology has provided important information during the last two decades. It is not surprising, therefore, that several books have appeared on the subject by eminent investigators recently. Nevertheless, new information about dermatoglyphics is accumulating every day. "Dermatoglyphics" the society publication of the International Dermatoglyphics Association is published for the dissemination of new findings in the field.

The present volume contains most of the lectures and several of the communications presented at the International Conference on Dermatoglyphics which was held in Athens, Greece, September 20-23, 1981. The 1981 conference, which was held under the auspices of the Ministry of Culture and Sciences of Greece, was jointly sponsored by the International Dermatoglyphics Association and the Second Department of Pediatrics of the University of Athens.

The subjects presented in the volume range widely from mathematical considerations to clinical applications of dermatoglyphics. The articles offer additional evidence that the field is not exhausted, that there is new information accumulating from recent research and that there is still ample ground available for further investigations.

The editor expresses his appreciation to the Ministry of Culture and Sciences of Greece for supporting the conference, to the many colleagues and contributors, who made this publication possible and to the publisher, Alan R.Liss, and his associates for meticulous attention and for the remarkably expeditious processing and publishing of this volume.

Christos S. Bartsocas, M.D.
Athens, Greece

Progress in Dermatoglyphic Research, pages 1–11

CHANGING TRENDS IN DERMATOGLYPHIC RESEARCH

CHRIS C. PLATO

Gerontology Research Center, NIA
Baltimore City Hospitals
Baltimore, Maryland 21224 USA

WLADIMIR WERTELECKI

Department of Medical Genetics
University of South Alabama
Mobile, Alabama 36617 USA

INTRODUCTION

Dermatoglyphics as an independent discipline and research tool has made great advances during the past fifteen years. Collection of dermatoglyphic data is no longer just a part of descriptive anthropology. Dermatoglyphic data are now collected specifically for population genetic surveys, for clinical and anthropological studies and are considered as an integral part of most pediatric case reports. The expanded spectrum in the utilization of dermatoglyphic data makes new demands and imposes greater responsibilities upon workers in dermatoglyphic research, the International Dermatoglyphic Association, the various National dermatoglyphic associations and on the participants of this gathering who are expected by the membership to provide leadership and direction. This is for all of us a time for soul searching. A time to look back and follow the progress in dermatoglyphics during the past one hundred and fifty years. It is also a time to evaluate the present status of dermatoglyphic research, to reasses our objectives and to formulate guidelines for future research.

It is not the intention of the present treatise to review the dermatoglyphic literature. This is not the proper forum for such undertaking. Besides, the recent publication of several outstanding reviews, such as those of

Mavalwala (1978) and Robert Meier (1980) to mention only two, render another review here redundant.

What I want to do during the next twenty-five minutes or so is, first to recall briefly four of the major milestones in dermatoglyphics established by the contributions of Johannes Purkinje, Sir Francis Galton, Harris Wilder and Harold Cummins. Second to take a look at the present status of dermatoglyphic research and finally to see where we can go from here and how. I will not provide many answers. I will only open the discussion by raising some questions, hoping that further discussion and answers would come from this meeting. I know that the two speakers after me, Dr. Mavalwala and Dr. Wertelecki, Presidents of the International and American Dermatoglyphics Associations, respectively, will follow with more specific discussions. I am sure other speakers will do the same.

Eventhough the term "dermatoglyphics" was coined by Cummins in 1926, interest in the papillary ridges and their patterns extends back to antiquity as Dr. Bartsocas will tell us on in another presentation of this conference (1982). It is generally accepted that the systematic study of papillary patterns began with the publication of Purkinje's thesis (1823). This means that the beginning of dermatoglyphics preceded the publication of the work of Gregor Mendel in Genetics (1865).

Purkinje, a Czech physiologist and biologist , wrote his thesis on the Physiological Examination of the Visual Organ and of the Cutaneous system ("Commentatio de Examine Physiologioc Organi Visus et Systematis Cutanei"). The thesis is only 58 pages long and only 23 of these are devoted to the study of the skin. The thesis was written in Latin with a number of Greek terms and from what the translators claim, it is far from being a work of literary art. Nevertheless, scientifically speaking, it represents a classic pioneering study of both the eye and the skin. According to Galton (1892), Purkinje's thesis has "been referred to by nearly all subsequent writers of whom there is reason to suspect never saw it, but contented themselves with quoting a very small portion at second hand". There were only three original copies in existence. One of them is presently in the United States and another one in the Library of the Royal College of Surgeons in London. The whereabouts of the third one are unknown. Partial translation of certain passages of Purkinje's thesis appear in Galton's book "Fingerprints" (1892). More recently Cummins and Kennedy (1940) published the English translation of the section on the "External Physiological Examination of the Integumentary System".

Purkinje's principle contribution to dermatoglyphics is the classification of fingertip patterns into nine types. Some time ago I was able to locate the United States copy of the thesis and reproduced the part of the plate (figures 7-15) which shows the nine types of fingerprint patterns (figure 1). These are very close to the present fingertip pattern classification (table 1).

After Purkinje the next milestone in dermatoglyphics was formed by the work of the genius of a scientist, Sir Francis Galton, who, among other contributions to science, wrote the classic book, "Fingerprints" (1892). Eventhough the primary objective of Galton's fingerprint work was to develop a personal identification system, he eventually reported on the biological variation as shown by fingerprints, the permanence of fingerprint patterns through longitudinal examinations, the inheritance and finally the racial variation of fingerprint patterns. Galton used Purkinje's classification as a model and proceeded to describe the various types of configurations in great detail as well as many of the transitional forms (1890). Galton's expended fingerprint pattern classification was based on the triangular plots or triradii, formed by the divergence of adjacent ridges. He coined many of the dermatoglyphic terms we use today. He defined the arch as the situation when the ridges travel paralled to each other from one side of the pattern to the other. In the loop the ridges have one recurving ridge, but no twist, while in the whorls, the ridges go at least over one circle or duplex spiral.

In addition to developing an elaborate fingerprint classification, Galton outlined detailed technical and methological procedures for taking prints and tracing key ridges from which patterns are classified (1892). He proposed a method for measuring the size of patterns either by absolute measurement from the center of the plot (pattern area) or by counting ridges per 1/10th of an inch. He recognized and studied the increased dermatoglyphic concordance among sibs and a limited number of twins as compared to unrelated individuals. He also reported briefly on

Figure 1. The nine fingerprint pattern types of Purkinje (from Purkinje 1823). See Table 1 for explanation.

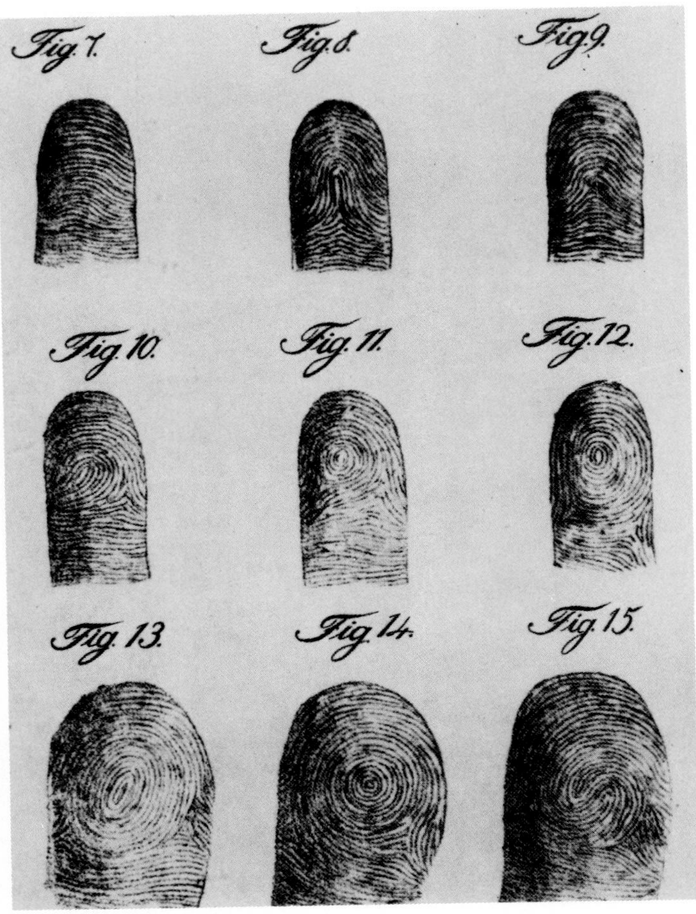

Table 1. The nine fingerprint pattern types of Purkinje (see figure 1).

Figure	Purkinje's Nomenclature[1]	English Translation[2]	Present Term[2]
7	Flexurae transversae	Transverse Curves	Arch
8	Stria centralis longitudinalis	Central Longitudinal Stripe	Tented Arch
9	Stria obliqua	Oblique Stripe	Loop, Ulnar or Radial
10	Sinus obliquus	Oblique Loop	Loop, Ulnar or Radial
11	Amygdalus	Almond	Almond Whorl
12	Spirula	Spiral	Spiral Whorl
13	Ellipsis	Ellipse	Elliptical Whorl
14	Circulus	Circle	Circular Whorl
15	Vortex Dupplicatus	Double Whorl	Twin Loop

[1] From J. Purkinge (1823)

[2] From Cummins & Kennedy (1940)

palmar ridges. However, it was Harris Wilder who pioneered comprehensive studies on the methodology, inheritance and racial variation of the palmar and plantar papillary ridges. The works of Wilder and his wife, the former Inez Whipple, published during the first quarter of the twentieth century, formed the next important milestone in dermatoglyphic research.

Wilder (1902) published the first serious study of palmar dermatoglyphics under the title "Palms and Soles." This was followed by several other elaborate reports in which he covered all aspects of palmar and plantar dermatoglyphics. (Wilder 1904; 1904a;1916) It was Wilder who: (1) identified the a, b, c and d (small letters) digital triradii; (2) named the Main Lines A, B, C, and D (large letters) to represent the paths of the ridges which travel from each triradius; (3) He assigned the numerical values at the periphery of the palm for qualifying the main line terminations of both the palms and the soles. (4) He introduced the mainline formulae and (5) he studied the palmar patterns in the hypothenar and thenar regions as well as the interdigital areas. He did the same with the soles. Eventhough all of these innovations are presently used widely in dermatoglyphics research, little credit is given to Wilder for his contributions. Many investigators give credit and reference for these methods to Cummins and Midlo instead. Wilder (1904), in his paper on the "Racial Differences in Palm and Sole Configuration", concluded that "eventhough there is much individual variation in all races, if one studies a large number of prints and averages, the occurence of the various features, these averages will be constant or nearly constant for a given race. Thus, such results will serve to distinguish peoples widely different from each other, but will not be reliable in comparing related tribes". In other words, he recognized the importance and limitations of dermatoglyphics to physical anthropology and population studies.

Wilder also reported on the palmar and plantar dermatoglyphic similarities in twins and triplets (1904a). During the same year that Wilder published his paper on racial differentiation (1904), his wife Inez Whipple (1904) published her classic treatise on "The Ventral Surface of the Mammalian Chiridium" which represents the first serious effort to study non-human epidermal ridges.

The next milestone in dermatoglyphic research is represented by the work of Cummins which started with his coining of the term "DERMATOGLYPHICS" in 1926 and culminated with the publication, with Charles Midlo, of the classic book "FINGER PRINTS, PALMS AND SOLES" (Cummins & Midlo 1943). Cummins introduced the term Dermatoglyphics at the 42nd annual meeting of the American Association of Anatomists in April 1926 and followed it up the same year in the publication "Palmar and Plantar Epidermal Configurations (DERMATOGLYPHICS) in European Americans" (Cummins & Midlo 1926). He proposed the term dermatoglyphics "both as a designation of the division of anatomy embracing the surface markings of the skin... and as a collective name for the integumentary features themselves... As a name for the skin markings, dermatoglyphics applies only to ridges and their arrangements. Flexion creases and other secondary folds being without the bonds of its intended meaning." Cummins also made some refinements to Wilder's main line termination definitions (cummins et al 1929). The propsed division of termination 5 into 5' and 5" and the acceptance of X and 0 as symbols for aberrant and absent C line. Cummins contributed to all aspects of dermatoglyphics research, methodology, anatomy, embryology, genetics and racial variation and medicine. His original observations on the dermatoglyphic stigmata of mongolism (Cummins 1936;1939) formed the springboard for the present surge in medical dermatoglyphic research. However, the most important contribution of Harold Cummins to the field of dermatoglyphics is that he refined the existing methodology, organized and consolidated most dermatoglyphic contributions up to his time, ranging from personal identification to medicine, and published them, with his long time collaborator Charles Midlo, into a simple well written book "FINGER PRINTS, PALMS AND SOLES" (Cummins & Midlo 1943).

During the post war years and especially during the past two decades, dermatoglyphics has entered into a new and very rapidly expanding phase. It attracted disciples from such diverse fields such as mathematics, embryology, computer science, anthropology, anatomy, genetics and medicine. The post war era of dermatoglyphic research was championed by David Rife, Sara Holt, Lionell Penrose, Margarite Weninger to mention only a few, and many of the participants of this symposium.

During the past ten to fifteen years, we witnessed new directions in dermatoglyphic research. Eventhough the collection and evaluation of descriptive data is still a primary task, we are looking into new ways to utilize these data for answering medical anthropological, genetic and evolutionary questions. There is no doubt that research is indeed changing and progressing at an impressive rate. What remains to be seen now is whether we as individual researchers, our laboratories, and the various national and international dermatoglyphics associations, are meeting the new challenges.

In some aspects we have met these challenges with considerable success. We have created new channels of communication and exchange of ideas through dermatoglyphic associations and several dermatoglyphics conferences. The International Dermatoglyphics Association has over 300 active members. The American Dermatoglyphics Association has almost 150 members. Other regional dermatoglyphics associations are also either active or are in the process of establishment. Dermatoglyphic papers appear regularly in a number of respected national and international journals, and dermatoglyphic description has become an integral part of many clinical reports. The International Dermatoglyphics Association has been publishing its own bulletin for the past two years and plans are now underway to convert that publication into a formal journal. During the past five years there have been nine dermatoglyphic conferences with international participation. Two of them took place within the past ten days. The American Dermatoglyphics Association has been holding annual meetings or symposia for the past six years. Other national associations also hold regular meetings.

As a result of these meetings and publications more scientists were attracted to dermatoglyphic research. This in turn resulted in collection of more data and consequently more publications. The expansion of dermatoglyphic research rekindled some old problems and created new concerns. Some of these concerns will be addressed in detail by speakers of this conferenc while others will have to be dealt by smaller committees. For the remaining five minutes I would like to comment briefly on some of these problems in order to get the discussion started.

The first problem is the issue of nomenclature and terminology. There are two major nomenclature schools, the Cummins and the Penrose. In addition to these two there are a number of other more specific notations introduced by various investigators during the past few years. For the sake of comparability, it is imperative that some sort of standardized nomenclature be established. Dr. Mavalwala and a commitee of the International Dermatoglyphic Association has been considering this issue recently, and hopefully a progress report will be forthcoming soon.

A second issue, somewhat related to the nomenclature is the training of technical personnel. Eventhough some of the introductory courses in physical anthropology and human genetics do make mention of dermatoglyphics, there are no formal sessions for training students in dermatoglyphic techniques. It is important that intensive efforts be made to formalize a short course for training students in collecting, reading and evaluating dermatoglyphic data. This is something the national organizations can do more efficiently. In addition to training technical personnel, seminars and workshops are needed to introduce professionals of related fields into the basic principles of dermatoglyphics, their advantages and their limitations. Because of its inherent advantages as a research tool, dermatoglyphics attracted professionals from several fields. While most of them made significant contributions to dermatoglyphic research, a few of them have been doing considerable damage by publishing papers of little or no scientific merit and making unsubstantiated claims. Those of you who review manuscripts for journals should do the utmost to prevent publication of manuscripts of poor quality.

The last issue I want to raise is that of collaboration and data sharing. The availability of computer facilities in some countries have enabled investigators not only to handle, store, retrieve and analyze large volumes of data in very short time but also to devise and employ very complex models. In other countries on the other hand, computer facilities are completely out of reach of many investigators who have collections of valuable data begging for analysis. This disparity needs to be narrowed by closer collaboration between those with facilities and those with data.

In clinical situations it is many times impossible for a single investigator to collect enough data of certain rare syndromes for meaningful analysis. Yet, if two or more investigators pool their material, a first rate study will result. What is needed in this case is some sort of organized effort to bring together data, facilities and research workers for maximum utilization of all three resources.

Dr. Wertelecki and I have been working towards the creation of a dermatoglyphics repository and we should have a report very shortly. Dr. Wertelecki will elaborate further on this issue later in this session.

In summary during the past thirty minutes, we tried to trace the major stages in the evolution of dermatoglyphics research and point to some of the issues which we are confronted with at the present. These are: (1) The establishment of a standardized nomenclature as well as a method for recording and analyzing dermatoglyphic data. (2) To promote collaboration and exchange of services among various laboratories and investigators. (3) To promote pooling of rare data. (4) To establish well defined guidelines for training dermatoglyphic associates and, (5) To establish strict criteria for reviewing and accepting manuscripts submitted for publication in national and international journals.

REFERENCES

Bartsocas C (1982). Paleodermatoglyphics. In Bartsocas C (ed): "Proceedings of the International Conference of Dermatoglyphics," New York: Alan R. Liss, p

Cummins H (1936). Dermatoglyphic stigmata in mongolian idiocy. Anat Rec 64:(suppliment 3) 11.

Cummins H (1939). Dermatoglyphic stigmata in mongoloid imbeciles. Anat Rec 73:407-415.

Cummins H, Keith HH, Midlow C, Montgomery RB, Wilder HH and Whipple-Wilder I (1929). Revised methods of interpreting and formulating palmar dermatoglyphics. Am J Phys Anthrop 6:415-743.

Cummins H and Kennedy WR (1940). Purkinje's observations (1823) on fingerprints and other skin features. Am J Crim Law and Criminology 31:343-356.

Cummins H and Midlo C (1926). Palmar and plantar epidermal ridge configurations (dermatoglyphics) in European-Americans. Am J Phys Anthrop 9:471-502.

Cummins H and Midlo C (1943). "Finger prints, Palms and Soles." Philadelphia: Blackiston Co.

Galton F (1890). The patterns in thumb and finger marks--on their arrangement into naturally distinct classes, the permanence of the papillary ridges that make them and the resemblance of their classes to ordinary general. Philosophical Transactions of the Royal Soc of London 182:1-23.

Galton F (1892). "Fingerprints." London: MacMillan and Co.

Mavalwala J (1978). A methodology for dermatoglyphics--fingers and palms. In Mavalwala J (ed): "Dermatoglyphics," The Haugue: Mouton, pp 19-54.

Meier RJ (1980). Anthropological dermatoglyphics: a review. Yearbook of Phs Anthrop 23:147-178.

Mendel GJ (1865). Versuche uber Pflanzenhybriden. Verhandlungen des Naturforschenden Vereins (Brunn).

Purkinje JE (1823). Commentatio de examine physiologico organi visus et systemtis cutanei. Vratislaviae Typis Universitat. Breslau.

Whipple IL (1904). The ventral surface of the mammalian chiridium. Z Morph Anthrop 7:261-368.

Whipple-Wilder I (1930). The morphology of the palmar digital triradii. J Morphol 49:153-221.

Wilder HH (1902). Palms and soles. Am J Anat 1:423-441.

Wilder HH (1904). Racial differences in palm and sole configuration. Am Anthropologist 6:244-293.

Wilder HH (1904a). Duplicate twins and double monsters (dermatoglyphics part only). Am J Anat 3:426-472.

Progress in Dermatoglyphic Research, pages 13-23

DERMATOGLYPHICS: LOOKING FORWARD TO THE 21st CENTURY

Jamshed Mavalwala

Department of Anthropology
University of Toronto
Toronto, Canada M5S 1A1

Every area of science is affected in its progress by many factors. The current state of the Art is the major factor; the level of communication and interaction with other areas of knowledge is another. The political, social, and economic context within which the scholar must junction also affects the outcome. Another factor that affects research in areas of science is the imputed status that scientists give to various areas. This status-giving is based on rewards available from doing research in the area and can change very quickly or remain static over a long period of time.

A major factor that can override all other considerations in the progress of a scientific field is the impact of a single scholar. It is quite common in science to observe a steady rate of progress for years, and then see a major step forward as the result of the work of a single scholar.

The progress of our knowledge in dermatoglyphics is best understood if we also understand the context within which researchers worked at the time. If we also realize that our progress is linked to society's attitudes toward scientific research and to the cooperation within separate areas of science, then we will be in a better position to improve our research methodologies in the future.

THE DESCRIPTIVE PHASE

The early descriptive phase of dermatoglyphics began with the work of Malphigi in 1686 and continued with the attempt of Purkinje in Czechoslovakia in 1823 to classify finger patterns into nine types. In 1892 Galton in England postulated a simplified system using only three types. The context of dermatoglyphic studies must take into account that, as the usefulness of anthropometric measurements as identification tools declined and Bertillon's work of 1882 came to be increasingly questioned, scientists were willing to look elsewhere for a human variation that would be unique to the individual. Finger prints filled the vacuum. As this major identification device was accepted across North America and Europe the stimulus was to produce efficient *classify-file-identify* systems that could be readily used by law enforcement agencies. Scores of systems appeared to satisfy this need. Bridges (1942) in his book, Practical Fingerprinting, describes some major systems of classifying finger prints: the Henry system, the Battley system, the Vucetich system and *forty-seven* other systems. At the same time that these systems were being devised and used, human anatomists were exploring their own interests, resulting in systems as elementary as the arches, loops, and whorls classification of Galton (1892) to the extraordinarily complex system of up to ninety-five patterns by Ökrös (1965). The motive for these classifications was not the identification of individuals but the identification of populations. Human biology was in the throes of a taxonomic fever and it was believed that human populations could be categorized as if they were both discrete and stable. Both premises have proved to be untenable in the light of current knowledge. No human population has a definite boundary and no human population is stable.

During this initial developmental phase of dermatoglyphics we were all significantly affected by a major work of Harold Cummins and his fellow anatomist, Charles Midlo. Their comprehensive work

'Finger Prints, Palms and Soles. An Introduction to Dermatoglyphics' first published in 1943, put into one volume material that would allow both anthropologists and geneticists to follow the clearly laid out methodology and would result in a larger number of research studies in dermatoglyphics than ever before.

In fact, even the name, dermatoglyphics, was coined by Harold Cummins and Charles Midlo in April 1926 at the 42nd annual meeting of the American Association of Anatomists. Reporting in the American Journal of Physical Anthropology in that same year they state, "The term *dermatoglyphics* (*derma,* skin + *glyphe,* carve) is used herein for the first time, barring its verbal introduction at the 42nd annual session of the American Association of Anatomists, April, 1926, It is proposed both as a designation of the division of anatomy embracing the surface markings of skin, within the limits defined below, and as a collective name for the integumentary features themselves. Manifestly, the literal sense of the word is more especially applicable to the skin of the palmar and plantar surfaces, with its configurations of sharply sculptured ridges. The intention of the proposal is that the term be limited in its regional application to skin surfaces thus marked, including not only the hand and foot but also such regions as the tails of certain forms which bear similarly specialized skin. As a name for the skin markings, dermatoglyphics applies only to ridges and their arrangements, flexion creases and other secondary folds being without the bounds of its intended meaning." However flexion creases have by usage come to be incorporated today under this rubric.

The descriptive phase of dermatoglyphics was a time when anatomists explored this aspect of the human body, often without much encouragement and the study of skin ridges did not carry the same academic prestige as other areas of anatomy. Research grants were few or non-existent, and it is not surprising that studies that did emerge during this phase were often the secondary work of a scholar and carried on because of personal interest. Under these circumstances the work of single scholars had a major impact and one should not underestimate those such as Cummins in the U.S.A., Geipel and Weninger in Europe, and Shiono and Furuhata in Japan.

THE ASSOCIATIVE PHASE

This phase of dermatoglyphics has its beginnings as early as 1926 when Cummins reported on the dermatoglyphics of developmental defects. Gradually, advances in human genetics, particularly in cytogenetics, coupled with a social and political consciousness of mental retardation, its causes and its effects, aided and abetted the interests of geneticists, human biologists, physical anthropologists, anatomists and embryologists among others, to examine varying aspects of dermatoglyphics.

The current literature of dermatoglyphics spans the gamut from physical anthropology to human genetics to pediatrics. The workers formalized themselves into an entity during the second International Congress of Human Genetics held in Rome in 1961 and on September 10th, 1961 the International Conferences on Dermatoglyphics was founded with Professor Harold Cummins as Honorary President. At the Fourth International Congress of Human Genetics held in Paris in September 1971 this organization changed its name to the International Dermatoglyphics Association and has continued to function under that name since. Formal dermatoglyphics associations now exist in the U.S.A. (The American Dermatoglyphics Association) and in India (The Indian Dermatoglyphics Association), and extensive groups of workers meet regularly in countries such as Austria, West Germany, Poland, Japan, England and Czechoslovakia.

It is of interest to note that while we have made major advances in understanding the mechanisms of human heretability our knowledge of the transmission of dermatoglyphics has not significantly improved since the earlier studies of workers such as Bonnevie (1927, 1931). Nor did our knowledge of the embryology of dermatoglyphics advance as rapidly as our knowledge of its phenotypic variability. Only a handful of workers, notably M. Okajima of Japan, come to mind.

Because dermatoglyphics became the prerogative of physical anthropologists, the aspects of populational variability were assiduously pursued. The underlying basic developmental principles are only now being brought to light as exemplified by the work of anatomists such as de Wilde (1980), and the growing influence of biological statistics initially propounded by pioneers such as Karl Pearson, followed by Haldane and Penrose are showing results in the work of scholars such as Jantz, Meier, Chopra and Malhotra, among many others. In spite of the efforts of Biegert and Brehme our knowledge of dermatoglyphics of non-human primates remains poorly documented. For an excellent review of anthropological dermatoglyphics see Meier (1980).

The current state of the Art in dermatoglyphics has changed over the past five decades in its nature as measured by its publications reported in 'Dermatoglyphics - An International Bibliography' (Mavalwala, 1977). In the earlier decades the bulk of the publications are on populational variability and are limited to using the arch/loop/whorl classification. Increasingly this aspect of dermatoglyphics will become of interest only as a recording of a variable with little or no genetic or taxonomic value. To even further erode the value of this section of dermatoglyphic literature is the fact that many of these studies were done on populations that may actually exist in terms of political states, such as Germans, Hungarians, British, Indians, etc., but are not specific enough to satisfy the geneticists need to delineate a breeding population. We are now aware that a breeding population is temporary (except for the Hindu caste structure which changes only slowly) and can be rapidly changed by social factors. All populations termed 'black', but who are really brown, do not breed with each other in the U.S.A. Class and regional factors play major roles in establishing exogamy. It is erroneous to conclude that the pink skinned populations of the U.S.A. are a homogeneous mass. The Roman Catholic/Protestant/Jewish dividing line is only one of many.Class,status, ethnicity, regionality and a large number of other factors create temporary breeding populations. Unfortunately until the social scientists can clearly understand and describe the ways in which communities hold themselves together and establish their boundaries within technologically complex societies the human biologist appears unable to clearly define the population from which samples are being drawn.

The next two decades will either convince us that populational variability in dermatogyphics is of little significance to us either in its use as a diagnostic tool in medicine or in aiding us in our understanding of its inheritance, or, if we are convinced of the importance of human population variability, the bulk of our populational studies will have to undergo a critical re-examination.

The major change that we perceive has been brought about by advances in fields other than dermatoglyphics. Dramatic advances in chromosomal variability and the great social change in attitudes towards the mentally handicapped have generated a mass of studies seeking dermatoglyphic associations with various conditions. The initial enthusiasm fired by the expectation that dermatoglyphics would provide an early and quick diagnosis quickly faded to be replaced by the more realistic attitude that dermatoglyphics of such patients do reflect the early trauma but may not do so specifically enough to be of specific diagnostic value. Dermatoglyphics is being seen more realistically as a screening device, and as the methodologies used to report clinical cases become internationally compatible and the actual numbers of cases mount, a realistic understanding of dermatoglyphics as a diangostic aid will be achieved. This phase of dermatoglyphics has benefitted greatly from the interest of the medical sciences.

THE ANALYTICAL PHASE

While some work has been done in the first two phases on how dermatoglyphics are formed in early foetal life, the mechanisms of ridge formation are only now beginning to attract major attention. Within the analytical area are also the newer studies on the transmission of those genetic codes that generate these embryological phenomena. But we have not made much progress in this area since the early work of Bonnevie. In spite of the fact that my international bibliography of dermatoglyphics cites 352 references under this heading all we have been able to establish is that dermatoglyphics are inherited. The problem has been dealt with by examing specific patterns in a pedigree, and also by looking for correlations between sibs and **between mother** and child. Twin studies have also attempted to use correlations to postulate genetic causality.

Two modes of inheritance for dermatoglyphics are in vogue today. The first proposes simple single factor inheritance for epidermal patterns and the second a polygenic transmission of quantitative dermatoglyphic traits such as total ridge counts.

Recent work postulating a monogenic mode of inheritance has been done on the Habbanite isolate of Israel by Statis and co-workers (1976). They postulate that a single gene effect alters a basal ulnar loop to other patterns depending on the dominance of the allele. Juberg (1977) also postulates a single gene mechanism and Morgan (1978) postulates a single gene effect for palmar patterns. But the etiology of dermatoglyphics is too complex for the majority of dermatoglyphic workers to accept a single gene hypothesis. Peristatic influence also can not be discounted.

The polygenic model first proposed by Lionel S. Penrose and extensively reported by Holt, has the support of C.A.B. Smith. Weninger has criticized this model for its indiscriminate use of total ridge counts as if they directly represented patterns and for ignoring individual digit and radial/ulnar variation. Armstrong (1978), de Wilde (1956), Froehlich(1976), Penrose (1969) and Matsukura (1967) also postulate varying degrees of polygenic inheritance.

We now have a large body of data showing the varying effects of early trauma on the development of dermatoglyphics. Rubella, the cytomeglovirus, thalidomide, and the fetal-alcohol syndrome are just some of the examples of maternal effect.

Knussmann (1977) has postulated extra nuclear inheritance for dermatoglyphics. Roberts and Coope (1975) extracted four fields. The field approach has to be refined to deal with interpopulation variability.

We must note with interest that Green and Thomas (1978) were able to culture human epidermal cells derived from human newborn foreskins. These were proliferated in petri dishes and they formed dermal patterns by cell movement going from arches into whorls by successive movement. Findlay and Harris (1977) also found dermatoglyphic patterns on skin other than volar areas on human foetuses.

LOOKING FORWARD

What, then, can we expect in the two decades that will bring us into the 21st century?

1. A growing understanding between biologists and statisticians will permit us to handle large bodies of data better than before.
2. This will increasingly lead to a demand for providing better data, better in terms of sampling and better in terms of methodology.
3. If human societies continue to coalesce due to advanced communication systems, then our science will benefit in that all dermatoglyphic work will become internationally available. This will clearly aid us in the clinical aspects of dermatoglyphics.
4. Population genetics appears unlikely to advance with the same velocity as biochemical genetics,

biochemistry and cytogenetics, and dermatoglyphics of populations will be proportionately reduced.
5. Even though only a few histologists/anatomists will work in dermatoglyphics their impact will be high, especially in the embryology of dermatoglyphics.
6. Working backwards from the phenotype it is unlikely that we will understand the heredity of dermatoglyphics but there is the possibility that workers examining how DNA sequences formulate cell structure and consequently tissue structure, will be able to complete the pathway from the genetic code in the DNA to the final dermatoglyphic pattern.
The likelihood remains however that the genetic code determines only the basic dermatoglyphic understructure, and that what we see as the final skin ridge is the result of considerable peristatic influence.

It does not appear to me that we are on the brink of a major advance in any area of dermatoglyphic research, rather that our advances are up a steady incline and that those of us who use dermatoglyphics solely for descriptive purposes need to closely examine the genetic hypotheses that are being currently postulated and to refine our descriptive terms.

I am discouraged by the repetitive and unanalytical papers that continue to appear but I am also encouraged, as I am sure we all are, by some of the increasingly sophisticated work appearing today. We can only hope that it gets the attention that it deserves.

REFERENCES

[For references to the work of significant scholars see listings in Mavalwala JM (1977). "Dermatoglyphics. An International Bibliography." Den Hague: Mouton.]

Armstrong R (1978) A curve-fitting method for estimating the number of loci in total finger ridge count and its implication for the number of loci involved in skin color. In Mavalwala J (ed): "Dermatoglyphics. An International Perspective," The Hague: Mouton, p 231.

Bertillon (1882). Identification anthropometrique. Annales de demographie internationale.

Bonnevie K (1927). Lassen sich die Papillarmuster der Fingerbeere für Vaterschaftsfragen praktisch verwerten? Zentralblatt für Gynakologie 51:539

Bonnevie K (1931). Was lehrt die Embryologie der Papillarmuster über ihre Bedeutung als Rassen- und Familiencharackter? III. Zur Genetik des quantitativen Wertes der Papillarmuster. Z f indukt Abst u Verebungslehre 59:1

Bridges BC (1942). "Practical Fingerprinting." New York: Funk and Wagnalls

Cummins H (1926). Epidermal-ridge configurations in developmental defects, with particular reference to the ontogenetic factors which condition ridge direction. Am J Anat 38:89

Cummins H, Midlo C (1943). "Finger prints, palms and soles. An intorduction to dermatoglyphics." Philadelphia: Blakiston.

Findlay GH, Harris WF (1977). The topology of hair streams and whorls in man, with an observation on their relationship to epidermal ridge patterns. Am J Phys Anthropol 46:427

Froehlich JW (1973).The usefulness of dermatoglyphics as a biological marker of human populations in Melanesia. Ph.D. dissertation, Harvard University, Cambridge, Massachusetts.

Galton F (1892). "Fingerprints". London:Macmillan.

Green H, Thomas J (1978). Pattern formation by cultured human epidermal cells: development of curved ridges resembling dermatoglyphs. Science 200:1385.

Juberg RC, Morgan LY, Faust CC (1977). The inheritance of digital dermatoglyphic patterns in 54 American Caucasian families. Paper presneted at Harold Cummins Memorial Dermatoglyphics Symposium, Gulf Shores, Alabama.

Knussmann R (1977). Differences between mother-child and father-child correlations in the human epidermal ridge system. J Hum Evol 6:123.

Malphigi M (1686). "De Externo Tactus Organo." London

Matsukura T (1967). Studies on the inheritance of fingerprints. Med J Osaka Univ 18:227.
Mavalwala,J (1977). "Dermatoglyphics. An International Bibliography." The Hague: Mouton.
Meier RJ (1980). Anthropological dermatoglyphics: a review. Yearbook Phys Anthropol 23:147
Morgan LY, Juberg RC, Faust CC (1977). The inheritance of palmar dermatoglyphic patterns in 54 American Caucasian families. Paper presented at the Harold Cummins Memorial Dermatoglyphics Symposium, Gulf Shores, Alabama.
Ökrös S (1965). "The Heredity of Papillary Patterns." Budapest: Akademiai Kiado.
Penrose LS (1969). Effects of additive genes at many loci compared with those of a set of alleles at one locus in parent-child and sib correlation. Ann Hum Genet 33:15.
Purkinje JE (1823). A physiological examination of the visual organ and of the cutaneous system. (Translated into English by H Cummins and RW Kennedy). Am J Crim Law and Criminology (1940) 31:343
Roberts DF, Coope E (1975). Components of variation in a multifactorial character: a dermatoglyphic analysis. Hum Biol 47:169.
Slatis HM, Bat-Miriam Katznelson M, Bonne-Tamir B (1976). The inheritnace of fingerprint patterns. Am J Hum Genet 28:280.
de Wilde AG (1956). Biologisch-mathematische Aspekte der Fingerbeerenmustervererbung. Deut Gesell f Anthrop 6:45.
de Wilde AG (1980). A theory concerning ridge pattern development. Dermatoglyphics 8:2.

Progress in Dermatoglyphic Research, pages 25-31

DERMATOGLYPHIC RESEARCH AND THE CLINICIAN

WLADIMIR WERTELECKI

Department of Medical Genetics
University of South Alabama
Mobile, Alabama 36617 USA

CHRIS C. PLATO

Gerontology Research Center, NIA
Baltimore City Hospitals
Baltimore, Maryland 21224 USA

H. Cummins (1939) published a classic paper delineating the dermatoglyphic stigmata of mongoloid imbeciles. At that time, medical cytogenetics did not exist and "mongolism" was ascribed to a bewildering array of obscure causes. Yet, decades before Trisomy 21 was to be found at the root of Down Syndrome, dermatoglyphic studies had pointed towards a single genetic causation. Although the growing edge of medical sciences is moving forward, it is still true that our understanding of human birth defects remains sketchy. In the last decade, Medical Genetics has reached most clinicians, and the general interest in human genetics and malformation syndromes is expanding. An increasing attention is paid by clinicians to developmental traits during medical examinations. Among these developmental traits is dermatoglyphics, and today, as in 1939, dermatoglyphics remain relevant to the study of human malformation.

The purpose of this presentation is to analyze the nature of the inter-relationships between those of us engaged in dermatoglyphic research, on one hand, and clinical geneticists, particularly general clinicians, on the other. The views expressed are, in part, determined by our experience of the past 15 years.

If the views that follow can stimulate further dialog

concerning the topic "Clinicians--Dermatoglyphic Research", our aim will be accomplished.

Briefly, we wish to formulate and elaborate on two basic questions. The first: "Is scientific progress concerning dermatoglyphics sufficient to warrant the attention of clinicians at large?" Our answer is "yes". Such a view is supported by selected examples concerning achievements in methodology, embryology, primatology and clinical studies.

Concerning methodology, it is sufficient to refer the reader to the contributions of our colleagues Drs. D. F. Roberts, and D. Loesch, as well as those of other colleagues contained in this volume or in "Dermatoglyphics--Fifty Years Later" (Wertelecki and Plato, 1979). The analytical approaches used in dermatoglyphic research have applications to major medical questions. For example, dermatoglyphic differences between offspring of identical twin sisters compared to the offspring of identical twin brothers are useful to assess maternal effects on the developing fetus (Nance, 1981).

In the realm of embryology, recently developed techniques for in-vitro culture of epithelial cells reveal cell migration patterns that may give clues to understanding the formation of dermatoglyphic patterns (Greene and Thomas, 1978). The extensive studies of human fetuses by W. Babler (1978,1979) demonstrate how a pool of novel data can provide clinicians with opportunities to test or generate hypotheses. A key observation by Babler is the correlation between dermatoglyphic patterns and general fetal growth. Fetuses resulting from spontaneous and induced abortions differ from one another in dermatoglyphics and growth patterns. The understanding of fetal wastage is currently limited. Babler's work, through the inclusion of dermatoglyphics, adds an important dimension to the study of abortions.

The contention that a basic pattern of development is stretched and pulled by various forces during embryonic life is not new to dermatoglyphic researchers. Recently J.B.L. Bard (1977) elaborates further on earlier principles held by D'Arcy Thompson. Focusing on zebras as a model of striping, Bard recognizes two basic facets: the first is a unity compelling striping; the second is that different temporal "windows" during embryogenesis result in different patterns. While each species of zebra has a different striping pattern and a different stripe count, it is proposed by Bard that such differences can be viewed as resulting from embryonal timing of the striping phenomena.

Returning to Babler's observations, differences in dermatoglyphic patterns of fetuses stemming from spontaneous or induced abortions could be viewed simplistically as genotypic differences. However, they also can be viewed as secondary to timing of embryonal development. It is interesting to think of Bard's postulates when considering the observations of L. Newell-Morris, detailed in part in this volume. Her studies of primates revealed dermatoglyphic alterations following the application of stress to the pregnant female. Maternal stress and fetal dermatoglyphic alteration can be accommodated by Bard's and Babler's views.

Lastly, it may be illustrative to single out several clinical observations that hold broad and direct interest to clinicians. The original report of Menser and Purvis-Smith (1969), concerning the association of childhood leukemia and Sydney creases has been followed by a series of complimentary observations. It appears that children with acute lymphocytic leukemia have an increased birth weight (Wertelecki and Mantel, 1973); that higher birth weights are also observed in Down Syndrome children who develop leukemia (Fabia et al., 1970); that Sydney creases are more frequently associated with leukemia if the disease develops at an early age (Oorthuys et al., 1979); that a leukemic child's siblings (known to have a higher risk to develop leukemia) also have a higher occurrence of Sydney creases (Anderman et al., 1981); that other childhood neoplasms diagnosed at an early age are also associated with Sydney creases (Oorthuys et al., 1979).

In teratology, dermatoglyphic traits can become a practical tool for the assessment of teratogens. Among common drugs with teratogenic potential are anti-convulsive agents such as those prescribed in epilepsy. Pregnant women in need of anti-convulsive drugs face the risk of producing defective fetuses. The issue is complex and difficult to assess, since subtle teratogenic effects must be detected. The recent report by Anderman et al. (1981) of dermatoglyphics being a subtle indicator of anti-convulsant maternal medication effects on the fetus, underscores this potential. Such observations as these in childhood neoplasia and teratology provide many departure points for clinical researchers.

The second basic question is: "Do clinicians incorporate

dermatoglyphic studies in their clinical protocols with a reasonable frequency?" Our opinion is that they do not.

In contrast to the vigorous growth of Medical Genetics and the training of young clinical geneticists, it is self-evident that neither the ranks of the American Dermatoglyphics Association (ADA) nor those of the International Dermatoglyphics Association (IDA) have captured significant numbers of these new specialists. The field of dermatoglyphics appears to be remote to most clinicians. The medical literature reveals an exponential growth of articles published in the area of Medical Genetics while those concerning dermatoglyphics, even if indirectly, have shown little, if any, growth.

Table 1. Number of Dermatoglyphic Articles (Medlar)

	Primary	Secondary
1966-68	160	145
1969-71	280	330
1972-74	220	385
1975-76	135	260
1977-78	160	140
1979-80	225	165

The remoteness of dermatoglyphics to key clinicians, like neonatologists and pediatricians, is illustrated further by the Pediatric Year Books of the last years which do not even list the word "dermatoglyphics" in their indices.

We believe that the major block between clinicians and the use of dermatoglyphic parameters relates mostly to difficulties with data collection and subsequent analysis. Collection of clinical dermatoglyphic data is complex, slow, expensive and must include thorough and accurate medical background information as well as carefully selected controls. Clinicians are aware that opportunistic collection of dermatoglyphics, even if pursued vigorously, is unlikely to generate sufficient material for comprehensive analysis. Indepth dermatoglyphic studies of clinical conditions have been relatively few. Often, such studies concern medical disorders of unknown or variable etiology and therefore, the results have frequently been inconclusive.

Table 2. Dermatoglyphic Studies of Medical Disorders. Prevalence Among 200 Studies Reviewed.

	Number of Reports	Number of Patients
Down Syndrome	17	2676
Cancer	6	1694
Leukemia	13	1647
Schizophrenia	7	1381
Heart Disease	6	950
Sex Chromosome Abnormality	8	529

Although representing an ideal group to include along with unrelated controls, first degree relatives are rarely used, even by our own ranks.

Table 3. First Degree Relatives in Medical Dermatoglyphic Studies

Studies Reviewed	175
Studies including Relatives	8/175
Number of Patients	671
Number of Relatives	855

Easy access to control populations is not within the scope of an average medical center. Even if accomplished, the clinician is still left with the difficulty of interpretation and analysis. Rather than engage in the slow and cumbersome acquisition of the dermatoglyphic methodology, clinicians prefer linkages to experts in our field. Relatedly, a scan of clinical dermatoglyphic literature reveals a prevalence of case reports rather than indepth studies.

Table 4. Case Reports Among Medical Dermatoglyphic Articles

Number of Controls	Number of Patients 10	10-99	100
None	70	15	5
100	4	10	4
100	5	26	36

Furthermore, our own ranks tend to study anthropologic or

genetic questions, rather than clinical ones (it is easier to find 200 Cypriots in Athens alone, than 200 leukemic children in the whole of Greece). We believe that a vigorous dermatoglyphic research requires an intimate involvement with medicine and that such linkage can be developed only by involving clinicians at large. Clinicians must perceive that collecting dermatoglyphic data, even if from a single patient, has the potential to contribute to the understanding of the disease in question. Therefore, a system for collaborative data collection, data pooling, selection of controls, analysis and interpretation which provides appropriate weight to medical variants must exist before clinicians can be expected to respond.

As a result of our opinion, we have become engaged in the development of a Dermatoglyphic Data Bank (DDB). We seek linkages with clinicians willing to contribute data or interested in collaborative studies. We offer technical assistance as well as existing control or clinical data already contained in the DDB.

We invite our colleagues to follow suit and hope that the ADA and IDA will develop policies concerning our relationship with clinicians. We are now at a challenging threshold because developments in Medical Genetics and Dermatoglyphic Research include strong indicators that the study of dermatoglyphic traits can become an integral part of the clinical process.

REFERENCES

Anderman E, Damsky L, Anderman F and Loughman P (1981). Increased Frequency of Dermal Arches: A Subtle Indicator of Anticonvulsant Effect on the Fetus. Sixth Int Congress Hum Genetics, abstract p 9.6.

Babler WJ (1978). Prenatal Selection and Dermatoglyphic Patterns. Am J Phys Anthrop 48:21-27.

Babler WJ (1979) Quantitative Differences in Morphogenesis of Human Epidermal Ridges. Birth Defects: Original Article Series XV No 6:199-208 and Personal Communication.

Bard JBL (1977) A Unity Underlying the Different Zebra Striping Patterns. J Zool, Lond. 183:527-539.

Cummins H (1939). Dermatoglyphic stigmata in mongoloid imbeciles Anat Rec 73:407-415.

Oorthuys AN, deVaan GAM, Behrendt H, Coris JA, Lion S and Helsper WM (1979) Dermatoglyphics in Childhood Leukemia in

"Dermatoglyphics--Fifty Years Later." Wertelecki W and Plato C (eds): Birth Defects: Original Article Series Vol XV No 6, 721-735.

Fabia J and Drolette M (1970). Malformations and Leukemia in Children with Down's Syndrome. Pediatrics 45:60-70.

Greene H and Thomas J (1978). Pattern Formation by Cultured Human Epidermal Cells: Development of Curved Ridges Resembling Dermatoglyphs. Science 200:1385-1388.

Menser MA and Purvis-Smith SG (1969). Dermatoglyphic Defects in Children with Leukemia. Lancet i:1076.

Nance W (1981) Personal Communication.

Wertelecki W and Plato CC (eds) (1979). "Dermatoglyphics--Fifty Years Later" Birth Defects: Original Article Series Vol XV No 6 p 721-735.

Wertelecki W and Mantel N (1973). Increased Birth Weight in Leukemia. Pediat Res 7:132-138.

Wertelecki W, Plato CC, Fraumeni JF and Nisewander JD (1973). Dermatoglyphics in Leukemia. Pediat Res 7:620-626.

Progress in Dermatoglyphic Research, pages 33-44

MEDICAL APPLICATIONS OF DERMATOGLYPHICS

Blanka Schaumann and Sue Barden Johnson

Veterans Administration Medical Center
Minneapolis, Minnesota, U.S.A.

Although scattered earlier dermatoglyphic reports exist on selected medical disorders such as mental retardation, schizophrenia, epilepsy, leprosy and psoriasis, widespread medical interest in dermatoglyphics developed only relatively recently, after it became apparent that individuals with some gross chromosomal aberrations had unusual epidermal ridge formations. During the last two decades, the area of clinical applications became one of the most active areas of dermatoglyphic research. As a result, dermatoglyphic analysis is now recognized as a useful diagnostic aid in some disorders and an effective research tool in many others.

Much of the clinical interest in dermatoglyphics stems from the fact that the epidermal ridge patterns are formed during early fetal development and thereafter remains unchanged for the rest of life except for an increase in size and possible distortions by disease or injury. Because of the close association between ridge differentiation and embryogenesis of the extremities, any disturbances of the limb growth during early fetal life are likely to be reflected by changes of the epidermal ridge configurations. Indeed, all anomalous extremities show an unusual epidermal ridge arrangement proportional to the skeletal defects. Although striking, dermatoglyphic patterns in grossly malformed hands and feet are of a limited diagnostic value as they only reflect the obvious anatomical defect which can be readily and more precisely identified by other means.

Of potentially higher clinical significance are abnormal epidermal ridge pattern formations and unusual pattern constellations without accompanying gross limb distortions such as those associated with certain chromosomal aberrations, single gene defects and environmental factors. The first disorders reported to be consistently associated with unusual dermatoglyphic traits were the autosomal trisomies (Table 1). In spite of some dermatoglyphic similarities shared by two or more of the trisomies, enough differences have been found to make dermatoglyphics a useful tool in their differential diagnosis.

No single dermatoglyphic feature has emerged as being diagnostic of a particular medical disorder; rather, the dermatoglyphic features must be considered in their combinations. Based on this fact, several diagnostically useful indices have been derived for Down syndrome (Walker 1957, Beckman et al. 1965, von Greyerz-Gloor et al. 1969, Reed et al. 1970, Bolling et al. 1971, Borgaonkar et al. 1971, Deckers et al. 1973, Rodewald et al. 1976, Preus 1977), utilizing the traits that account for most of the total dermatoglyphic variation between Down syndrome and controls. Although simple and easily applicable, the indices can differentiate the two groups of subjects fairly accurately.

Sex chromosome aberrations have been found to have less influence on ridge formation than autosomal chromosome anomalies, with dermatoglyphic deviations being mainly of quantitative value. Nevertheless, several indices using dermatoglyphics in combination with other physical characteristics have been proposed for Turner syndrome (Dallapiccola et al. 1972, Milcu and Ciovîrnache 1976, Preus 1976). Their discriminating power is, however, less effective than that achieved for Down syndrome.

The development of new cytogenetic techniques in recent years now allows the identification of chromosomal aberrations less pronounced than trisomies, i.e., small deletions, partial trisomies, translocations, inversions, etc. As a result, numerous associations between newly recognized chromosomal syndromes and dermatoglyphic anomalies were reported. These have been reviewed recently by Reed (1981) who also pointed out that the reported dermatoglyphic anomalies should be considered tentative because in many instances only a few patients have been studied while in others the dermatoglyphic findings are variable or insufficiently documented. For the same reasons, attempts to correlate specific dermatoglyphic characteristics with particular

TABLE 1

DERMATOGLYPHIC FEATURES IN AUTOSOMAL TRISOMIES

FEATURE	TRISOMY 21	TRISOMY 18	TRISOMY 13	TRISOMY 8
Fingertip patterns (%)				
Arch	0.4- 2.7	81.4	26.6	26.0
Radial loop	0.8- 5.2	5.6	14.9	4.3
Ulnar loop	75.1- 85.2	7.2	38.0	42.8
Whorl	12.1- 20.1	0.7	16.1	26.9
Palmar patterns (%)				
Thenar/I_1	1.3- 2.4	16.1	37.5	53.6
I_2				19.2
I_3	68.0- 79.2	41.7	69.2	80.8
I_4	8.6- 21.5	36.4	31.6	89.3
Hypothenar	58.3- 74.3	33.3		42.9
Mean TFRC	92.2-130.3	4.9		90.2
Mean *a-b* ridge count	39.0- 42.7		50.0	49.3
Mean *atd* angle (%)		70.6	95.2	61.7
Distal axial triradius (%)	81.2- 90.0	52.6	93.9	55.3
Main lines (%)				
A (thenar exit)		21.0	78.8	11.1
C (abortive or missing)	30.8- 36.8			
Single transverse crease (%)	31.3- 85.9	57.7	63.4	34.6
Single crease, fifth digit (%)	10.8- 27.0	56.3		
Hallucal area (%)				
Arch tibial	43.8- 59.6			
Arch fibular, A^f-S pattern			43.6	
Loop distal (small)	32.1- 47.9			

I_1, I_2, I_3, I_4.....first, second, third, fourth interdigital area

TABLE 2

DERMATOGLYPHICS IN CHROMOSOME 9 PARTIAL TRISOMES

EXTRA CHROMOSOME MATERIAL	FINGERTIP PATTERNS (%)				TFRC	*a-b* RIDGE COUNT	*atd* ANGLE	DISTAL AXIAL *t*	DIGITAL TRIRADII *b,c,d*		SIMIAN CREASE
	A	R	U	W	(mean)	(mean)	(mean, °)	(%)	Absent (%)	Fused (%)	(%)
p(24→21)	15	0	75	10	63			100	100	0	100
p(ter→14)											100
p(ter→13)	75	8	18	0		64	66	75	40	40	83
p(ter→12)	38	4	58	0	82		46	70	60	20	68
p(ter→11)	0	10	90	0	76	84	50	43			70
(pter→q11)	14	6	67	12	36		55	80	62	12	60
(pter→q12)	14	1	80	4	71	77	43	83	40	20	92
(pter→q13)	50	5	38	7	47		46	83	83	17	83
(pter→q21)	13	33	53	0				0	0	100	50
(pter→q22)	44	4	50	2	35		52	62	75	0	75
(pter→q31)	10	15	65	10				0	100	0	100

chromosomal segments (e.g. Table 2) have so far not been successful. It is expected, however, that the new, more accurate cytogenetic methods will contribute toward better understanding of the relationship between chromosomal sites and dermatoglyphics.

Encouraged by the results of the dermatoglyphic studies in chromosomal syndromes, researchers broadened the scope of their investigations to include non-chromosomal medical disorders. Among these are inborn and postnatal disorders with and without an established genetic basis (e.g. de Lange syndrome, Smith-Lemli-Opitz syndrome, Rubinstein-Taybi syndrome, Poland syndrome, microcephaly, neurofibromatosis, phenylketonuria, tuberous sclerosis, Wilson disease, celiac disease, cleft lip and/or palate, congenital heart disease, malignant neoplasias, leukemia, cerebral palsy, diabetes mellitus, epilepsy, leprosy, myocardial infarction, psoriasis, schizophrenia and many others) as well as disorders caused by environmental factors such as viruses (e.g. rubella, cytomegalovirus) or drugs (thalidomide, phenytoins, alcohol, etc). When present, dermatoglyphic anomalies in these disorders are similar, although usually less pronounced than those in chromosomal aberrations. Numerous associations between the investigated disorders and dermatoglyphics have been established. However, there still exist many unconfirmed or contradictory claims of such relationships. Reasons for these failures range from inappropriate patient samples or controls to erroneous data interpretation. Nonchromosomal disorders without limb malformations and without any deleterious factors acting during the period of dermal ridge differentiation will probably have normal dermatoglyphics. In other disorders, dermatoglyphic changes might be too subtle and elude analysis, particularly when only selected dermatoglyphic features are considered. Problematic diagnosis, small patient samples and high dermatoglyphic variability are among the factors diminishing the value of the results of many dermatoglyphic studies. Furthermore, it is unlikely that consistent dermatoglyphic deviations will be found in disorders of heterogeneous etiology because different etiological factors are apt to influence dermatoglyphics in various ways. Even in disorders where dermatoglyphics are obviously unusual in a group of patients (Table 3), dermatoglyphics may be of uncertain, if any, diagnostic value due to the lack of a specific dermatoglyphic stereotype in individual patients (Table 4). Problems of nomenclature and statistics in the clinical interpretation of dermatoglyphics as they were discussed for chromosomal aberrations by Reed (1981), pertain to non-chromosomal disorders as well. Finally, the selection of controls is of crucial importance as numerous factors such as sex, race and ethnic origin may significantly influence data interpretation. Whenever possible, unaffected first-degree relatives should be used as one of the control groups in order to distinguish between familial dermatoglyphic traits and dermatoglyphic features truly associated with a specific disorder.

TABLE 3

DERMATOGLYPHICS IN RUBINSTEIN-TAYBI SYNDROME

Fingertip patterns (%)	
Arch	18.4
Radial loop	5.8
Ulnar loop	46.4
Whorl	29.3
Mean TFRC	
Males	120.3
Females	99.7
Mean *atd* angle (^{o})	50.2
Distal Axial triradius (%)	60.2
Palmar patterns (%)	
Thenar/I_1	48.3
I_2	27.9
I_3	50.5
I_4	41.7
Hypothenar	37.4
Simian crease (%)	32.6

The role of dermatoglyphics in medicine has been changing along with the evolution of diagnostic techniques. At the time of their discovery, for example, abnormal dermatoglyphics in Down syndrome would have been of considerable practical diagnostic use. Similarly, prior to the availability of accurate chromosomal identification, dermatoglyphics would have played a significant role in distinguishing between the deletions of the short arm of chromosome four and five (Table 5) in patients when the clinical picture was unclear. Availability of modern cytogenetic methods, however, makes a positive identification of chromosomal aberrations mandatory, a task which dermatoglyphic analysis cannot successfully fulfill. Nevertheless, dermatoglyphics have retained their place in medicine, particularly in medical

TABLE 4

DERMATOGLYPHICS IN SELECTED PATIENTS WITH RUBINSTEIN-TAYBI SYNDROME

FINGERTIPS						P A L M S					
A	R	U	W	TFRC	*atd* ANGLE	Hy	Th/I_1	I_2	I_3	I_4	SIMIAN CREASE
6	0	3	1	34	81	-/-	-/-	+/+	-/-		
0	0	5	5	213	99	-/+	+/-	-/+	+/+		
8	0	2	0	25	93	+/-	+/+	-/-	-/-		
0	0	3	7	216	130	-/-	-/-	-/-	+/+		
0	1	7	2		68	-/+	+/-	-/-	-/+		
0	0	9	1		95	+/?	-/-	-/-	+/+		
0	2	8	0	121	115	+/+	-/-	-/-	+/+	-/-	-/-
4	0	6	0	56	198	+/-	+/+	-/-	+/+	-/-	
2	0	8	0	70	58	-/-	+/+	+/-	-/+	+/-	-/-
6	0	4	0	9		-/-	-/-	-/-	+/+	+/+	-/-
0	1	4	5	172		-/-	+/+	+/+	-/-	+/+	-/-
0	0	2	8		77	-/-	-/-	-/-	-/-	-/+	+/+
9	0	1	0		89	-/-	+/-	-/-	-/+	-/+	-/+
7	0	3	0	13		-/-	-/-	-/-	-/-	-/-	-/-

research with the emphasis shifting toward more general and theoretical implications.

TABLE 5

COMPARISON OF DERMATOGLYPHIC FEATURES IN 4p- AND 5p- SYNDROMES

FEATURE	4p-	5p-
Fingertip patterns (%)		
Arch	40.1	10.1
Radial loop	1.6	4.3
Ulnar loop	41.7	49.8
Whorl	16.6	35.8
Mean TFRC	45.6	115.9
Mean *atd* angle (^{o})	58.2	50.0
Distal axial triradius (%)	43.2	84.7
Palmar patterns (%)		
Thenar/I_1	13.3	26.9
I_2	0.0	1.8
I_3	20.8	40.3
I_4	70.8	72.7
Hypothenar	25.0	27.4
Simian crease (%)	57.1	71.0
Ridge dissociation (%)	83.3	0.0

Dermatoglyphic analysis cannot be used as a substitute for either a careful physical examination, a critical chromosomal analysis or other available means of diagnosis. However, in some disorders, dermatoglyphics may help to confirm a suspected diagnosis or to signal a disorder which might otherwise be overlooked or discovered much later. Aberrations of dermatoglyphics or flexion creases may also provide an incentive to re-examine the results of tests thought to be normal (Reed and Hodes 1979, Reed 1981).

Dermatoglyphics are also of interest in genetic counseling, especially in spontaneous abortions, stillbirths or early deceased children with malformations that cannot be easily diagnosed and where tissue cultures were not obtained or failed to grow.

One of the most useful applications of dermatoglyphic analysis is in screening for autosomal aberrations. For example, individuals with multiple congenital malformations, mental retardation and abnormal dermatoglyphics were found to be excellent candidates for karyotyping (Higurashi et al. 1977). The usefulness of dermatoglyphic screening of potential parents to identify otherwise undetected carriers of Down syndrome was demonstrated in several independent studies (Pospíšil 1977, Ayme et al. 1979, Rodewald et al. 1980, Rodewald et al. 1981).

Dermatoglyphics are known to reflect subtle morphological disturbances in the developing fetus such as in the process of separation of fingers. They are sensitive indicators of syndactyly and have been used as such to trace the gene for type II syndactyly within families. While cutaneous syndactyly of a minor degree may be difficult to diagnose, the fusion of the triradius at the base of the digits is good evidence that the basic defect leading to syndactyly was present during the dermal ridge differentiation even if the syndactyly is not obvious at birth. Dermatoglyphics may also be useful as means of precise identification of other types of digital anomalies. In the absence of a scar, they may provide the only permanent evidence of a surgically removed or spontaneously amputated supernumerary digit (Cummins 1932). They may sometimes replace an x-ray examination for the diagnosis of preaxial polydactyly or be used to differentiate between congenital ring constrictions and absence deformities or syndactyly (Temtamy and McKusick 1969, Temtamy et al. 1981).

Examination of dermatoglyphics may help to determine the time during embryogenesis when the causative agents such as teratogens were acting or the time of onset of a disorder. Thus, for example, the unusual longitudinal ridge configurations in many patients with congenital arthrogryposis multiplex suggest that the defect was present in these individuals at least as early as the process of ridge formation. Similarly, dermatoglyphic studies demonstrated that in some individuals with undifferentiated mental retardation, a developmental defect rather than a birth trauma is implicated. Using dermatoglyphics, an attempt has been made to separate patients with cleft lip and/or palate by the etiology of the disorder, i.e., teratogens and inheritance (Deshmukh et al. 1979).

Recently developed methods of computerized dermatoglyphic analysis using sophisticated statistical methods are opening new possibilities of application of dermatoglyphics in medicine. The first indications of the potential of this type of analysis in syndrome discrimination have been demonstrated in disorders in which previously no abnormal dermatoglyphics or only minor, diagnostically non-applicable variations were recognized (Wong et al. 1977).

Considering the relatively short period of active research in medical aspects of dermatoglyphics, impressive results have been achieved. Because progress in dermatoglyphics is parallel to that in other fields of human genetics, it is to be expected that the changing concepts and present uncertainties encountered in human genetics will be reflected in dermatoglyphic studies. It is obvious now that dermatoglyphics cannot fulfill their originally envisioned role as a decisive medical diagnostic tool. Nevertheless, dermatoglyphic research should contine to contribute significantly to better understanding of embryonal development and its influencing factors as well as to theoretical genetic concepts.

REFERENCES

Ayme S, Mattei MG, Mattei JF, Aurran Y, Giraud F (1979). Dermatoglyphics in parents of children with trisomy 21. Clin Genet 15:78-84.

Beckman L, Gustavson KH, Norring A (1965). Dermal configurations in the diagnosis of the Down syndrome: an attempt at a simplified scoring method. Acta Genet (Basel) 15:3-12.

Bolling DR, Borgaonkar DS, Herr HM, Davis M (1971). Evaluation of dermal patterns in Down's syndrome by predictive discrimination. II. Composite score based on the combination of left and right pattern areas. Clin Genet 2:163-169.

Borgaonkar DS, Davis M, Bolling DR, Herr HM (1971). Evaluation of dermal patterns in Down's syndrome by predictive discrimination. I. Preliminary analysis based on the frequencies of patterns. Johns Hopkins Med J 128:141-152.

Cummins H (1932). Spontaneous amputation of human supernumerary digits: pedunculated postminimi.Am J Anat 51:381-416.

Dallapiccola B, Bagni B, Pistocchi G (1972). Dermatoglyphic and skeletal hand abnormalities in Turner's syndrome. A tentative scoring method. Acta Genet Med Gemellol (Roma) 21:69-78.

Deckers JFM, Oorthuys AMA, Doesburg WH (1973). Dermatoglyphics in Down's syndrome. III. Proposal of a simplified scoring method. Clin Genet 4:381-387.

Deshmukh RN, Grewal MS, Sidhu SS (1979). Dermatoglyphics in cleft lip and cleft palate anomaly: familial and teratogenic groups. Indian J Med Res 70:814-818.
Higurashi M, Segawa M, Matsui I, Ihnuma K, Nakagome Y (1977). Screening for autosomal aberrations. Acta Paediatr Scand 66:501-504.
Milcu SM, Ciovîrnache M (1976). Dermatoglyphics in the diagnosis of Turner's syndrome. Rev Roum Med Endocrinol 14:35-38.
Pospíšil J (1977). Vyhledávání potencionálních nosiček Downovy choroby pomocí kožních kreseb na rukou. Čs Gynekol 42:98-101.
Preus M (1976). A screening test for patients suspected of having Turner syndrome. Clin Genet 10:145-155.
Preus M (1977). A diagnostic index for Down syndrome. Clin Genet 12:47-55.
Reed T (1981). Review: Dermatoglyphics in medicine - Problems and use in suspected chromosome abnormalities. Am J Med Genet 8:411-429.
Reed TE, Borgaonkar DS, Conneally PM, Yu P, Nance WA, Christian JC (1970). Dermatoglyphic nomogram for the diagnosis of Down's syndrome. J Pediatr 77:1024-1032.
Reed T, Hodes ME (1979). Single crease on the 5th finger in medical disorders and in normal population (Letter to the editor). J Med Genet 16:407.
Rodewald A, Zang KD, Zankl H, Zankl M (1981). Dermatoglyphic peculiarities in Down's syndrome detection of mosaicism and balanced translocation carriers. In Burgio GR, Fraccaro M, Tiepolo L, Wolf U (eds): "Trisomy 21". An International Symposium, Berlin:Springer-Verlag, pp. 41-56.
Rodewald A, Zang KD, Ziegelmayer G (1976). Bilateral symmetry of qualitative dermatoglyphic patterns in the Down syndrome. Z Morphol Anthropol 67:333-344.
Rodewald A, Zankl M, Zankl H, Zang KD (1980). Dermatoglyphs in carriers of a balanced 15;21 translocation. J Med Genet 17:301-305.
Temtamy SA, El-Mazny A, Hussein FH, Abdel Salam M, Moussa AA, Zaki ME (1981). Diagnostic significance of dermatoglyphics in certain birth defects. This volume.
Temtamy S, McKusick VA (1969). Synopsis of hand malformations with particular emphasis on genetic factors. Birth Defects 5(3):125-184.
von Greyerz-Gloor RD, Auf der Maur P, Riedwyl H (1969). Beurteilung des diagnostischen Wertes der Finger- und Handleistenmerkmale von Mongoloiden unter Anwendung einer Diskriminanzanalyse. Humangenetik 8:195-207.

Walker NF (1957). The use of dermal configurations in the diagnosis of mongolism. J Pediatr 50:19-29.

Wong AKC, Vogel MA, Steg NL (1977). Syndrome discrimination by computerized dermatoglyphic analysis. Birth Defects 13(3A):61-66.

Progress in Dermatoglyphic Research, pages 45–77

GENETIC STUDIES OF DERMATOGLYPHICS - ADVANCES AND LIMITATIONS.

DANUTA Z. LOESCH

Department of Genetics, Psychoneurological Institute,
Warsaw, Poland

INTRODUCTION

Francis Galton summarized progress in earlier studies on finger patterns with the following words:"... I made inquiries, and was surprised to find, both how much had been done, and how much there remained to do ..."(Galton, 1892). This is precisely how, nearly one hundred years later, one could comment on the advances in studies on genetics of dermatoglyphic patterns. Besides evidence for polygenic inheritance for some dermatoglyphic traits, such as ridge counts, with indications of genetic non-additivity, the data on genetics of dermatoglyphs are fragmentary and often contradictory. No adequate model of inheritance has yet been presented, despite rapid progress in recent years in the statistical and genetical methods of analysis of the data and the widespread availability of computers.

Apart from the complexity of factors and processes underlying the ridge formation, the reasons for inadequacy of the models hypothesized to explain the inheritance and development of ridge patterns are related to the difficulties in classification and scoring of dermatoglyphic characters for the purpose of genetic analysis. On the other hand, statistical methods are often deficient if applied to this kind of data;these two aspects are, naturally, closely interrelated.

DERMATOGLYPHIC CHARACTERS IN GENETICAL ANALYSIS

The main difficulty is in what way patterns should be classified in order to obtain characters equivalent to biological entities. In any patterned area of the palm or of the sole, as shown in Fig. 1, we can consider percentage frequencies of traditionally classified patterns, such as loops, whorls, vestiges, or their various combinations. If, however, we apply topological approach where only true patterns are considered and they are expressed in the form of elementary discontinuities (see Penrose and Loesch, 1969;Loesch 1982), we can record the occurence of specified loops or triradii in percentage frequencies or in the ratio scale;alternatively, we can sum up these discontinuities within the area to form a new character, pattern intensity. Pattern intensities on individual areas of the palm, of the sole or on individual fingers may be combined. This way of formulating characters enables the methods of biometrical genetics to be applied,although the distributions of some of these traits may be inconvenient for statistical analysis. The distributions for pattern intensities on individual fingers and in the palm and sole, which are shown in Table 1, clearly deviate from normality and in palms and soles they are, for most areas, positively skewed. In spite of it, however, a suitability of methods of quantitative genetics to study patterns must not be questioned considering the factors that influence the formation of ridges and of discontinuities in the field of parallel ridges, represented by loops and triradii. These are mainly size and shape of the embryonic volar eminences and time of their subsidence (see Cummins and Midlo, 1943;Penrose, 1971a; Loesch, 1982). The variation of these traits is evidently continuous and, consequently, the assumption of continuity of variation underlying the presence or absence as well as the number of pattern elements in a given area is probably justified.

At a practical level it can easily be demonstrated, by simply inspecting palmar of sole patterns in individual pedigrees that similarity between various relatives is evidently greater if they are compared for pattern intensities in individual areas, instead of comparing the occurence of specified loops or their numerous combinations (see Fig. 2). But it would be even more difficult to perceive any significant similarity between relatives, if patterns were formulated in the traditional way (according to Cummins and Midlo, 1943). The results of such an inspection also indicate that, in classifying patterns for the purpose of genetical analysis, the possibility of chance variation should be eliminated as much as possible in that the fewer morphological varieties of a given basic pattern are distinguished, the less chance influence on their variability there is to be expected.

A concept of pattern intensity as the fundamental dermatoglyphic characteristics, which can be further subdivided into single, mutually exclusive pattern elements, sufficiently meets these requirements. But some classifications are incompatible with these principles, such as, for instance, a system suggested by Bhanu (1975), where various subtypes of whorls are distinguished according to the direction of ridge course.

The traditional way of classifying patterns (see Cummins and Midlo, 1943) distinguishes, particularly in the hypothenar area, a great number of apparently different types of pattern, so that the chance is low for one and the same type to occur more than once in a family. At the same time it may be asked how such a trait as the main line formula can represent a biological entity, and, consequently, in what way it could be interpreted genetically. Similar objections may be raised if, in some genetical analyses, the presence of true patterns, that is loops, is combined, with an absence of true patterns, that is arches on fingertips, to form a single trait, as opposed to whols, which, again, represent true patterns (De Wilde and Amesz-Voorhoeve, 1979).

Another group of relevant problems is in making a clear distinction between discrete and continuous variables, on the basis of their phenotypic expression. This can be illustrated by closer inspection of a vestige of ladder configuration, or any local disarrangement in a parallele course of the ridges (Fig. 3). Traditionally, these have been considered typical discrete variables and combined, in one and the same formula, with true patterns (see Cummins and Midlo, 1943). However, we can approach it in a different way by observing that this type of configuration is characterized by the increased intensity of minutes, such as ends or junctions, as compared with the adjacent field of parallel ridges and thus represents a typical metrical character. Similarly, a loop may be scored as present or absent, but it can also be considered in respect of its size and thus represented by the number of ridges between its centre and the associated triradius;after all, these two aspects are closely intercorrelated and display a parallel factor (Lin et al., 1979;Reed et al., 1978a).

Although the size of pattern typical metrical and easy to calculate trait, should not present any difficulties in genetical analysis, it raises the problem in selection of subjects to be included in the sample. The more commonly adopted way of selecting is random and the absence of true pattern simply scores zero. This, however seems illogical and causes a considerable distortion of the distribution, particularly if patterns in some areas, such as of the palm, are rare.An alternative way is to select only the individuals with the presence of pattern in a given area so that zero counts would, more correctly, represent only very small loops or tented loops. But such a procedure cannot also be fully satisfactory, as it would result in a truncated distribution which may modify the values of genetic parameters.

Finally, an important source of difficulties in formulating characters is related to the well known phenomenon of interdependence either of elementary, specified pattern elements that is loops, or pattern intensities on individual fingers or on respective areas of the palm or on the sole. Should intercorrelated characters be considered jointly or separately in genetical analyses? The use of the total ridge count (TRC) (as summarized in Holt, 1968) was much criticized, especially by Weninger (1964, 1965) and Weninger et al. (1976) as representing a combination of the very different traits. However, considering either the individual counts alone or, alternatively, their sum, means unnecessary loss of information. Clearly, including both alternatives in one and the same study is advantageous and can provide evidence for the presence of negative environmental covariance between individual traits. At the same time, various genetic models can be applied to covariance structure (both these approaches will be demonstrated in the next section of this paper).

It is doubtful however if these procedures would be at all appropriate for the total palmar pattern ridge count (TPPRC), as defined by Malhotra et al. (1980) because, as these authors themselves point out, it is a combination of different traits, which may represent quite distinct gical units;this is also indicated by the distribution of individual values. Indeed, no accosiations have been found between ridge counts of patterns on individual areas of the palm and the count of the interdigital loops III and IV are negatively correlated (Malhotra et al., 1980).

GENETICAL METHODS AND DERMATOGLYPHIC RESULTS

It is thus understood that, regardless the way of recording dermatoglyphic traits, their most efficient analysis should be based on the methods of quantitative genetics, considering the alleged underlying continuity of variation. Besides, no convincing evidence for single gene character has been obtained for any dermatoglyphic pattern or configuration. Evidently, the choice of a suitable method of quantitative genetic analysis for a particular study considers its purpose as well as the type of characters included, although the way of dealing with a deviation of their distributions from normality has not yet been established. The same is true for the problem of applying an appropriate scale and of selecting samples.

The most common choice has been that of regression (or correlation) between relatives. Correlation coefficients have been, however, often wrongly interpreted as representing the degree of genetic determination of a given trait, although they are merely a measure of resemblance within pairs of relatives, as was already pointed out by Fisher (1918). If the environmental effects are negligible, such as, for instance, in the finger ridge count (Holt, 1956, 1957, 1968;Vogelius-Andersen, 1963;Loesch, 1971;Matsuda and Matsunaga, 1971; Jelisiejew and Marcinkiewicz, 1972; Mi and Rashad, 1975) of finger pattern intensity (Mukherjee, 1966; Loesch, 1971, 1974), the equality of parent-child and sib-sib correlations, observed in these studies, with mid-parent-child correlation approximating 0.71 indicate additivity of a large number of genes (as summarized in Holt,1968). Lowered value of parent-child correlation as compared with sib-sib correlation would generally indicate dominance, but no evidence for this has been obtained for most dermatoglyphic traits so far investigated. The only exception have been the t triradius on the palm, the hallucal distal loop I (Loesch, 1974), and the hallucal counts (Orczykowska-Swiatkowska, 1972).

Correlations have also been applied to estimate heritability, sex linkage or maternal influence. By using Penrose's formulae based on parent-child and sib-sib correlations (see Penrose, 1971b) the highest heritability that is, approximating one, was found for the total ridge count, the total pattern intensity on fingers, the number of whorls and of ulnar loops on fingers, the total pattern intensity on palms and the a - b palmar ridge count (Loesch, 1971, 1974, 1982), for the total palmar ridge count it is 0.60 on the basis of correlations given by Malhotra et al. (1981). On soles the highest heritability was found for the hallucal ridge counts (Orczykowska-Swiatkowska, 1972) and distal hallucal loop, while this value for the other sole characters was low (Loesch, 1974). Heritability approximating 0.5 was found for thenar loops, hypothenar H loop, interdigital loop III and triradius t.

However, simple comparisons of correlation coefficients from various pairs of relatives can only be a rough guide, as the conventional genetical methods are not efficient enough either to estimate heritability accurately or to detect the mode of inheritance. Correlations can be used much more effectively in testing various alternative models, as was shown, for instance, by Morton (1974), Morton et al. (1974) or Rao el al. (1974), but these modern techniques of genetical analysis have not yet concerned dermatoglyphic traits. On the other hand, various genetic models can be fitted to a set of correlations following Mather's biometrical genetical concepts (Mather, 1973), which has already been performed for the pattern intensity on fingers (see below).

Whatever is the purpose of calculating family correlations, the question arises as to which estimate can be considered more reliable. Several methods have been worked out to allow for varying family size, based on analysis of variance, such as those by Fieller and Smith (1951), Cochran (1954), Smith (1957), or ensuring greater precision of the results as well as the least standard error by means of maximum likelihood procedures (see, for example,

Patterson and Thompson, 1971;Smith, 1980a and b). The efficiency of all these methods was recently compared, using the simulated as well as observational dermatoglyphic data, by Bener (1979a). He concludes that methods based on maximum likelihood give the best estimates and smallest standard error;but, in fact, there is not much difference between the results obtained by either of these methods, including the simplest one, without any correction for a varying family size. This remarkable consistency, particularly between the simplest and the most sophisticated method, is shown in Table 2 for the total finger pattern intensity (PIF), but has also been observed for most other dermatoglyphic traits in sib-sib as well as parent-child pairs.

A comparison between the results of the three methods: the simplest pairwise estimator, semi-weighted analysis of variance according to Cochran (1954) and of maximum likelihood estimate according to Patterson and Thompson (1971), based on the like and unlike-sexed sib pairs, also show their considerable consistency for finger and palmar patterns (Table 3a);however, the correlations for sole patterns, based on lower number of pairs, are much less consistent (Table 3b). An underestimation of the values of standard error in the simplest way of calculating correlations is evident for most characters, but this should not be unexpected. Otherwise, it seems that, having a sufficiently large sample of relatives, the extra labour of using sophisticated statistical methods for estimating correlations is not worthwhile. Moreover, any deviation of the distribution from a normality, which is common with dermatoglyphic traits, or a departure from an assumption of polygenic additive inheritance, make estimates based on the maximum likelihood procedures much less reliable.

Information of genetical interest has also been obtained, for a majority of dermatoglyphic traits, from the within and between pair variances and mean squares in two types of twins:monozygotic (MZ) and dizygotic (DZ). Two studies were concerned with estimates of heritability based on the conventional formulas, using one or both variances, or of genetic variance, such as the combined estimate, G_{CT}, according to Christian et al. (1974). The results of these analyses were, for finger patterns, generally consistent with the earlier data based on correlations between non-twin relatives in that they indicated a predominant genetic component in finger ridge counts, particularly in TRC, for the total finger pattern intensity, the palmar pattern intensity and for the hallucal patterns and counts (Reed et al., 1975;Loesch, 1979). But for some palmar loops, particularly in the interdigital and hypothenar areas, they were incompatible with heritability estimates, based on familial correlations in that its value was relatively lower;such an incompatibility concerned also a majority of individual loops and pattern intensities on soles, where the results based on twins showed much higher degree of genetical determination than indicated by the data based on other pairs of relatives.

Although the reason for these discrepancies has not yet been specified, it must be related to the fact of inadequacy of the conventional methods of estimating heritability or genetic variance,because they do not test various models concerning the sources of variation, so that it is impossible to say which of these models is most appropriate for a given trait. This is especially important considering the fact that many factors, partly identified for dermatoglyphic characters by means of these methods, may introduce a bias to estimates based solely on twins. These are:maternal influence (Reed et al., 1979), inequality of MZ-DZ total variances (Reed et al., 1975; Loesch, 1979), probably partly related to the heterogeneity of MZ twin sample with regard to a chorion type (Reed et al., 1978b) or other environmental effects specific for MZ twins, and various forms of genotype-environmental interactions.

However, more efficient methods of biometrical genetics, as advocated by Jinks and Fulker (1970), have recently been applied to finger dermatoglyphic data, namely, to the mean squares obtained in twins and sibs. These methods, elaborated and described by Eaves and Eysenck (1975), have allowed the testing of alternative hypotheses of the causes of variation and estimation (by the method of weighted least squares) of environmental, additive and non-additive genetic components of variation. The test for the equality of the total variances between MZ and DZ twins is also included in the model fitting procedure.As a result more accurate heritability measures have been obtained from the estimated (additive) genetic and non-genetic components which, for the ridge counts on individual fingers, total finger ridge count (TRC), total finger pattern intensity (PIF) and for right-left bilateral asymmetry in respect of each of these traits, are shown in Table 4. These heritability estimates are based on the E_1D_R model, that is, on the assumption that the only sources of variation for these traits are individual environment and genetic, additive factors, which does not necessarily have to be true, as will be shown below.

Heritability of the TRC and PIF is somewhat higher than estimated by means of conventional methods, particularly for the latter trait. As concerns heritability of ridge counts on individual fingers, its values are, in males, almost equally high on all fingers, except for left fingers II and III;but in females, they are the lowest for fingers I and III and the highest for finger V.

The results obtained for a bilateral asymmetry of finger ridge counts, whose genetics has been the subject of some controversy (see results of Holt, 1954; Singh, 1970; Mi and Rashad, 1977, Bener, 1979b) are noteworthy. They indicate that, after all, directional asymmetry in finger ridge counts may be affected by genetical influences, particularly in males.

The problem of genetics of the ridge count asymmetry is, however, not yet closed, as more complex models are needed to fit the data, mainly in order to explore a possibility of an influence of the common environment, which might have been confounded with the genetic (additive) component. It would be most interesting to apply modern techniques to test bilateral asymmetry in respect of the other dermatoglyphic characters, particularly of total pattern intensities and ridge counts on palms and soles.

It is also evident from the results, presented in Table 4 that heritability for the total ridge count as well as for the total signed difference (the latter only in males) is higher than for ridge counts or differences taken individually;the same applies to the total pattern intensity, as compared with the values for right and left taken separately. This phenomenon, which has also been noticed for heritabilities of palmar pattern intensities on individual areas or specified loops, as compared with heritability of the total palmar pattern intensity, estimated by conventional methods of quantitative genetics (Loesch,1979) indicates the presence of negative environmental covariance between individual fingers or between different palmar areas, respectively. On the other hand, however, heritability for some individual traits may be as high as for the total count or total pattern intensity;this has been observed for some digits with left and right counts added (Holt, 1968;Reed et al., 1975), as well as for some individual pattern elements (also with left and combined) on palms or soles (Loesch, 1979). This suggests that there may be genetic or environmental factors specific to these individual traits.

But the problem of a genetical basis of the interrelationships between various dermatoglyphic traits or their combinations can be approached in more efficient ways. Factor analytic techniques applied to finger ridge counts, with subsequent genetical analysis of identified factors have not been adequate for testing sources or pattern of covariation (Chopra, 1977; Rostron, 1977;Reed and Young, 1979;Reed et al., 1978a). These can be specified by fitting different models to the data, as has recently been done for covariation between ridge counts on individual fingers in twins and sibs (Martin, Eaves and Loesch, in preparation), by means of the method adapted from Jöreskog (1973). The preliminary results indicate that the individual environmental component is mainly specific for each finger, with small negative covariances while genetic (additive) component is represented by one common factor for all digits and independent factors for individual digits. This approach should be extended to study the sources and pattern of covariation between individual palmar or sole areas, in respect of pattern intensities or ridge counts, or between specified loops within one and the same areas, although already mentioned inconvenience related to distributions of these traits may present some problems. We already know that, while individual patterns, pattern intensities and pattern ridge counts on individual areas of the palm are weakly associated or even negatively correlated (Loesch, 1974; Malhotra et al., 1981), a majority of sole patterns are significantly intercorrelated (Loesch, 1974).

In modern genetic analysis of the data the estimate of a degree of genetic derermination is followed by the attempts at partitioning genetic component into its additive and non-additive aspects. It may seem absurd to try and do so for such a character as the total count which, on the basis of the results of correlations or regressions or regression between various relatives, has long been regarded as determined by perfectly additive genes (see Holt, 1968). However, some more recent studies of Spence et al. (1977) who used the efficient technique of pedigree analysis to reexamine the Holt's ridge count data, or the results of Robson and Parsons (1967) and Singh (1979) on the hybrids between Australian Aborigines and Europeans suggested some deviation from perfect additivity for this trait. These findings are not inconsistent with the skeweness of its distribution. Finally, a genetic model fitting approach, as described by Eaves and Eysenck (1975) has been applied to twin and sibling data, models being fitted to the mean squares by the procedure of iterative weighted least squares. This was in order to define the components contributing to the total variance of the total ridge count, as well as to ridge counts on individual fingers (Martin, Loesch, Jardine, Berry, in preparation). As a result, large and positive values of dominance variance were estimated. In the same study negative regression of DZ and sibling pair variances on pair means was found, which apparently suggested the action of dominant genes, tending to increase finger ridge count (as explained in Martin et al., 1978); this result cannot be related to presence of genotype-environmental interaction, because no such regression has been found in MZ twin pairs (see Jinks and Fulker, 1970). But the fact of almost perfect equality of parent-child and sib-sib correlations, as discussed above, has not been compatible with the hypothesis of dominance and this inconsistency is yet to be explained.

Some relevant information of importance has been obtained from similar procedures applied, in the same samples, to the total finger pattern intensity (PIF), which is highly correlated with the total finger ridge count a strong suggestion of genetic non-additivity has been obtained as a result of fitting various models of variation to the mean squares from twins and sibs (Table 5). Computation of the expected mean squares from the least-squares parameter estimates provides a chi-square test of goodness-of-fit of the model. As can be seen in the Table, both environmental models, E_1 and E_1E_2, fail badly for all three pattern intensity measures in both sexes and the E_1D_R model also fails in males, where the model containing a dominance as well as additive component gives best fit. Because there is no heterogeneity of fit over sexes (tested after

Clark et al., 1981), fitting the model to the full data set, including the opposite - sex sibs is valid and, as in males alone, the $E_1D_RH_R$ model gives the best account of the data. The results of polynomial meanvariance regression, presented in Table 6 show, consistently, significant coefficients in both male and female DZ twins and in opposite sex sibs, in the absence of genotype-environmental interaction.

Interpretation of these results in terms of dominance was, again, difficult to accept considering, similarly as in the ridge count, identical parent-child and sib-sib correlations, calculated in large sample of families (Loesch, 1974). It was thus necessary to apply more complex models, which included an epistatic as well as dominant type of genetic interaction. Because these require considering relatives other than twins, where these two types of interactions are confounded, hypotheses concerning the type of genetic interaction were tested on the basis of the entire set of correlations between parents and children, as well as between like-sexed and opposite-sexed sibs and two types of twins and spouses (Loesch et al., 1981). It was evident that the model including epistatic interaction gave much better account of the data than the model assuming dominance. This result is not incompatible with all the other previous findings, as this type of interaction is equally confounded with additive genetic effects in both parent-child and sib-sib correlations.

It should be noted that, for total pattern intensity, the correlation in MZ twins is higher than would be expected on the assumption of additivity. However, although it is compatible with evidence for epistatic interaction, it could also result from MZ - specific environmental effects; this being true, the possibility could not be excluded that these might be confounded with the estimates of genetic non-additivity. Thus, still more complex models are required to be tested to distinguish these alternative hypotheses for the finger pattern intensity as well as the ridge counts. On the other hand, comparison of monochorionic and dichorionic MZ twins may reveal the size of any intrauterine environmental effects specific to MZ twins. I want to draw your attention to the fact that higher than expected correlations in MZ twins can be found for some other dermatoglyphic characters, as shown in Table 7, which indicates that this problem is not confined to finger patterns.

The data presented here show clearly that twins, particularly monozygotic pairs, represent very specific material for genetic analysis in that the results do not fit with hypotheses postulated by the data from other relatives. It is not unjustified to believe that, by adopting the model fitting approach to dermatoglyphic data, it may be possible to identify all the factors, genetic and non genetic, which account for the peculiarities of twin material. It has already been revealed, on the basis of a simple estimation of within - twin pairs concordance of the palmar and sole total configurations in MZ and DZ pairs that unexpectedly high concordance in MZ pairs, as compared with DZ twins, is proportional to a greater bilateral symmetry of patterns (Loesch and Swiatkowska, 1978). Although no explanation of this finding in genetical terms can yet be given, it shows the potentialities of dermatoglyphic data in better understanding of fundamental problems of development and inheritance of phenotypic traits in the humans.

Concluding remarks

This account of difficulties in classifying and recording characters for genetic analysis and of problems in obtaining and interpretation of genetic results is far from complete. My intention has been, however, to indicate especially these applications of genetical methods to certain dermatoglyphic data and their results, which I consider particularly important for future studies.

In spite of a great number and variety of works, our knowledge of genetics of ridge patterns is limited and can be summarized as follows:

Nearly all dermatoglyphic traits are determined by polygenic systems, but some, such as patterns in area I and V of the sole may be determined by a small number of genes or a major gene, which has been indicated by the result of linkage test (Bener et al., 1980), as well as by some earlier data, based on analysis of correlation coefficients (Loesch, 1974). Generally it appears that there is no universal model which could explain the pattern of inheritance of dermatoglyphic traits, as they may largely differ not only with respect to the mode of inheritance, but also, evidently, with respect to heritability, from its highest value for finger patterns and counts, a - b palmar and hallucal ridge counts, to the lowest for some palmar patterns and palmar minutiae. There are also some indications that the action of genes on the total ridge count and finger pattern intensity is not perfectly additive. As concerns the relationships between individual fingers, the covariation and diversity from finger to finger in respect of ridge count is largely under genetic control, but bilateral asymmetry is influenced mainly by environmental factors, particularly in the females.

The information of genetical interest is still to be obtained for a great majority of dermatoglyphic features, especially for patterns on palms and soles, by using efficient methods of analysis. Future investigations need, in particular, precisely define these factors, genetic and non-genetic, which influence the formation of ridges and ridge patterns and the way they act and interact in various stages of early embryonic development; a specificity of influences which affect estimates based on monozygotic twins is also to be explained. It is important to include, in genetic models, the sources and patterns of covariation on one hand and of diversity on the other between patterns on different areas of the palm, of the sole, on individual fingers or on left and right side of the body. The problem of genetic basis of dermatoglyphic sexual dimorphism is also to be elucidated.

The future prospects for this kind of investigations are good considering the fact that in recent years many alternative ways of analysis of twins combined with other pairs of relatives, as well as nuclear families, have been introduced, based on path analysis, segregation analysis or the biometrical genetical approach, where different models of variation can be fitted to the data. It is important that these modern approaches combine classical segregation analysis with methods of quantitative genetics which is particularly convenient considering the type of characters represented by ridge patterns.

References

Bener A (1979a). "Statistical Analysis of the Genetics of Quantitative Characters in Man". Ph. D. Thesis, University of London.

Bener A (1979b). Sex differences and bilateral asymmetry in dermatoglyphic pattern elements on the fingertips. Ann Hum Genet Lond 42:333.

Bener A, Loesch DZ, Smith CAB (1980). Simplified formulas for detecting linkage with a quantitative character. Ann Hum Genet Lond 43:249.

Bhanu BV (1975). Ridge course of the whorles: classification and methods. Am J Phys Anthrop. 42:263.

Chopra VP (1977). Inheritance of dermatoglyphic characters (Presented at Harold Cummins Memorial Dermatoglyphic Symposium, Gulf Shores, Alabama, March 28-31).

Christian JC, Kang KW, Norton JAJr (1974). Choice of an estimate of genetic variance from twin data. Am J Hum Genet 26:154.

Clark P, Jardine R, Jones P, Martin NG, Walsh RG (1981). Directionnal dominance for low IGM and IGA levels. Amer J Hum Genet (in press).

Cochran WG (1954). The combination of estimates from different experiments. Biometrics 10:101.

Cummins H, Midlo C (1943). "Finger Prints, Palms and Soles". Philadelphia:Blakiston.

De Wilde AG, Amesz-Voorhoeve WHM (1979). Fingerprints: Classification, correlations, and inheritance. In Wertelecki W, Plato C (eds)"Dermatoglyphics-Fifty Years Later", New York: Alan R. Liss, p. 95.

Eaves LJ (1970). The genetic analysis of continuous variation: A comparison of experimental designs applicable to human data. II Estimation of heritability and comparison of environmental components. Brit J Math Statist Psych 23:189.

Eaves LJ, Eysenck HJ (1975). The nature of extraversion: A genetical analysis. J Person Soc Psych 32:102.

Fieller EC, Smith CAB (1951). Note on the analysis of variance and intraclass correlation. Ann Eugen Lond 16:97.

Fisher RA (1918). The correlation between relatives on the supposition of Mendelian inheritance. Trans Roy Soc Edinbg 52:399.

Galton F (1892). "Finger Prints". London: Macmillan, p.2.

Holt SB (1954). Genetics of dermal ridges: bilateral asymmetry in finger ridge counts. Ann Eugen Lond 18:211.

Holt SB (1956). Genetics of dermal ridges: parent-child correlations for total finger ridge count. Ann Hum. Genet Lond 20:270.

Holt SB (1957). Genetics of dermal ridges: sib-pair correlations for total finger ridge count. Ann Hum Genet Lond 21:352.

Holt SB (1968). "The Genetics of Dermal Ridges". Springfield, Illinois: Charles C Thomas.

Jelisiejew T, Marcinkiewicz S (1972). Numbers of cutaneous ridges on the finger and their heredity in the Polish population. Folia Morphol 31:219.

Jinks JL, Fulker DW (1970). Comparison of the biometrical genetical, MAVA and classical approaches to the analysis of human behavior. Psychol Bull 73:311.

Jöreskog KJ (1973). Analysis of covariance structures. In Krishnaiah PR (ed): "Multivariate Analysis III". Proceedings of the Third International Symposium on Multivariate Analysis, New York: Academic Press.

Lin PM, Crawford MH, Oronzi M (1979). Universals in Dermatoglyphics. In Wertelecki W, Plato C (eds): "Dermatoglyphics-Fifty Years Later", New York: Alan R. Liss, p. 63.

Loesch D (1971). Genetics of dermatoglyphic patterns on palms. Ann Hum Genet Lond 34:277.

Loesch D (1974). Genetical studies of sole and palmar dermatoglyphics. Ann Hum Genet Lond 37:405.

Loesch D (1979). Genetical studies of the palmar and sole patterns and some dermatoglyphic measurements in twins. Ann Hum Genet Lond 43:37.

Loesch D (1982). "Quantitative Dermatoglyphics: Normal Variation, Genetics and Pathology". London:Oxford University Press (in press).

Loesch D, Martin NG (1981). Asymmetry of digital ridge counts (submitted for publication).

Loesch DZ, Martin NG, Heath AC, Eaves LJ (1981). Evidence for polygenic epistatic interactions in man (submitted for publication).

Loesch D, Swiatkowska Z (1976). Topologically significant dermatoglyphic patterns in twins. Acta Genet Med Gemellol 26:247.

Loesch D, Swiątkowska Z (1978). Dermatoglyphic total patterns on palms, finger-tips and soles in twins. Ann Hum Biol 5:409.

Malhotra KC, Karmakar B, Vijayakumar M (1981). Genetics of palmar pattern ridge counts. Technical Report No Anthrop I, Calcutta: Indian Statistical Institute.

Martin NG, Eaves LJ, Kearsey MJ, Davies P (1978). The power of the classical twin study. Heredity 40:97.

Martin NG, Loesch DZ, Jardine R, Berry HS (1981). Evidence for directional dominance in the genetics of finger ridge counts (submitted for publication).

Mather K (1973). "Genetic Structure of Populations". London: Chapman and Hall.

Mather K, Jinks JL (1971). "Biometrical Genetics". London: Chapman and Hall.

Matsuda E, Matsunaga E (1971). Inheritance of total finger ridge count. Ann Rep Nat Inst Genet (Japan) 21:101.

Mi MP, Rashad MN (1975). Genetic parameters of dermal patterns and ridge count. Hum Hered 25:249.

Mi MP, Rashad MN (1977). Genetics of asymmetry in dermatoglyphic traits. Hum Hered 27:273.

Morton NE (1974). Analysis of family resemblance. I Introduction. Am J Hum Genet 26:318.

Morton NE, MacLean CJ (1974). Analysis of family resemblance. III Complex segregation of quantitative traits. Am J Hum Genet 26:489.

Mukherjee DP (1966). Inheritance of total number of triradii on fingers, palms and soles. Ann Hum Genet Lond 29:349.

Orczykowska-Swiatkowska Z (1972). Variability and inheritance of ridge count on soles (in Polish). Miscellanea, Mat Prace Antrop 83:291.

Patterson HD, Thompson R (1971). Recovery of interblock information when block size are unequal. Biometrika 58:545.

Penrose LS (1971a). Dermatoglyphics and medicine. Acta Clinica, Documenta Geigy 13:11.

Penrose LS (1971b). Notes on the interpretation of intrafamiliar correlation coefficients (Appendix). In Loesch D: Genetics of dermatoglyphic patterns on palms. Ann Hum Genet Lond 34:277, p. 291.

Penrose LS, Loesch D (1969). Dermatoglyphic sole patterns: a new attempt at classification. Hum Biol 41:427.

Rao DC, Morton NE, Yee S (1974). Analysis of family resemblance. II A linear model for familial correlation. Am J Hum Genet 26:331.

Reed T, Evans MM, Norton JAJr, Christian JC (1979). Maternal effects on fingertip dermatoglyphics. Amer J Hum Genet 31:315.

Reed T, Norton JAJr, Christian JC (1978a). Fingerprint pattern factors. Hum Hered 29:351.

Reed T, Sprague FR, Kang KW, Nance WE, Christian JC (1975). Genetic analysis of dermatoglyphic patterns in twins. Hum Hered 25:263.

Reed T, Ushida IA, Norton JAJr, Christian JC (1978b). Comparisons of dermatoglyphic patterns in monochorionic and dichorionic monozygotic twins. Amer J Hum Genet 30:383.

Reed T, Young RS (1979). Genetic analyses of multivariate fingertip dermatoglyphic factors with corresponding individual variables. Ann Hum Biol 6:357.

Robson MK, Parsons PA (1967). Fingerprint studies in four Central Australian Aboriginal tribes. Archae Phys Anthrop Ocean II, 1:69.

Rostron G (1977). Multivariate studies on the genetics of dermal ridges. Ann Hum Genet (Lond) 41:199.

Singh S (1970). Inheritance of asymmetry in finger ridge counts. Hum Hered 20:403.

Singh S (1979). Evidence of dominance in the finger ridge counts uisng multivariate analysis. In Wertelecki W, Plato C (eds): "Dermatoglyphics-Fifty Years Later". New York: Alan R. Liss, p. 495.

Smith CAB (1957). On the estimation of intraclass correlation. Ann Hum Genet (Lond) 21:363.

Smith CAB (1980a). Estimating genetic correlations. Ann Hum Genet (Lond) 43:265.

Smith CAB (1980b). Further remarks on estimating genetic correlations. Ann Hum Genet Lond 44:95.

Spence MA, Westlake J, Lange K (1977). Estimation of the variance components for dermal ridge count. Ann Hum Genet Lond 41:111.

Vogelius-Andersen CH (1963). On the genetics of certain dermatoglyphic traits. Proc IInd Internat Cong Hum Genet 3:1509, Roma: Istitúto G. Mendel.

Weninger M (1964). Zur "polygenen" (additiven) Vererbung des quantitativen Wertes der Fingerbeerenmuster. Homo 15:96.

Weninger M (1965). Dermatoglyphic research. Hum Biol 37:44.

Weninger M, Aue-Hauser G, Scheiber U (1976). Total finger ridgecount and the polygenic hypothesis: a critique. Hum Biol 48:713.

Table 1. Distributions of pattern intensities in all specified areas of the palm, of the sole and on individual finger-tips and of overall pattern intensities (PIP, PIS and PIF respectively) in two European samples.

Pattern intensities	Area	Polish sample: Males $\bar{x}$	σ	g_1	Females $\bar{x}$	σ	g_1
Fingertips	N	227			273		
	I	1.32	0.53	0.14	1.34	0.57	-0.13
	II	1.26	0.56	0.16	1.28	0.58	-0.14
L	III	1.19	0.47	0.59	1.16	0.52	0.18
	IV	1.41	0.52	0.25	1.38	0.54	-0.08
	V	1.17	0.40	1.32	1.11	0.37	1.30
	I	1.49	0.51	-0.07	1.39	0.53	0.00
	II	1.30	0.55	0.00	1.23	0.60	-0.15
R	III	1.26	0.50	0.42	1.10	0.49	0.24
	IV	1.56	0.50	-0.24	1.48	0.52	-0.14
	V	1.21	0.43	1.07	1.11	0.39	1.03
Palms	N	226			273		
	I	0.24	0.62	2.52	0.16	0.52	3.64
	II	0.01	0.09	10.47	0.01	0.10	9.36
L	III	0.31	0.46	0.82	0.35	0.48	0.62
	IV	0.76	0.51	-0.33	0.67	0.54	0.13
	V	0.28	0.50	1.49	0.46	0.66	1.20
	I	0.11	0.41	3.90	0.05	0.32	6.43
	II	0.06	0.23	3.78	0.02	0.15	6.51
R	III	0.61	0.50	-0.34	0.53	0.50	-0.12
	IV	0.47	0.52	0.31	0.49	0.53	0.33
	V	0.36	0.55	1.21	0.43	0.65	1.38
Soles	N	109			125		
	I	1.21	0.56	0.02	1.12	0.47	0.39
	II	0.30	0.50	1.29	0.32	0.56	1.60
L	III	0.78	0.69	0.31	0.70	0.66	0.42
	IV	0.20	0.40	1.48	0.09	0.28	2.90
	V	0.39	0.49	0.43	0.50	0.50	0.00
	I	1.14	0.48	0.37	1.14	0.48	0.36
	II	0.33	0.53	1.27	0.38	0.59	1.27
R	III	0.85	0.68	0.18	0.71	0.68	0.43
	IV	0.17	0.40	2.12	0.13	0.34	2.22
	V	0.41	0.49	0.35	0.48	0.52	0.25
PIF		13.18	3.21	0.24	12.58	3.47	-0.18
PIP		3.20	1.52	0.91	3.18	1.47	1.17
PIS		5.80	2.30	0.70	5.57	2.18	0.60

Table 1. continued

Pattern intensities		Area	British sample					
			Males			Females		
			$\bar{x}$	σ	g_1	$\bar{x}$	σ	g_1
Fingertips		N	138			164		
		I	1.20	0.49	0.46	1.24	0.56	0.03
		II	1.20	0.54	0.11	1.23	0.58	-0.06
	L	III	1.07	0.50	0.48	1.10	0.52	0.42
		IV	1.33	0.50	0.39	1.31	0.54	0.08
		V	1.13	0.38	1.34	1.11	0.40	0.89
		I	1.30	0.53	0.13	1.32	0.54	0.06
		II	1.13	0.61	-0.08	1.26	0.61	-0.21
	R	III	1.03	0.42	0.19	1.09	0.45	0.37
		IV	1.45	0.55	-0.06	1.42	0.53	-0.05
		V	1.13	0.36	1.70	1.13	0.37	1.46
Palms		N	138			164		
		I	0.19	0.55	2.75	0.14	0.43	3.14
		II	0.04	0.19	4.95	0.02	0.13	7.17
	L	III	0.38	0.49	0.48	0.41	0.49	0.37
		IV	0.62	0.54	0.05	0.67	0.59	-0.10
		V	0.36	0.55	1.21	0.36	0.49	0.73
		I	0.06	0.31	5.55	0.07	0.32	4.72
		II	0.07	0.26	3.29	0.04	0.19	4.92
	R	III	0.58	0.50	-0.32	0.52	0.50	-0.10
		IV	0.44	0.53	0.53	0.55	0.53	0.17
		V	0.42	0.60	1.11	0.47	0.64	1.16
Soles		N	138			164		
		I	1.28	0.55	0.04	1.25	0.52	0.46
		II	0.35	0.54	1.20	0.29	0.52	1.59
	L	III	0.81	0.63	0.17	0.66	0.66	0.50
		IV	0.20	0.44	1.98	0.11	0.31	2.49
		V	0.51	0.50	-0.03	0.54	0.50	-0.17
		I	1.21	0.50	0.32	1.22	0.50	0.31
		II	0.26	0.49	1.64	0.28	0.46	1.16
	R	III	0.83	0.64	0.16	0.77	0.65	0.26
		IV	0.27	0.46	1.27	0.14	0.37	2.44
		V	0.43	0.51	0.46	0.44	0.50	0.25
PIF			11.96	3.13	0.21	12.21	3.57	-0.10
PIP			3.17	1.55	1.17	3.25	1.42	0.96
PIS			6.14	2.30	0.50	5.70	0.96	0.74

Table 2. Sib-sib and parent-child correlations for the total finger pattern intensity (PIF) calculated in the simplest way (pairwise estimator) by Loesch (1974) and by means of more efficient methods (Bener, 1979).

Methods	Pairs										
	b - b			t - t			s - s			p - c	
	N	r	S.E.	N	r	S.E.	N	r	S.E.	N	r
Pairwise estimator	465	0.40	0.05	309	0.33	0.06	1631	0.34	0.02	2010	0.36
Analysis of variance according to Fieller and Smith /1951/	530	0.49	-	356	0.44	-	1837	0.41	-	-	-
Semi-weighted analysis of variance according to Smith /1957/	530	0.42	0.05	356	0.34	0.05	1837	0.34	0.04	-	-
Maximum likelihood estimate according to Patterson and Thompson /1971/	530	0.42	0.18	356	0.34	0.25	1837	0.34	0.31	-	-
Maximum likelihood estimate according to Smith /1979/	530	0.42	0.05	356	0.33	0.05	1837	0.34	0.03	1284	0.36

Table 3. Sib-sib correlations for some finger, palmar (a) and sole (b) patterns calculated in the simplest way (pairwise estimator) by Loesch (1974), by means of semi-weighted analysis of variance (SWV) according to Cochran (1954) and of maximum likelihood estimate (MLE), according to Patterson and Thompson (1971) (Bener, 1979).

Characters	Pairs	Estimate of r			
		Loesch (1974)[x]	Bener (1979)[+]		
			SWV	S.E.	MLE
Fingertips					
ΣW	b-b	0.42	0.41	0.05	0.41
	t-t	0.37	0.36	0.05	0.35
	s-s	0.39	0.37	0.03	0.37
ΣU	b-b	0.35	0.37	0.03	0.37
	t-t	0.33	0.31	0.06	0.30
	s-s	0.36	0.33	0.04	0.32
ΣR	b-b	0,15	0.10	0.06	0.10
	t-t	0.19	0.14	0.06	0.14
	s-s	0.15	0.10	0.04	0.10
Palms					
I+I[r]	b-b	0.25	0.19	0.05	0.20
	t-t	0.11	0.12	0.06	0.12
	s-s	0.25	0.24	0.04	0.34
II	b-b	0.09	0.19	0.05	0.20
	t-t	0.08	0.00	0.07	0.00
	s-s	0.18	0.13	0.04	0.13
III	b-b	0.15	0.20	0.06	0.21
	t-t	0.28	0.25	0.06	0.25
	s-s	0.24	0.24	0.04	0.25
IV	b-b	0.18	0.21	0.06	0.21
	t-t	0.22	0.24	0.06	0.24
	s-s	0.19	0.22	0.04	0.22
PIP	b-b	0.25	0.29	0.06	0.29
	t-t	0.25	0.17	0.06	0.17
	s-s	0.28	0.25	0.04	0.34

Characters	Pairs	Estimate of r			
		Loesch (1974)[xx]	Bener (1979)[++]		
			SWV	S.E.	MLE
Soles					
I	b-b	0.41	0.32	0.08	0.32
	t-t	0.30	0.17	0.10	0.18
	s-s	0.50	0.32	0.06	0.32
$\widehat{I}$	b-b	0.18	0.27	0.09	0.27
	t-t	0.28	0.16	0.10	0.17
	s-s	0.21	0.19	0.06	0.20
II	b-b	0.06	0.26	0.09	0.24
	t-t	0.15	0.03	0.11	0.03
	s-s	0.20	0.04	0.07	0.04
$\widehat{II}$	b-b	-0.08	0.14	0.09	0.14
	t-t	0.11	0.24	0.10	0.25
	s-s	0.05	0.13	0.07	0.14
III	b-b	0.19	0.18	0.09	-
	t-t	0.40	0.20	0.10	0.20
	s-s	0.15	0.15	0.07	0.15
$\widehat{III}$	b-b	0.08	0.38	0.08	0.37
	t-t	-0.01	0.02	0.10	0.03
	s-s	0.10	0.28	0.06	0.27
IV	b-b	0.22	0.31	0.08	0.30
	t-t	-0.02	0.28	0.09	0.28
	s-s	0.17	0.19	0.06	0.20
$\widehat{IV}$	b-b	-0.03	0.27	0.09	0.21
	t-t	-0.02	0.05	0.10	0.06
	s-s	0.19	0.26	0.06	0.26
$\widehat{V}$	b-b	0.06	0.10	0.09	0.10
	t-t	0.17	0.28	0.09	0.38
	s-s	0.21	0.21	0.06	0.21
PIS	b-b	0.03	0.30	0.08	0.29
	t-t	0.21	0.29	0.09	0.29
	s-s	o.07	0.21	0.06	0.21

x N° of brother-brother (b-b) pairs:465;S.E.approxim.0.05
N° of sister-sister (t-t) pairs:309;S.E. approxim. 0.06
N° of sib-sib (s-s) pairs:1631;S.E. approxim. 0.02

\+ N° of (b-b) pairs:530
N° of (t-t) pairs:356
N° of (s-s) pairs; 1837

xx N° of (b-b) pairs:179;S.E. approxim. 0.07
N° of (t-t) pairs:70;S.E. approxim. 0.13
N° of (s-s) pairs:494;S.E. approxim. 0.03

++ N° of (b-b) pairs: 253
N° of (t-t) pairs: 116
N° of (s-s) pairs: 725

Table 4. Heritability, h_n^2, of finger ridge counts (from Martin et al. 1981), of bilateral asymmetry in finger ridge counts (from Loesch and Martin, 1981) and overall finger pattern intensities, including right-left differences (from Loesch et al., 1981). Standard errors are calculated after Eaves (1970). Decimal points omitted.

	Males			Females		
	R	L	R-L	R	L	R-L
Ridge count						
I	79±04	86±03	36±10	73±06	74±06	16±12
II	76±05	82±04	40±10	79±05	58±08	-02±13
III	63±07	83±04	10±38	80±05	83±04	38±11
IV	87±03	84±03	20±11	82±04	76±05	12±13
V	79±04	80±04	43±09	83±04	92±02	19±12
Total	-	-	51±08	-	-	12±13
TRC	94 ± 01		-	97 ± 01		
Pattern Intensity						
Total	84±03	85±03	13±11	85±03	81±04	27±02
PIF	94 ± 01		-	91 ± 02		

Table 5. Results of fitting models to the observed mean-squares for the total finger pattern intensity on the left (PIL), on the right (PIR) and for PIF, according to Eaves and Eysenck (1975).

Variable	Model	Data Set	E_1	E_2	D_R	H_R	X^2	df
PIL	E_1	F	3.3···	-	-	-	34.75···	3
		M	2.9···	-	-	-	36.31···	3
		M+F	3.1···	-	-	-	73.47···	7
		T+OSS	3.1···	-	-	-	78.67···	9
	E_1E_2	F	1.5···	1.9···	-	-	17.06···	2
		M	1.5···	1.4···	-	-	28.80···	2
		M+F	1.4···	1.6···	-	-	47.00···	6
		T+OSS	1.7···	1.3···	-	-	47.76···	8
	E_1D_R	F	0.7···	-	5.6···	-	0.83	2
		M	0.5···	-	5.3···	-	6.48·	2
		M+F	0.6···	-	5.4···	-	8.22	6
		T+OSS	0.6···	-	5.2···	-	15.50·	8
	$E_1D_RH_R$	F	0.6···	-	3.4	4.3	0.32	1
		M	0.5···	-	0.6	9.1	2.27	1
		M+F	0.5···	-	1.7	7.8	4.58	5
		T+OSS	0.5···	-	0.4	9.2···	6.59	7
PIR	E_1	F	3.0···	-	-	-	36.57···	3
		M	2.8···	-	-	-	32.86···	3
		M+F	2.9···	-	-	-	70.41···	7
		T+OSS	2.7···	-	-	-	77.69···	9
	E_1E_2	F	1.3···	1.7···	-	-	21.01···	2
		M	1.6···	1.7···	-	-	32.04···	2
		M+F	1.5···	1.4···	-	-	57.26···	6
		T+OSS	1.6···	1.2···	-	-	52.79···	8
	E_1D_R	F	0.5···	-	5.4···	-	1.32	2
		M	0.5···	-	5.4···	-	12.49··	2
		M+F	0.5···	-	5.4···	-	13.88·	6
		T+OSS	0.5···	-	5.2···	-	17.04·	8
	$E_1D_RH_R$	F	0.5···	-	2.8	4.8	0.51	1
		M	0.5···	-	-2.4	14.7··	1.59	1
		M+F	0.5···	-	-0.2	10.5··	3.98	5
		T+OSS	0.5···	-	0.4·	9.1··	4.96	7

Table 5. continued

Variable	Model	Data Set	E_1	E_2	D_R	H_R	X^2	df
PIF	E_1	F	11.4···	-	-	-	40.92···	3
		M	9.9···	-	-	-	42.40···	3
		M+F	10.6···	-	-	-	85.63···	7
		T+OSS	10.4···	-	-	-	91.96···	9
	E_1E_2	F	4.6···	6.9···	-	-	29.96···	2
		M	4.6···	5.1···	-	-	43.41···	2
		M+F	4.8···	5.9···	-	-	75.00···	6
		T+OSS	5.6···	4.9···	-	-	66.74···	8
	E_1D_R	F	1.1···	-	22.2···	-	2.04	2
		M	0.7···	-	21.6···	-	9.89··	2
		M+F	0.9···	-	21.8···	-	13.63·	6
		T+OSS	0.9···	-	21.4···	-	19.89·	8
	$E_1D_RH_R$	F	1.1···	-	10.3·	22.1	0.77	1
		M	0.7···	-	-1.3	41.7·	2.45	1
		M+F	0.9···	-	3.6	33.4·	6.31	5
		T+OSS	0.9···	-	1.9	35.6···	7.29	7

· $p < 0.05$
·· $p < 0.01$
··· $p < 0.001$

Table 6. Second degres polynomial mean-variance regression coefficients for finger pattern intensities (linear regression model was not appropriate for the data).

Pairs	MZ Males		MZ Females		DZ Males		DZ Females		Opposite Sex Sibs	
Regression coefficients	b_1	b_2	b_1	b_2	b_1	b_2	b_1	b_2	b_1	b_2
PIL	0.05	0.00	-0.10	0.00	1.42···	-0.05··	0.41	-0.02	1.52·	-0.05·
PIR	0.03	0.00	0.10	0.00	1.77··	-0.06·	0.91·	-0.04·	1.20·	-0.04·
PIF	0.19	0.00	-0.25	0.01	1.42·	-0.02	0.63	-0.01·	0.97·	-0.01
R-L	0.16	-3.46	-0.01	0.00	0.25·	-0.07	-0.13	-0.01	-0.04	0.08··

Table 7. Examples of dermatoglyphic traits with MZ correlations higher than expected from correlations in DZ twins or in parent-child (p-c) and sib-sib (s-s). Left and right are combined. Male and female pairs are combined considering consistent tendencies in both sexes (from Loesch and Swiatkowska, 1976, for twins and Loesch, 1974, for other relatives).

Characters	Correlations			
	MZ·	DZ··	p-c···	s-s····
Fingers				
Total pattern intensity(PIF)	0.92	0.31	0.36	0.34
Total ulnar pattern intensity	0.50	-0.03	-	-
Pattern intensity on finger I	0.77	0.16	-	-
Pattern intensity on finger II	0.71	0.17	-	-
Palms				
Interdigital loop II	0.43	-0.04	0.10	0.18
Hypothenar palmar H loop	0.73	0.09	0.14	0.14
Sum of digital triradii D	0.69	0.02	-	-
Distally displaced t triradii	0.76	0.24	0.16	0.18
Total palmar pattern ridge count+	0.80	0.29	0.14	0.22
Soles				
Hallucal loop I	0.85	0.29	0.29	0.21
Loop III	0.86	0.29	0.20	0.15
Loop III	0.73	0.25	0.21	0.10
Loop IV	0.76	0.29	0.23	0.17
Triradius z'	0.78	0.22	(0.29)	(0.22)
Total pattern intensity (PIS)	0.87	0.30	0.23	0.07

· 110 pairs, 60 males and 50 females

·· 111 pairs, 62 males and 49 females

··· 2010 pairs for fingers and palms, 773 pairs for soles

···· 1631 pairs for fingers and palms, 494 pairs for soles

x correlations estimated by Malhotra et al. (1981), where the number of pairs was as follows: 52 for MZ, 50 for DZ, 617 for p-c and 554 for s-s.

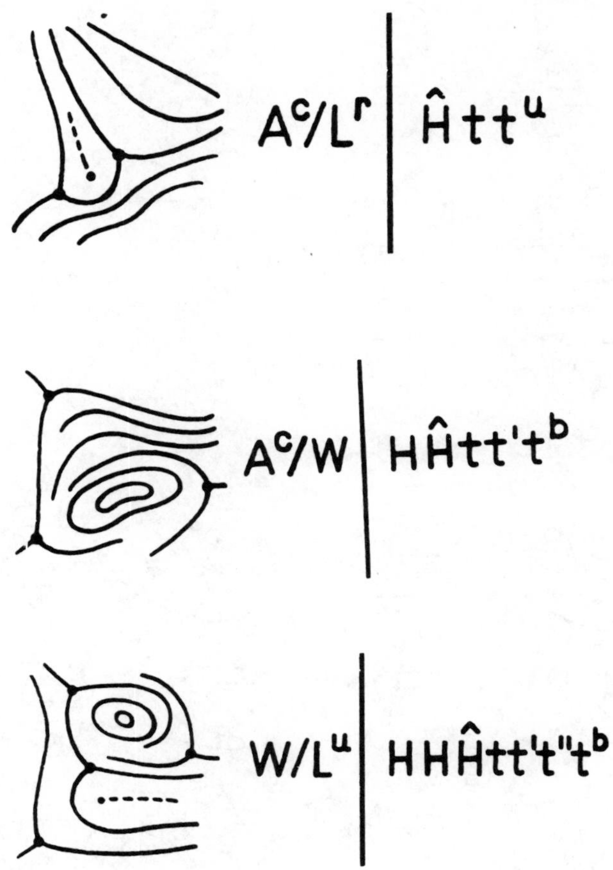

Fig. 1. Three different types of pattern in the right hypothenar area with their traditional and topological descriptions.

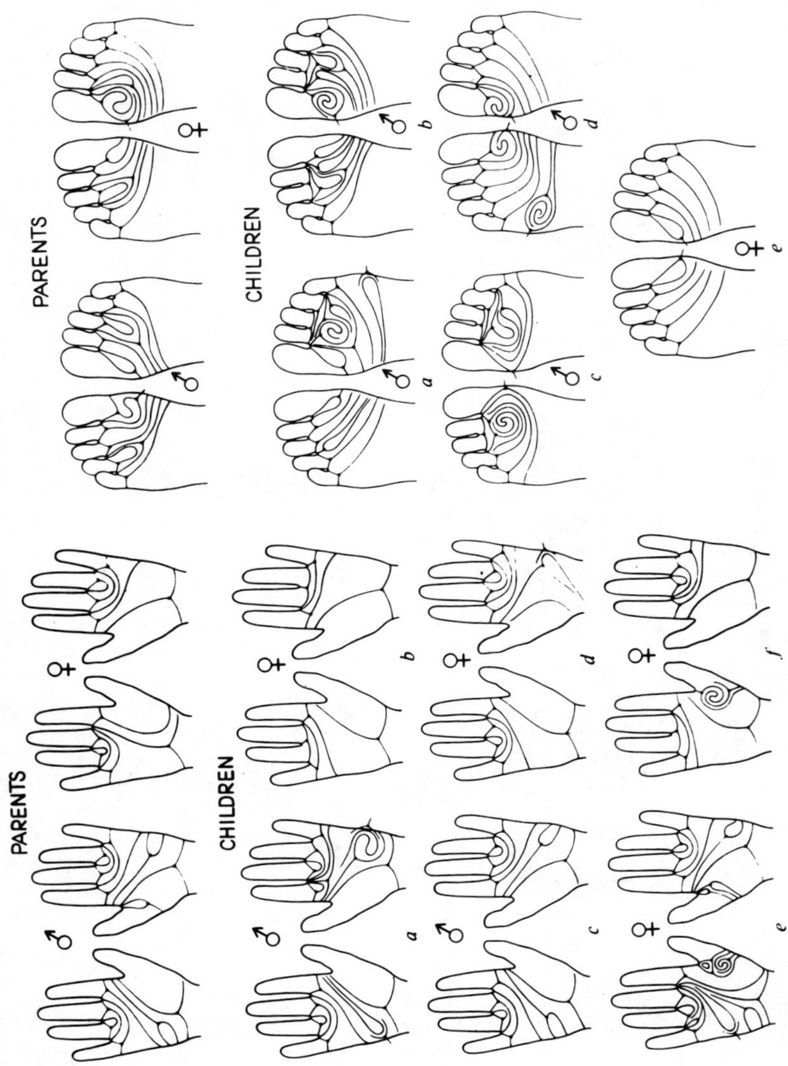

Fig. 2. Examples of palmar (a) or sole (b) ridge configurations within families (from the sample of Polish origin).

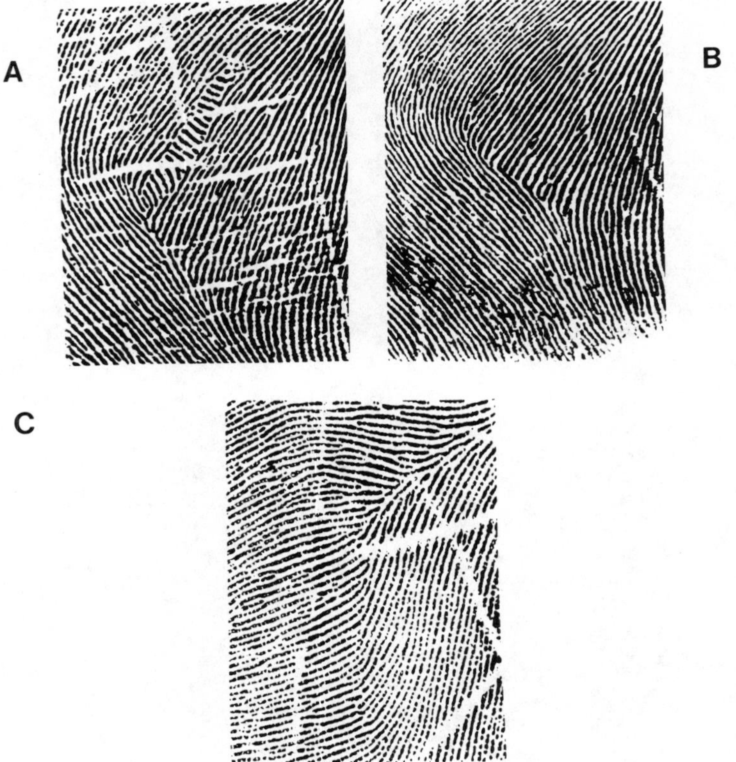

Fig. 3. Three types of vestigial configurations in the left thenar (a and b) and hypothenar (c) area, which represent the local disarrangement in the parallel course of ridges. These configurations can alternatively be expressed by the intensity of minutiae, whose number (particularly of "ends") is evidently increased within the vestige area as compared with the adjacent field of parallel ridges (Modified from Loesch D, 1982:"Quantitative Dermatoglyphics: Normal Variation, Genetics and Pathology", Oxford University Press (in press).

Progress in Dermatoglyphic Research, pages 79–91

POPULATION VARIATION IN DERMATOGLYPHICS: FIELD THEORY

D. F. ROBERTS

Professor and Head, Department of Human Genetics, University of Newcastle upon Tyne, England.

POPULATION VARIATION IN DERMATOGLYPHICS: FIELD THEORY

SUMMARY

Identification of principal components of digital dermatoglyphic variation in several populations of varying degrees of genetic affinity suggests close correspondence or universality of the components. Each component varies from one population to another in the amount of the variance for which it accounts, and so may come to vary in rank between populations and between sexes. Slight differences in loading on the different digits also occur. Differences tend to be less between populations geographically and genetically similar than between those more distant.

The first population studies of dermatoglyphics were those of Galton (1892) who examined fingerprints of different races in a search for evidence of hereditary transmission. He hoped to find some distinguishing peculiarity in each race, but was led to conclude "the only differences so far observed are statistical, and cannot be determined except through patience and caution, and by discussing large groups." Certainly by the time Bonnevie wrote in 1924, there were a number of series available for different human populations from India (Schlaginhaufen, 1906), for Italy (Gasti, 1907; Falco, 1908), from Sumatra and Indonesia (De Zwaan, 1911), from Japan and Korea (Furuse, 1913; Kubo, 1918; Hasebe, 1918) and to these Bonnevie added her magnificent Norwegian material. Today there are in the literature data on several hundred populations.

The earliest analyses were by simple frequencies of digital pattern types. These remain useful in the differentiation of continental populations, and if, say, one were given a hundred finger and palm prints with the information that they came from a random indigenous sample somewhere in Africa, South America, or northwest Europe, one would be able to assign it without difficulty to one or the other continent. But it is in the geographical distributions of such frequencies that the most interesting developments are occurring. These appear to show the existence of clines, that is to say gradients, of frequency across continents, with breaks in the gradients at particular points. One needs to enquire into the reasons for these gradients, and for the breaks of slope, and why they are located where they are.

Useful though they are, analysis of pattern frequencies is restricted by the lack of precision of knowledge of their inheritance. With the development of quantitative methods, particular by Bonnevie, Penrose and Holt, it seemed that at last one was dealing with a phenotypic character very closely related to the underlying genotype. From the systematic series of studies by Holt in which she examined the distribution of ridgecounts in the normal population (1949, 1954), the correlations between ridgecounts on different fingers (1951a, 1951b), the inheritance of total ridgecount (1952), bilateral asymmetry (1954), and the intrafamilial correlations (1957a, 1957b, 1958, 1961a, 1961b, 1968), she concluded that "the results of these investigations leave no doubt that pattern size, as determined by total ridgecount, is strongly determined by heredity. "From these and other studies the heritabilities have been calculated on the grounds that the pattern of the correlations is very similar to that expected in a polygenic situation. For total ridgecount, for example Huntley (1967) obtained a heritability of 98% from twin correlations, and a similar figure from sib correlations. Dominance is virtually absent, as shown by the linearity of the regression of children on midparent, and of the values of the regression coefficients, whereas the similarity of the mother/child and father/child correlations supports the view that the effect of maternal environment on total ridgecount is minimal (Holt, 1961). Holt also suggested that the negative skewness of the frequency distribution in a population indicated a fairly small number of genes having any appreciable effect. Altogether these intensive investigations indicated that the genetic basis of the total ridgecount was polygenic, with heritability very high indeed.

Unfortunately, total ridgecount is much less informative for population studies. For example, females of northeast Cumbria have a mean total ridgecount of 132.0, urban Mexicans of 132.1; females of northern Cumbria have a mean total ridge count of 130.4, rural Mexicans 130.5; the mean from Faringdon males in Berkshire is 112.5, from tribal Guarani in Brazil 112.7; of Lunana in Bhutan 136.1, of males from the east Downs in Berkshire 136.6; of males from Chipping Norton in north Oxfordshire 137.2, of Greeks from Tinos 137.5. Thus a mean TRC in one population can be matched by that in another which is genetically quite distinct. On the other hand, total ridge counts have proved particularly useful in local differentiation of populations, for example in the south midlands of England (Roberts & Coope, 1972) or between tribal samples in southern Brazil (Roberts et al, 1971).

These types of analysis using total ridge count consistently overlook one important feature of digital dermatoglyphics. This is the fundamental interdependence of dermatoglyphic traits, and in particular the close interrelationship between the digits, known since Galton originally pointed this out. The genes influencing the tissues of each finger must be identical initially; the overall consistency of ridgecount and pattern type between the fingers suggests that somatic mutation is an unlikely phenomenon. A more complex scheme of inheritance requires to be formulated to take into account the variation in expression of the genotype on the several fingers, the differential occurrence of particular pattern forms on certain digits, and the relationship between pattern type, shape and size. That is to say, the total ridgecount is not a homogeneous biologically meaningful character (Weninger, 1976). Individuals with the same total ridgecount may have quite different distribution of counts on different fingers. Total ridgecount, in summing the values on the ten fingers, disregards information relevant to individual and population differences. Fingers differ from each other in pattern frequency, mean ridgecount, its variability, pattern size, and other features, variation in all of which may be completely obscured by close similarity in total ridgecount.

Yet there is a basic biological similarity of digital dermal traits in the majority of populations sampled. For instance, the largest mean ridgecounts tend to occur on the thumb and fourth finger, and the smallest on the index finger; furthermore, the index and middle fingers carry the highest frequencies of radial patterns. Hence it seems that although each finger is subject to the same spectrum of hereditary factors, each digit appears to be influenced to a differing extent and in a different context. The extent of these influences may vary from one population to another. Whereas genotype expresses itself on all ten finges, each finger exerts its own modifying influence to produce its characteristic features. It seems therefore that just as to summate all fingers in total ridge count discards information, so to deal with particular fingers individually also discards information. A method of analysis is required suited to the analysis of multiple related measurements. Some form of multivariate analysis seems appropriate. It has been applied in the analysis of other biological data, including body build, the differentiation of crania, sex determination, and evolutionary studies. Howells (1969) pointed out that an individual is a unit, "not a discrete assembly of independent measurements. Accordingly a specimen should be treated as a vector of measurements, as an integrated whole, not as an inventory of separate figures. Any measurements must have a context of other measurements of the same specimen ...... in fact, a matrix of variation and co-variation is the mathematical basis for such analysis." The same approach is relevant to digital dermatoglyphics (Roberts & Coope, 1975).

Principal Components Analysis

To meet these requirements, principal components analysis was chosen. Its object was to reduce the 20 counts on the fingers (i.e. 10 fingers each with radial and ulnar count) to several uncorrelated components, to be explored subsequently for their biological interpretation. The analysis is effected through the variance/covariance matrix of the original variables. There is first computed that linear function of the variables that accounts for the largest proportion of their variation, then a second component independent of the first accounting for the largest fraction of the remaining variance and so on until all the variance is exhausted. No detailed theoretical structure is postulated initially, and the components are extracted from the analysis as mathematical formulations only. Among the necessary conditions, the multivariate distribution curves should be approximately normal, though slight departures from normality will not invalidate the analysis. Initial exploration indicated that several of the 20 counts met this condition fully, and the majority of the remainder sufficiently. A second requirement is that the variability and covariability in the populations examined should be relatively similar in form. The little information in the literature that there is on correlation matrices within populations indicates their essential similarity, and this was confirmed by the correlation patterns observed in all the material used.

i. Berkshire

The first application was to dermatoglyphic data from a large sample from Berkshire in the south of England, about 800 males and 800 females divided in two two subsamples, urban and rural, for each sex (Roberts & Coope, 1972). The four subsamples showed impressive consistency in the components extracted. First the variances (eigenvalues) for the first 10 components, together with the cumulative proportion of the total variance for which they account, are very similar in all four subsamples. Each showed that an appreciable number of components influenced the digital ridge count matrix, since eight components were required to account for 80% of the total variance and 15 to account for 95%. However, it was the distributions of the eigenvectors over the digits that were particularly informative. There is a characteristic distribution of the weighting of each component over the variates in each subsample. The first component appears to represent some factor determining the general magnitude of the finger ridge counts. The second appears to differentiate between the radial and ulnar sides of the fingers, the radial side of the finger generally having a positive weighting and the ulnar side a negative, with the index finger (and possibly the adjacent radial side of the mid finger) having a lower weight than the other digits. The third component, whle again to some extent involved in ulnar/radial contrasts on each digit, takes the general form of a gradient across the fingers from radial to ulnar side of the hand. It is remarkable for its strong effect on the thumb, high positive ratings being attached to individuals who have much larger counts on the thumb than the remaining fingers. Component 4 contrasts strongly the radial and ulnar sides of the index finger, the thumb is apparently also influenced by the radial element, and contrasted with this are the remaining mesial digits including the radial side of the little finger. The fifth component has a clearly defined effect on the fifth finger and is expressed by very high weightings on its radial and ulnar sides.

The great similarity between the Berkshire subsamples was shown first by graphical representation of the distribution of the components. Secondly, each component was described in terms of an arbitrary arithmetic value (obtained by subtracting, for a given individual, his ridge count in the variates of greatest negative loading from those of greatest positive loading). These arithmetic values were then plotted against the component weightings for individuals in each of the four subsamples, and these showed very close linear associations. This was almost exact for component number 1, but the association progressively diminished thereafter. Despite the crudity of the procedure, the analysis obviously produced results that were consistent between samples of appreciable size, showing the first five components extracted to be essentially similar in effect in the different subpopulations. It was clearly necessary to examine other populations.

ii. Oxfordshire

The next population examined was that from Oxfordshire, the adjacent county to Berkshire. Again a very large sample was analysed of 1,083 subjects, divided into four samples, male and female, rural and urban, the urban containing rather fewer than the rural. The eigenvalues were very similar to those in Berkshire, perhaps slightly less variable over the four subsamples, but eight components again being required to account for 80% of the total variance. The eigenvectors show that there is no doubt at all about components 1 and 2, where the pattern and extent of the differentiation are virtually identical to the Berkshire material. The gradient across the hand that describes the Berkshire component 3 occurs, however, in Oxfordshire as component 5, except in the urban male sample. The mesial/laterial contrast represented by Berkshire component 5 occurs as component 3 in rural males, and component 5 in urban males. It thus appears that in these adjacent populations the same components are identified, but the order in which they occur is slightly different.

iii. Cumbria

A similar analysis was carried out of 1,002 Cumbrians, in north-west England, distant some 250-300 miles from the other samples. The initial eigenvalues account for a greater proportion of the variance, only five being required for over 80% in both males and females (Table 1). Component 1 is easily identified, but it shows a much lower loading than in the previous samples. Component 2 again as identifiable, but here the thumb shows much lower loadings and apparently draws down with it the loading on the radial side of the index finger, but the contrast between radial and ulnar sides of digits 1, 3, 4 and 5 remains pronounced. The gradient across the hand shown in Berkshire component 3 now appears as component 4 in Cumbrian males, but with less of a contrast between the ulnar and radial sides of the digits, and with a heavier positive loading on the radial side of the thumb; in females component 3 shows the same heavy loading on the thumb, but digit 5 tends to positive loadings instead of negative. Components 3 in Cumbrian males, 4 in Cumbrian females, contrast the ulnar and radial sides of the index finger, but otherwise this component only appears to reflect the contrast between the ulnar and radial sides of each finger. The fifth component in both sexes is similar to that in Berkshire in that its maximal loadings occur on the fifth finger with high weightings on both the radial and ulnar sides in both sexes; in the males the thumb is clearly involved in this contrast, but much less so in the females. In view of the genetic differences between the population of Cumbria and the South Midlands, it is not surprising that some differences occur between the digital loading patterns; what is of interest is that essentially the same components occur and that the slight differences in each can be identified.

iv. The Basques

From farther afield samples tend to be smaller. In Europe, a population distinct genetically from those so far examined in Britain is that of the Basques, and here a sample of 335 was analysed, 200 males and 135 females. The cumulative proportions accounted for by the first ten eigenvalues were very similar to those of rural Oxfordshire. Components 1 and 2 are the same as in the British series, the loadings in component 1 and the loadings in component 2 on the thumb and the radial side of the index finger being much more similar to those in the Berkshire and Oxfordshire samples than in the Cumbrians. The Basque component 3 with its firm contrast of the radial and ulnar sides of the index finger and strong positive loading on the ulnar side of the little finger corresponds clearly to component 4 of the Oxfordshire female and total Berkshire samples, component 3 in Berkshire rural males and component 5 in the urban male. Basque component 4 is Berkshire component 3, but with particularly heavy loadings on the thumb which apparently do not affect the index finger. Basque component 5 is as expected, contrasting the mesial with the lateral digits. In all of these, the eigenvector loadings appear generally more similar to those in the Berkshire and Oxfordshire data than to the Cumbrian.

v. The Hehe of Tanzania

From farther afield and genetically quite distinct from the European populations is a sample of Hehe from central Tanzania. It is unfortunately rather smaller, consisting of 107 males and 89 females, so random variation in the eigenvalues and eigenvectors would be expected to be greater. The eigenvalue for component 1 appears to be elevated over that in the European populations, and the fact that this occurs in both sexes suggests that it is real rather than random variation. Only six components are required to account for 80% of the total variance. The distribution of component 1 is very similar to that seen in all the other populations, and its general level also is similar to all the others except the Cumbrians. Component 2 carries a lower loading on the thumb and a higher on the radial side of the index finger than all except the Cumbrians but its essential contrast of the ulnar and radial sides of the digits remains. The rank of the next two components appears to be interchanged in the two sexes. Component 3 in females and 4 in males corresponds to Berkshire component 4, with its pronounced contrast of the radial and ulnar sides of the index finger, its principal difference being a much stronger negative loading on the radial side of the little finger, enhancing the pronounced contrast of the two sides of this digit. Component 3 in males and 4 in females consists of very little else than the gradient across the digits, corresponding to Berkshire component 3 but with much less variation about this gradient particularly in males; in females digit 5 has a lesser negative loading. The fact that the two sexes differ suggests that random effects are beginning to manifest, so further components were not characterized.

vi. West Africa

A recent sample from West Africa is sufficiently large to provide estimates of principal components for comparison with the Hehe and so give an idea of the variation within the African continent. It consists of 364 Buzu males. Only five components are required to account for over 80% of the total variance. Distribution of component 1 is similar to that in the other populations, but at a rather lower level than in the Hehe. Component 2 is equally identifiable, but the positive loadings on the thumb are rather higher than in the Hehe, and resemble those of Oxfordshire and Berkshire. Component 3, the gradient across the hand, is rather more variable than in the Hehe, and is more reminiscent of the Berkshire distribution. In component 4 the contrast of the sides of the index finger is less pronounced than in the Hehe males, and the radial side of the thumb has a heavier positive loading. Component 5 contrasts the mesial with the lateral digits, but digit 4 appears to participate more with digit 5 as in the Berkshire series.

DISCUSSION

This comparison of several digital dermatoglyphic analyses shows quite clear correspondence among the principal components identified in the different populations. An identified component may well vary from one population to another in the amount of the variance for which it accounts, so it will not necessarily occupy the same rank in the contribution to the total variance. Slight differences in loading on the different digits may also occur, together with some random variation. But from the general correspondence in the several populations, it is tempting to suggest that the components are in fact universal.

It has been pointed out elsewhere that the present components are not to be equated with biological entities, but they may not be far removed, however, from mathematical representations of such entities (Roberts & Coope, 1975). Evidence from the study of fetal limb formation and particularly of the principal axes of growth suggests the existence of several growth factors. There is first a general size factor, whereby growth in each segment keeps pace with that in every other. A second factor differentiates radial and ulnar sides of the fingers and hands. Then parallel to the main axes of development there is a third influencing the mesial digits, and a fourth the lateral digits. Further evidence comes from disturbance in limb development (Penrose, 1963, 1965) and the congenital limb malformations to which they give rise. Such defects point to the independence of development of the radial side from that of the ulnar side of the hand, while the reduction or absence of central rays in one type of ectrodactyly suggests the independence of mesial development. Some of these defects appear to be influenced by major genes, for instance in the families showing apparently dominant hypoplasia of radial or ulnar rays. The components extracted in the present analysis bear a general resemblance to this scheme, in that the first component can be equated to the general size factor, the second with the differentiation of radial and ulnar counts on the fingers, the fifth contrasting the sides of the hand, and the fourth contrasting the lateral and mesial digits. There thus appears to be a general association between the components governing digital ridge counts, and the factors affecting general development of the distal end of the limb, and this leads one to speculate that the growth factors may also influence the appearance of the dermal patterns on the fingers.

These results can be explained in terms of field theory. Dahlberg (1945) recognised the possible existence of a complex of induction fields influencing the forming teeth to give a pattern of relatedness in general size and structure, yet with regionally distinct morphologic classes. There would be the possiblity of fields overlapping and of 'field polarisation' (that individual teeth may be the foci of particular fields). Butler (1963) developed the theory to describe the genetic control of tooth development when he envisaged each tooth as a modification of those next to it. "One could imagine a continuous (morphogenetic) field which has been sampled at intervals represented by the positions of the tooth germ. If the sampling is done at a slightly diffeent place, the results of the pattern will be slightly different." One can apply the same reasoning to the digital ridges, the characters of each digit being due to a development at a particular point in the field across the extremity of the limb bud.

The components emerging from the principal components analysis can be seen as the reflection of biological factors inducing gradients, with each finger at a different point in relation to others in the multidimensional space produced by these factors. The thumb, for instance, would sample this field at a quite different point from the fourth finger, since these digits have different positions in the series. These biological gradients would thus explain both the matrix of interdigital correlation coefficients, as well as the general similarity and detailed differences between such correlation matrices in different populations (Jantz, 1977). They would also agree with the present analysis, where fingers adjacent to each other tend to be more similarly weighted in a given component than fingers physically distant from each other, which according to the field theory would be further apart in the field. Field polarisation would explain the phenotypic peculiarities characteristic of a given digit. Field theory would account for the observation that correlations between relatives seem to be higher for total ridge count than for the separate fingers.

The correspondence in, or indeed universal occurrence of, the components in the different populations here reviewed, would on field theory indicate similar communality of the development fields which they reflect. The fields, and the sampling thereof by the developing digits, would be expected to be similar in populations genetically and geographically close to each other, and the great similarity between the subsamples within Oxfordshire and Berkshire shows this. The Cumbrian sample, genetically different from these, shows slight differences in the loadings, for example the lower loadings of the thumb and the radial side of the index finger of component 2, suggesting that the positions of the first and second finger buds sample the underlying field at a slightly different position, or that the intensity of the underlying field is rather less. The suggestion from the Hehe that fewer components account for more of the variation than in the United Kingdom Midland and Basque samples is supported by the West African sample, and also by the analysis of Jantz and Owsley (1977) of American Whites, Blacks and West African Yoruba, though it is of interest that the Cumbrian sample shows a similar increase in the proportion of the variance accounted for.

TABLE 1: Eigenvalues of the first 10 components in Buzu (Nigeria) and Cumbrians (N.W. England)

Component	BUZU MALES		CUMBRIAN MALES		CUMBRIAN FEMALES	
	Eigen-values	Cumulative Proportion	Eigen-values	Cumulative Proportion	Eigen-values	Cumulative Proportion
1	8.52	52.0	7.76	50.0	8.27	53.4
2	2.03	64.4	1.67	60.8	1.62	63.8
3	1.55	73.8	1.29	69.1	1.21	71.7
4	0.99	79.9	1.13	76.3	1.00	78.1
5	0.75	84.4	0.86	81.9	0.85	83.6
6	0.68	88.6	0.63	86.0	0.58	87.3
7	0.41	91.1	0.51	89.2	0.38	89.8
8	0.34	93.1	0.40	91.8	0.38	92.2
9	0.24	94.6	0.31	93.8	0.31	94.2
10	0.23	96.0	0.29	95.7	0.20	95.5

These differences in eigenvalues suggest different intensities of effect of the batteries of polygenes responsible for each induction field.

By field theory can be explained much of the complexity that must be involved in gene action in dermal traits. By it can also be understood gene action on the 'digital complex' as a whole, seeing each finger as a discrete part of this complex and not as a separate unit acted on independently by the genes involved. To slight variation in the fields can be attributed the variation observed beween different populations. Field theory does not, of course, discredit the polygenic hypothesis of quantitative dermatoglyphics, it merely adds a further dimension to their perception.

REFERENCES

Butler PM (1963) Tooth morphology and primate evolution. In Brothwell DR (ed): "Dental Anthropology." Oxford University Press.

Dahlberg AA (1945) The changing dentition of man. J Am Dent Assoc 32: 676.

Falco G Ricerche sulla frequenza e simpatia dei diversi tipi di figure papillari su 1579 individui. Atti della Soc Med Leg I.

Furuse Y (1913) Untersuchungen über Verbrecher in Sugamo. (Mentioned by Kubo, 1918, exact title not known.)

Gasti G (1907) Sui disegni papillari. Att del Soc Rom Anthrop, vol. XIII.

Hasebe K (1918) Uber das Hautleistensystem der Vola u. Planta der Japaner u. Aino. Arb Anat Inst Kais, Japan, Univ. Sendai, H. l.

Holt SB (1949) A quantitative survey of the fingerprints of a small sample of the British population. Ann Eugen 14: 329.

Holt SB (1951a) The correlations between ridge-counts on different fingers. Ann Eugen 16: 287.

Holt SB (1951b) A comparative quantitative study of the fingerprints of Mongolian imbeciles and normal individuals. Ann.Eugen. 15: 355.

Holt SB (1952) Genetics of dermal ridges: Inheritance of total finger ridge-count. Ann Eugen 17: 140.

Holt SB (1954) Genetics of dermal ridges: bilateral asymmetry in finger ridge-counts. Ann Eugen 18: 211.

Holt SB (1957) Genetics of dermal ridges: Sib-pair correlations for total finger ridge-count. Ann Hum Genet 21: 352.

Holt SB (1957) Quantitative genetics of dermal ridge-patterns on fingers. Acta Genet (Basel) 6: 473.

Holt SB (1958) Genetics of dermal ridges: the relation between total ridge-count and the variability of counts from finger to finger. Ann Hum Genet 22: 323.

Holt SB (1961a) Dermatoglyphic patterns. In "Genetical Variation in Human Populations." Harrison GA (ed) Oxford: Pergamon Press, p.79.

Holt SB (1961b) Quantitative genetics of finger-print patterns. Br Med Bull 17: 247.

Holt SB (1968) "The Genetics of Dermal Ridges." Illinois: Thomas.

Howells WW (1969) The use of multivariate techniques in the study of skeletal populations. Am J Phys Anthropol 31: 311.

Huntley RMC (1967) Some problems in the study of quantitative variation in man. In Spickett SG (ed): "Endocrine Genetics." Cambridge: Camb Univ Press.

Jantz RL (1977) Sex and race differences in finger ridge-count correlations. Am J Phys Anthropol 46: 171.

Jantz RL & Owsley DW (1977) Factor analysis of finger ridge-counts in Blacks and Whites. Ann Hum Biol 4: 357.

Kubo T (1918) Beitr.zur Daktyloskopie der Koreaner. Mitteil Med Fachschule zu Keijo.

Penrose LS (2963) Finger-prints, palms and chromosomes. Nature (Lond.) 197: 933.

Penrose LS (1965) Dermatoglyphic topology. Nature (Lond.) 205: 544.

Roberts DF, Chavez J, Salzano FM & Fernando J da Rocha (1971) Dermatoglyphics of Caingang and Guarani Indians Man, 6: 61.

Roberts DF & Coope E (1972) Dermatoglyphic variation in the South Midlands. Heredity 29: 293.

Roberts DF & Coope E (1975) Components of variation in a multifactorial character: a dermatoglyphic analysis. Hum Biol 47: 169.

Schlagenhaufen O (1906) Zur Morphologie d. Palma u. Planta der Vorerindier u. Ceyloner. Zeitschr J Ethnol H 4-5.

Weninger M, Aue-Hauser G, Scheiber V (1976) Total finger ridge-count and the polygenic hypothesis: a critique. Hum Biol 48: 713.

de Zwaan, Kleiweg (1911) Daktyloskopisch Onderzoek bij de Niassers. Nederl Tijdschr v Geneeskunde.

Progress in Dermatoglyphic Research, pages 93–104

PARENTAL INFLUENCES ON FINGERDERMATOGLYPHICS

André G. de Wilde and Harmien W.M. Amesz-Voorhoeve
State University Groningen

The Netherlands

Introduction

During the last 3 years several studies appeared (Bener (1979, 1980), de Wilde (1980)) pointing to the existence of different parental influences on the fingerpatterns. De Wilde and Bener even found arguments that some underlying sex linked inheritance might exist. Our own findings here were based on rather small samples and published in a preliminary report. Since then, thanks to the cooperation of our dear colleagues, we were able to enlarge our data extensively. The results will be given here; we publish here some new findings, on other biological influences than the sex-determining ones too.

The Between Tribes Correlationmatrix

In order to get enough comparable patternscores of individuals from different populations, patterns were classified into whorls and non-whorls (=loops and arches). Working with percentages, to which a 0-1 classification inevitably leads, implies difficulties in the statistical interpretation. Working with individual records, an arcsintransformation cannot be applied , as a between individuals covariancematrix is needed. The majority of frequences being not far from .50, invalidates most of the strength of the argument in favour of an arcsinus transformation.

Four different sets of data were at our disposal: the

data of Plato and Wertelecki; of de Wilde and Julien; of Dankmeijer and of Salomé. In order to omit the implication of interclassification variances the first was dicarded. The remaining sets comprise 26 different ethnic groups of males and 23 groups of females (Table 1).

	male	female	
DUTCH	1000	539	Dankmeyer
SURINAM	118	148	Salomé
INDIA			Julien
CHENCHU	71	54	
SIKH	50	51	
TAMIL	73	62	
WEDDA	80	71	
TODA	54	48	
GAUDA	73	37	
MALDHARI	60	19	
INDIA			Julien
6 groups	64	54	
	59	44	
	65	83	
	89	21	
	51	15	
	21	4	
W. IRIAN			de Wilde
11 (8)	41	8	
groups	106	19	
	96	59	
	23	8	
	13	4	
	7	-	
	47	6	
	66	13	
	61	6	
	26		
	17		

Table 1: 49 groups of data on which the between-group-correlation-matrix was calculated.

The patterns in all groups were classified in whorls and non-whorls, according to the rules given by Dankmeijer (1934). The importance of working with the between correlation matrix, and not with the total one or the within groups matrix, rests on the argument that the BCM is more likely to show the effects of differences in genfrequences of the groups than the T or W matrices.

Principal components were calculated from the between groups correlation matrices for the right hands and left hands separately. After this a varimax rotation was applied. For both hands the Eigenvalues for the first two factors were more than 90%. The results did not differ substantially from those, obtained from five factors for R and L hands taken together in one 5 * 5 matrix. For the fingers (1 to 5), the 5 factor coefficients were found at .3659; .8165; .8508; .7636; .3128 respectively. There is a tendency towards symmetry around the third finger. The fifth and first fingers have the lowest loadings, the second and fourth have two or three times this weight, and the third one still more.

Data on Parents and Children

The following symbols were used: F=father; M=mother; S1=first sib is a son; D1=first sib is a daughter; S2=second sib is a son; D2=second sib is a daughter; SS=S2 after S1; SD=D2 after S1; DS=S2 after D1; DD=D2 after D1. Data were obtained on classified fingerpatterns from 7 different ethnic groups. From all groups the families were selected with two children. If more children were present in one family, both eldest sibs were selected. This was only possible if all the birth dates were known. In those groups where this was not the case, both presumably eldest children were elected. The data were: families from the Netherlands (Woubrugge, collected by IJdens, published by de Wilde, 1953), America I and II (from Plato/Wertelecki), Uruguay (from Kolski), Brasil (from Perreira da Silva), from the Netherlands (surroundings of Tiel, Bringmann, Huizinga), Belgium (Suzanne). The classification criteria for whorls/non-whorls probably are not identical for all groups. For this reason all parents/offspring correlations between the scores for the first factor of all 7 groups were tested on inconsitencies (Table 2 and 3). The correlations between the right or left hands of the parents and the first or second children in the combinations SS, SD, DS, DD were investigated. This means that 16 χ^2's each for 7 r-values were calculated. One chi-square was significant at the 5% level, what is nearly what might have been expected if no heterogeneity exists. Thus there is no serious indication for heterogeneity in the r-values between the 7 ethnic groups.

			1st children							
			S1		S2		D1		D2	
			r	n	r	n	r	n	r	n
Dutch I	R	F	.353*	43	.199	42	.314	29	.512***	37
		M	.310	49	.416**	44	.462*	30	.331	37
	L	F	.191	50	.044	44	.319	30	.597***	37
		M	.452***	49	.504***	44	.320	30	.288*	36
Amer. I	R	F	.374**	105	.407***	106	.344***	96	.353***	92
		M	.275*	105	.344***	106	.304*	96	.259	92
	L	F	.410***	105	.392***	106	.538***	95	.246**	92
		M	.242*	105	.310**	106	.208	95	.289*	92
Amer. II	R	F	.144	14	.072	22	.443	19	.321	11
		M	.444	14	.186	22	.348	19	.136	11
	L	F	.362	14	.097	22	.471	19	.497	11
		M	.343	14	.160	22	.393	19	.247	11
Urug.	R	F	.485***	52	.264	41	.166	43	.331*	54
		M	.491***	52	.510***	41	.266	43	.218	54
	L	F	.245	52	.202	41	.337	43	.418**	54
		M	.474***	52	.634***	41	.497*	43	.355*	54
Bras.	R	F	.336***	123	.270	130	.309***	145	.281***	138
		M	.390***	123	.563***	130	.454***	145	.469***	138
	L	F	.248*	123	.314***	130	.390***	145	.291***	138
		M	.412***	123	.454***	130	.401***	145	.429***	138
Dutch II	R	F	.582***	38	.396**	44	.228	50	.411**	42
		M	.614***	37	.319*	44	.434**	50	.689***	41
	L	F	.568***	37	.232	42	.250	51	.437**	43
		M	.628***	37	.057	42	.364**	49	.530***	42
Belg.	R	F	.324	30	.460**	32	.258	37	.590***	36
		M	.601***	30	.404*	32	.306	37	.507**	36
	L	F	.181	31	.348	32	.290	37	.257	36
		M	.484**	30	.579***	31	.370*	37	.542***	36

Table 2: Correlation tables for parents and 1st and 2nd sibs in seven ethnic groups; F=father; M=mother; S1=1st sons; D1=1st daughters; S2=2nd children if sons; D2=2nd children if daughters; SS=S2 after S1; SD=D2 after S1; DS=S2 after D1; DD=D2 after D1; r=correlation coefficient; n=number of pairs; *=significant at 5%; **=1%, ***= 1°/oo level. Dutch I=Dutch, Woubrugge; Dutch II=Dutch, Tiel; Amer. I=American whites; Amer. II=American blacks; Urug.=Uruguayans; Bras.=Brasilians; Belg.=Belgians.

2nd children							
SS		SD		DS		DD	
r	n	r	n	r	n	r	n
.158	31	.400*	16	.483	10	.683***	19
.444*	31	-.070	17	.304	12	.512*	18
.024	32	.431	17	.101	12	.666	13
.444**	32	.140	16	.704**	12	.416	18
.533***	60	.298	42	.258	46	.404***	50
.279*	60	.355	42	.382**	46	.209	50
.393**	60	.134	42	.430**	45	.354***	50
.342**	60	.304	42	.310	45	.281	50
.159	11	-.277	3	.023	11	.575	8
-.037	11	-.149	3	.453	11	.112	8
.089	11	.933	3	.239	11	.445	8
.120	11	-.570	3	.094	11	.295	8
.427*	26	.245	26	-.283	15	.537***	28
.713***	26	.279	26	.469	15	.171	23
.294	26	.225	26	-.197	15	.628***	28
.717***	26	.346	26	.621**	15	.416*	29
.326	58	.166	65	.226	72	.388***	73
.586***	58	.482***	65	.548***	72	.464***	73
.383*	58	.158	65	.254	72	.398***	73
.499***	58	.414***	65	.414**	72	.441***	73
.392	17	.657**	19	.407*	27	.227	23
.460	17	.710***	18	.206	27	.714***	23
.099	15	.324	19	.382*	27	.518**	24
.344	16	.738***	19	-.207	26	.458*	23
.742**	12	.693***	18	.242	20	.575*	17
.319	12	.569*	18	.461*	20	.420	17
.719**	12	.613**	19	-.060	20	.016	17
.517	10	.682***	19	-.610**	20	.332	17

Table 2: Continuation

		SS	SD	DS	DD
R	F	7.14	9.28	5.24	4.67
	M	10.35	8.45	3.96	9.23
L	F	7.53	5.20	6.67	7.19
	M	12.08	8.37	14.39*	1.26

Table 3: Values of χ^2_6 as results of the test on the homogeneity of the correlationcoefficients (after z-transformation) between parents and second children. 5% level is χ^2_6 = 12.59.

The r-value for all groups combined are given in Table 4.

		S1		S2		D1		D2		SS		SD		DS		DD	
		r	n	r	n	r	n	r	n	r	n	r	n	r	n	r	n
R	F	.378	410	.321	417	.292	419	.371	410	.408	215	.308	189	.218	201	.438	218
	M	.398	410	.430	419	.379	420	.396	409	.417	215	.414	189	.443	203	.381	217
L	F	.310	412	.285	417	.392	420	.344	411	.313	214	.249	191	.253	202	.420	218
	M	.400	410	.404	416	.353	418	.396	409	.438	214	.423	190	.371	201	.384	217

Table 4: Values of the parent/offspring correlation coefficients for all 7 ethnic groups combined. All r-values are significant at the .001 level.

Differences in Parent/Offspring, Dependent on Sex and Birth Order

Comparison of the P/O correlations gives significant (5% level) differences between father/2nd son correlations on the right hands, dependent on the sex of the 1st child; rF/SS = .408; rF/DS = .218. Another significant difference is found on the left hands of father/daughter correlations: rF/SD = .249; rF/DD = .420. In mothers the difference between the correlations mother/2nd child with respect to the sexes of 1st and 2nd children are insignificant ($\bar{r}$ = .419); these observations are indicative for an influence of the first child on the patterns in the second child. The correlations F/2nd child, where the sex of the 2nd child is the same as that of the 1st one, are on the same level ($\bar{r}$ = .396) as the $\bar{r}$ in mothers. However, the "heterosex" childrenpairs have 2nd partners with significant lower correlations with the fathers. This is true for both hands ($\bar{r}$ = .262).

Partial Correlations

Even when the first sib exerts no influences on the second one, then they remain correlated by their common parents. In a polygenic system the correlation coefficient is expected at .50. If the influences of the parents are eliminated by means of partial correlation analysis, then the sib-sib correlation must be zero.

	Corr. between			controlling for			
				Father	Mother	F+M	
		r	n	r'	r''	r'''	
R	S1/SS	.454	(215)	.331 ***	.323 ***	.175 *	sibs with the same sex
L	S1/SS	.380	(215)	.307 ***	.221 ***	.213 -	
R	D1/DD	.438	(219)	.349 ***	.343 ***	.235 ***	
L	D1/DD	.338	(219)	.192 **	.262 ***	.095 -	
R	S1/SD	.369	(190)	.308 ***	.266 ***	.195 **	sibs with different sexes
L	S1/SD	.392	(191)	.346 ***	.275 ***	.231 ***	
R	D1/DS	.417	(203)	.379 ***	.298 ***	.241 ***	
L	D1/DS	.380	(202)	.319 ***	.262 ***	.194 **	

Table 5: Correlations between first and second child; r=full correlation; r'=correlation after controlling for fathers (F); r''=correlation after controlling for mothers (M); r'''=correlation after controlling for fathers and mothers (F+M). S1=first son, D1=first daughter etc. All 7 groups combined.

Table 5 gives the results of these calculations. Both parents evidently influence the correlation between the sibs; sibs with different sexes show on both hands significant partial correlations; sibpairs with equal sexes have lower partial correlations, which are even insignificant on the left hands. On right hands also the D1/DD and S1/SS correlations are significant. Without further analysis we can only conclude that first sibs influence second sibs. Possibly all later born children undergo influences by all their older sibs. These influences must work along nongenetical, parental ways. For example, some change in the maternal body,

correlation between		controlling for: cases	d.f.	F	d.f.	M	d.f.	F + M	d.f.	DIFF1	d.f.	DIFM1	d.f.
S1/SS	R	.360***	102	.224*	99	.284**	99	.125	98	.358***	99	.356***	99
S1/SS	L	.441***	103	.390***	100	.362***	100	.288**	99	.441***	100	.441***	100
S1/SD	R	.257*	62	.228	58	.208	58	.181	57	.247	58	.234	58
S1/SD	L	.382**	62	.336**	58	.330	58	.279*	57	.348**	58	.328	58
D1/DS	R	.351**	69	.290*	64	.273*	64	.192	63	.322**	64	.324**	64
D1/DS	L	.347**	68	.214	65	.260*	65	.117	64	.335**	65	.318**	65
D1/DD	R	.478***	77	.355**	73	.419***	73	.2[illegible]1*	72	.490***	73	.487***	73
D1/DD	L	.411***	77	.231*	73	.374***	73	.196	72	.417***	73	.410***	73
S1/SS	R+L	.439***	102	.347***	99	.350***	99	.230*	98	.437***	99	.437***	99
S1/SD	R+L	.357**	62	.299*	57	.301*	57	.245	56	.326*	57	.303*	57
D1/DS	R+L	.399***	68	.291*	63	.303*	63	.172	62	.371**	63	.359**	63
D1/DD	R+L	.513***	76	.298**	71	.451***	71	.220	70	.520***	71	.513***	71

correlation between		DIFF1 + F	d.f.	DIFM1 + F	d.f.	DIFF1 + M	d.f.	DIFM1 + M	d.f.	DIFF1 + F + M	d.f.	DIFM1 + F + M	d.f.
S1/SS	R	.214*	98	.222*	98	.281**	98	.277**	98	.113	97	.120	97
S1/SS	L	.388***	99	.390***	99	.361***	99	.361***	99	.286**	98	.288**	98
S1/SD	R	.209	57	.200	57	.193	57	.183	57	.157	56	.152	56
S1/SD	L	.280*	57	.267*	57	.300*	57	.278*	57	.225	56	.216	56
D1/DS	R	.267*	63	.264*	63	.265*	63	.262*	63	.184	62	.174	62
D1/DS	L	.190	64	.165	64	.269*	64	.253*	64	.121	63	.096	63
D1/DD	R	.374***	72	.372***	72	.433***	72	.430***	72	.291*	71	.289*	71
D1/DD	L	.233*	72	.231*	72	.388***	72	.381***	72	.195	71	.195	71
S1/SS	R+L	.341***	98	.346***	98	.347***	98	.345***	98	.223*	97	.227*	97
S1/SD	R+L	.251	56	.239	56	.274*	56	.255	56	.194	55	.187	55
D1/DS	R+L	.266*	62	.245	62	.304*	62	.290*	62	.172	61	.148	61
D1/DD	R+L	.311**	70	.308**	70	.465***	70	.458***	70	.231	69	.229	69

Table 6: Correlations and partial correlations between first and second children of the Dutch, Americans I and Americans II combined.

caused by an earlier child, might influence the development (and thereby the ridgepatterns) of a later sib. Another possibility may be found in an immune reaction of the mother on the sperm of the husband, or on the X or Y chromosomes of the husband, etc.

The Age of the Parents at Time of Birth of the 1st Child

In the data Dutch I, Americans I and II, ages of parents and children are given. In Table 6 the sib-sib correlations given seem to be independent of the agedifference between parent and first child. The ages of the parents are correlated with fingerpatterns in the second sons in the D<u>S</u> pairs. This holds for both parents. In Table 7 the partial correlations are given for the agedifference between parent and first child with the fingerpatternscores in 1st and 2nd sibs (all with respect to sexes), controlling for the other parent/child agedifference. None of the correlations is significantly different from zero.

Corr.	S1		D1		S<u>S</u>		S<u>D</u>		D<u>S</u>		D<u>D</u>		control-
between	R	L	R	L	R	L	R	L	R	L	R	L	ling for
DIFF1	-.045	.030	-.016	.029	.001	-.051	.060	-.080	-.092	-.046	.090	.154	DIFM1
DIFM1	.013	.034	-.099	.082	-.049	.029	-.131	.058	-.138	-.221	-.068	-.076	DIFF1
d.f.	165	166	143	142	99	100	59	59	66	65	74	74	

Table 7: Partial correlations between agedifference from parent and first child (DIFF1=father-1st child; DIFM1=mother-1st child) and fingerpatterns in first and second sibs, based on Dutch I, Amer. I and Amer. II combined.

Realising that the ages of both parents are highly positively correlated, controlling for father/1st sib-ages in the case of correlation mother/1st sib-age with factorscores 2nd sib, will eliminate the age influences. This means that, all correlations not being significantly different from zero, the age of the parents at the time of birth of the first child seems to be the over all important factor.

In Table 8 the partial correlations between parent/1st sib-agedifferences and the factorscores of 1st and 2nd sibs are given, controlling for the factorscores of the parents. As expected, no correlation seems to exist between agedifferences and the factorscores in the first children. However, in the 2nd children, positive correlations exist for the D<u>S</u> and S<u>D</u> sibs, with the ages of parents minus age first sibs.

	S1	D1	SS	DS	SD	DD	control-ling for
DIFF1	.037	-.086	-.090	-.345**	.377***	.206	F
	.040	-.074	-.058	-.212	.299*	.095	M
	.045	-.036	-.090	-.218	.379**	.225	F+M ←
d.f.	162	136	98	62	56	70	
DIFM1	.070	-.120	-.036	-.412***	.347**	.146	F
	.058	-.119	-.072	-.318**	.311	.026	M
	.072	-.082	-.053	-.336**	.337**	.166	F+M ←
d.f.	162	136	98	62	56	70	

Table 8: Partial correlations between agedifference from parent and first child and fingerpatterns in first and second sibs. ← = row with "cleant up" correlation.

These correlations are in general still significant after controlling for the factorscores of one or both parents. Another interesting fact lies in the signs of the correlations: DS correlations are all negative, SD correlations are all of comparable magnitude as the DS correlations, but positive.

Influences Agedifferences Sibs

The correlations between the agedifference of both sibs and the factorscores of the 2nd sibs, controlling for the parental age-1st sib-age, are all non significant. In other words: the time lapse between the births of 1st and 2nd sibs, has no influence on the ridgepatterns of the latter.

Discussion

Many studies have shown that fingerpatterns are for the greater part influenced by genetic factors (Bonnevie (1924), Holt (1968), de Wilde (1953)). This is in accord with the parent/offspring correlations found in the data presented here, varying between .20 and .44 (Table 4). However, when the influences of father and mother are eliminated by partial correlation techniques, significant sib/sib correlations remain (Table 5). The sib/sib correlations lie between .34 and .45. Controlling for both parents significant (at 1% level) correlations remain for D1/DD. D1/SD combinations. This implies that, the first sib influences the second one in its ridgepatterns. Of course such influences must exert themselves by means of the maternal organism. A common environmental cause, eventually working via the mother, seems improbable. In that case all sibpairs should have the same correlations with the parents. In Table 4 it comes out that the SD and DS second sibs are significantly lower correlated with their fathers than the SS and DD 2nd sibs. In the SD, DS, SS and DD correlations with the mothers such differences were not observed.

An earlier publication (de Wilde (1980)) suggested an sex-linked + autosomal genetic background. In this publication another linear transformation of the individual patterns was applied (an error in the sorting program gave other factorscorecoefficients than applied now). The results point in the same directions as the studies of Bener. At this moment we think it better not to enter into an eventual sex-linked or sex-linked + autosomal model. Some other phenomena must first be analysed.

The age of the mother at the time of birth of the first child has an important influence on the patterns in the 2nd sib, in the "heterosexual" sibpairs SD and DS (Table 7). In the older mothers the second child undergoes more influences of its precursor. The agedifference between both sibs has no effect. The correlation of the DS sibs with the parent/1st sib-agedifference is negative, that of SD sibs positive. The absolute magnitudes of both correlations do not differ ($\bar{r}$ = .37). The genetic influences of both parents seem to be without importance in the SD sibs. In DS sibs the father seems to have some influence, together with the agedifference-factor. It may be such, that in the older maternal organism the first male child evokes some reaction which to a greater extent determines the patterns in the female second sib. When the second sib is a male, this reaction has no effect. The first female child in the younger mother determines by some maternal reaction the patterns in the second male sib.

The factorscores can also be reinterpreted into patterns; the younger the mother, the more loops and/or arches in the DS sib; the older the mother, the more whorls in the SD sib.

Further analysis of the qualitative aspects of the results mentioned above is going on. This analysis goes into the pattern combinations in individual sibs and is supported by the topological pattern classification given by the author in the Amsterdam symposium in April 1981.

We believe that our results open new fields of research

in Dermatoglyphics. Since decennia it was generally accepted that the ridgepatterns of the skin were "completely" genetically determined. Our results indicate socio-economic and demographic factors do influence the patterns too. It is very probable that with more refined classification techniques and a better understanding of the underlying biological process, dermatoglyphics become important monitoring characters for other environmental factors too.

Acknowledgements

We are deeply indepted to the following colleagues who made this study possible: Dr. J. Dankmeijer†, Dr. A.J. Salomé, Dr. P.F.J.A. Julien for the population data put at our disposal. Very specially we are indepted to those colleagues who gave us full access to their unique collections of family data: Dr. W. Wertelecki and Drs. C. Plato (U.S.A., also population data), Dr. R. Kolski (Uruguay), Dr. M. Perreira da Silva (Brasil), Dr. C. Suzanne (Belgium) and Dr J. Huizinga (Utrecht). We are also indepted to Mrs. J.G. Benjamins and Mr. B. Deddens for their invaluable assistance.

References

Bener A (1979). Correlation Between Relatives, Their Theoretical Values for Autosomal and Sex-linked Characters with Respect to Dermatoglyphic Characters. Coll Antrop 3/2: 211-224.

Bener A (1980). Grandparental Influences in the Expression of Dermatoglyphic Pattern Elements (Loops and triradii) on Fingertips and Palms. Coll Antrop 4/2: 151-154.

Bonnevie K (1924). Studies on papillary patterns of human fingers. J Genet 15: 1-111.

Holt SB (1968). "The Genetics of Dermal Ridges." Springfield: Thomas.

De Wilde AG (1953). De grondslagen der overerving van het vingerpatroon. Thesis.

De Wilde AG (1980). Fingerpatterns in families, a preliminary report. Bull Soc roy belge Anthrop Préhist 91: 103-109.

Progress in Dermatoglyphic Research, pages 105–109

PARAMETERS USED TO DESCRIBE LESS COMMON SINGLE MAJOR GENES EXPRESSED IN DERMATOGLYPHIC FEATURES.

H. Warner Kloepfer, Ph. D
Department of Anatomy, Tulane University
New Orleans, Louisiana, USA.

In a recent informal discussion with Dr. Aue-Hauser of Vienna, Dr. A. DeWilde of Groningen, and Dr. E. R. Iagolnitzer of Paris, it was suggested that the term glyphogenetics might be a useful term to describe the study of genes associated with dermatoglyphic features. Dr. Harold Cummins used the Greek term "glyphics"for carvings when he suggested the term dermatoglyphics to describe the study of ridges of the hands and feet. We use the terms neurogenetics and pharmacogenetics to describe genes associated with neurological and pharmaceutical implications. Why not use the term glyphogenetics to describe genes associated with dermatoglyphic features? Whereas most geneticists have directed attention to multiple gene effects, all my studies in clinical genetics have been unique to the extent that they have dealt only with single major gene effects. With this particular background experience it is logical that my efforts in glyphogenetics also should be concerned with the study of single major gene effects.

For months I have had in my possession an OUTPOST 11 home computer, with 64 K of memory, two 8" disk drives, and a printer, which were made available by the CENTER FOR THE STUDY OF MULTIPLE BIRTH and the TANO CORPORATION. With the help of various Mothers of Twins Clubs and twin organizations, I now have in my possession dermatoglyphic prints from some 3000 sets of twins and families of twins. It is my intention to extend this body of data to include 4000 sets of twins and as many relatives as possible.
This effort to obtain prints began some six years ago.

As I work with the formulations of these prints I am aware of some 6 to 12 different single major genes that I feel can be described. This presentation will be limited to a progress report. My computer program to store 78 items of dermatoglyphic feature information in a 126-digit string for each person is working beautifully and I have recorded information from over 2000 persons. Actually, recordings take much less time than the formulations. Eventually I expect to record three times this amount of information for each person, especially when the person is in a family used to identify carriers of major genes.

I will review briefly what I consider to be some of the most important parameters involved when one begins the description of a less common major gene, whether the gene be in glyphogenetics or clinical genetics. First it should be emphasized that there is a negative correlation between the amount of information needed to describe a major gene that is very rare compared to the amount of information needed for a gene that is less rare; the less frequently a gene is encountered, the fewer the number of families needed. I suggest that the more rare genes be described first, and the ones that are less rare be described later. However, it takes a lot of data to locate relatively rare major genes, which explains why my study involves so many families.

Before one attempts to describe a major gene, it is necessary to determine whether or not a major gene is associated with a trait under consideration. When I encounter a rare feature in a family, I make a real effort to get prints from as many relatives as possible to learn if the feature is distributed in the kindred according to a recognizable genetic pattern. The higher the occrrence of bilateral expression of the feature the greater the likelihood the feature can be described genetically.

A first step involved to describe a relatively rare major gene is to determine its penetrance and expressivity. It happens that a very small percentage of the major dominant genes in human clinical genetics based on animal genetics or they have been taught by professors with more research experience in animal genetics than human clinical genetics. When students with this kind of background experience in elementary genetics learn that major genes in clinical genetics typically are not 100% penetrant, they often are confused. Textbook examples of human genes most often are limited to genes that are 100% penetrant such as genes for Huntington's chorea, albinism, dwarfism, and the blood groups. When various major genes in glyphogenetics are described fully the will be found to be more typical of the types of genes a medical student will encounter in human clinical genetics. One should not attempt to describe any major gene without first understanding the percentage of time the gene is expressed when the genotype is present. One also needs to know the frequency with which various expressions of the gene occur that do not represent the "full-blown"syndrome or expression of the genotype. Usually textbook descriptions of clinical syndromes are limited to full-blown expressions only. I do not expect to find 100% penetrance in any of the 6 to 12 major genes in glyphogenetics that I feel may most easily be described.

Dermatoglyphic features are especially advantageous for the determination of this first important parameter of penetrance and expressivity. Much time is spent in clinical genetics to locate a sufficient number of sets of identical twins in which one member of each set has a particular major gene expressed. Since all cells in a set of MZ twins are derived from the same zygote, one can ask the question, when a particular genotype is expressed in one member of the set, how frequently is the same expression seen in the other member of the set. The answer to this question is an estimate of penetrance. Estimate of penetrance also may be obtained from family data.

When the late Dr. Franz Kallmann at Columbia University studied the psychiatric features seen in the opposite member of a set of identical twins when one member had developed schizophrenia, he was describing the penetrance and expressivity of the genotype involved. In glyphogenetics the two hands and the two feet are genetically homologous to a set of identical twins. We can ask the question when a major gene is expressed in one hand or foot, how frequently is the gene also expressed in the other hand or foot, even though characteristic left/right asymmetry may also be involved. The various clinical expressions of the genotype in the opposite member of a set of identical twins and the various dermatoglyphic expressions of genotype in the opposite hand or foot each represent variations in expressivity of the genotype.

After one is certain that a major gene is involved and after one has learned the penetrance of a gene, a second parameter to be described is how to detect the carrier of the gene. To detect the carrier actually is an extended aspect of the expressivity of the gene. Most clinical genes have expressions in more than one tissue or organ of the body. Although a presenting symptom may be limited to a particular organ, all tissues share the same genotype and may have minor manifestations. It will be interesting to learn at some time in the future non-dermatoglyphic features which also are expressions of the glyphogenetic genes. In my studies thus far, carrier detection is limited to variations in other dermatoglyphic or anthropometric features of the hands and feet. When the various blood group genes were first described, it was not known that they also had various clinical effects involving other systems of the body. In the major gene for absent c-triradius, it was found in a certain sample of material (Kloepfer, 1979) that the presence of the gene not only was expressed in other dermatoglyphic features, but also that these other features could be used to detect the apenetrant carrier of the gene 95% of the time.

A third parameter involved when a major gene is described is heterogeneity. I recall my first experience with a major recessive gene for the occurrence of Marchesani syndrome (Kloepfer and Rosenthal, 1955;Rosenthal and Kloepfer, 1956), where the presenting clinical feature was a spherical shaped lens of the eye. In the Louisiana area two families with this condition were located. When the literature was reviewed, it was learned that the syndrome had been described in 12 previous families to be recessive, but instead two of the 12 families involved clear-cut autosomal dominant genes with clinical features indistinguishable from the features found in families with the autosomal recessive gene. When different genes are found to have similar expressions, one has heterogeneity. One should expect the possibility of heterogeneity when attempts are made to describe a gene involving data from unrelated families.

Parameters mentioned thus far to describe a major gene are, first, penetrance; second, expressivity which is an aspect of carrier detection; and third, heterogeneity. A fourth parameter to be considered is the frequency of the gene in the population. Without understanding specific major genes involved, physical antrhopologists know feature frequency varies from population to popylation, from ethnic group, to ethnic group, whether they be in hands or feet.

There are many similarities between variations in gene frequency from one population group to another population group whether a major gene be associated with a dermatoglyphic feature or some particular clinical syndrome.

The parameters reviewed briefly to describe a particular less common major gene whether in glyphogenetics or in clinical genetics are penetrance and expressivity, including ability to detect apenetrant carriers, heterogeneity, and gene frequency. In my studies I have not included other important parameters. A fifth parameter involves various biochemical pathways in the expression of a gene down to the level of DNA. Eventually, a sixth parameter will be the precise location of a gene on a particular chromosome.

REFERENCES

Kloepfer H.W.: The detection of the genotype for absent c-triradius in individuals with Main Line Sequence CBD. BIRTH DEFECTS: Original Article Series, THE NATIONAL FOUNDATION, Vol. XV, No. 6, pp. 511-527, 1979.

Kloepfer H.W. and J.W. Rosenthal: Possible genetic carriers in the Spherophakia-Brachymorphia Syndrome. Am. J Human Genetics 7: 398-425, 1955.

Rosenthal J.W. and H.W. Kloepfer: The Spherophakia-Brachymorphia Syndrome. A.M.A. Arch. of Ophthalmology 55: 28-35, 1956.

Progress in Dermatoglyphic Research, pages 111-128

PROGRESS IN GENETICS OF PALMAR PATTERN RIDGE COUNTS IN MAN

K.C. MALHOTRA, B. KARMAKAR AND M. VIJAYAKUMAR

Anthropometry and Human Genetics Unit, Indian Statistical Institute
203 B.T. Road, Calcutta 700035, INDIA

INTRODUCTION

Genetics of finger patterns, using quantitative ridge counting methods have been extensively studied since Bonnevie's (1962) work on 'mean ridge count' and Newman's (1931), Giepel's (1941) and several others on total ridge count, TRC. The extensive genetical studies of Holt (see, among others 1952, 1956, 1958) have established that the patterns of finger balls, as determined by ridge counts, are strongly determined by almost additive polygenes.

Despite the spectacular success registered by Holt, it is strange that no serious attempt has been made to extend the ridge counting technique to the palmar patterns. Instead, a great deal of attention has been paid to a number of other palmar characters. Family correlations have been estimated for interdigital ridge counts ab, bc and cd (Fang 1950, Pons 1964; Tiwari 1965; Pateria 1974; Sciulli and Rao 1975; among others), atd angle (Penrose 1954), main line index (Pons 1954, 1959); pattern intensity (Mukherjee 1966); A'd ridge count (Glanville 1965a) and palmar patterns and triradii based on topological principles (Loesch 1971, 1974).

Curiously enough, and despite the doubtful evolutionary significance of interdigital ridge counts, they continue not only to receive increased attention but have led to a measure unfortunately designated as 'total palmar ridge count TPRC' (Dennis, 1977). The implied meaning in TPRC is that it is analogous to total finger ridge count, TFRC.

Clearly TPRC has nothing whatsoever to do with the palmar patterns, not even interdigital patterns, instead it is a measure which simply conveys inter-digital triradial distances, expressed in terms of ridge counts. In contrast, TFRC is a measure of the size of the patterns of finger tips. These two measures, therefore, have nothing in common and are not comparable. Any measure on palm comparable to TFRC undoubtedly has to be based on ridge counts of the palmar patterns.

It appears that such a measure in respect to palmar patterns has not been possible to develop because as Holt (1968) writes : "Quantifying palmar pattern is far from straight forward. Difficulties arise from such causes as deep flexion creases and the fact that some pattern do not lend themselves to measurement by ridge counting". It is true that compared to digital patterns, palmar patterns, especially those in the hypothenar area, do pose certain difficulties, but to our knowledge, in fact, no attempt has so far been made to extend application of ridge-counting technique to palmar patterns- and which proved unsuccessful. It is, therefore, not known whether these difficulties can not be resolved; whatever evidence that is available, on the contrary, is an affirmative. As a matter of fact, Ford Walker (1957) successfully studied quantitatively patterns in the hallucal area by means of ridge counts and Smith (1964) has shown that the ridge count of hallucal patterns is determined by multifactorial additive genes. Glanville (1965a) made an original attempt in applying ridge count technique to patterns in the palmar inter-digital areas, and defined a measure, total inter-digital pattern ridge-count (combined total for left and right hands). Unfortunately Glanville's technique suffers from the fact that he counted the ridges at the greatest width of the patterns instead from the recognized practice of triradii to core. Moreover, Glanville did not consider hypothenar and Thenar/I interdigital patterns. Using familial correlation method and twin pair analysis Glanville concluded that the character "appears to be determined by additive genes...."

In the pages to follow we report results of our attempt to develop suitable ridge count techniques for application to the true palmar patterns. Based on palmar pattern ridge counts, we defined a new measure, analogous to TFRC, called 'total palmar pattern ridge count TPPRC'. The sum of the single counts on the ten palmar configurational areas of an individual is the TPPRC. The reasons for using single counts rather than double or triple count (theoretically a hypothenar whorl has three triradii, thus three counts are made) are those put forward by Holt (1968 : 41-42). If, however, all counts (double or triple as the case may be) are taken into consideration we arrive at a measure, 'absolute palmar pattern ridge count, APPRC' which is analogous to absolute finger ridge count, AFRC. The palmar pattern ridge counts also now open up an exciting possibility of developing a new measure which could combine ridge counts of both palmar and finger balls. This measure could be designated as 'total manus pattern ridge count, TMPRC' when single (higher) counts are used, and when all counts (double or triple as the case may be) on the hand are used the measure be called as "absolute manus pattern ridge count, AMPRC".

Recently, using population, family and twin data we have carried out extensive genetic studies on the character TPPRC (studies on other measures APPRC, TMPRC and AMPRC are in progress), including distributions, correlation between individual configurational areas, familial correlations (between parents and children, between sibs) and correlations between pairs of monozygotic (MZ) and dizygotic (DZ) twins (Malhotra et al 1981a, b, c, d, e; Karmakar and Malhotra 1981; Malhotra and Rao 1981). In this paper we report the salient features emerging out of the series of studies referred to above.

RIDGE COUNTING OF THE TRUE PALMAR PATTERNS : METHODS

Since it is for the first time that ridge counting of the true palmar patterns has been developed by us, it is appropriate that we give a detailed description of the methods adopted.

The basic rules of ridge counting as advanced by Henry (1901) for digital loops, and extended for application to other digital patterns by Bonnevie (1924) and Holt (1958) were adopted for counting ridges of true palmar patterns.

The true palmar patterns-loops, whorls, tented arches-are though morphologically similar to the digital patterns, they, in fact, are formed, in a majority of the cases, quite unlike the digital patterns. For example a whorl in the hypothenar area is formed by three triradii, instead of two as in the case of digital whorls. Again, loops on the palm could be formed by a single triradius (as in the digital loops), quite often, in the interdigital areas loops are also formed by two triradii. Often hypothenar patterns, in particular loops formed by the main lime A, lack a triradius, which in fact is extralimital.

These morphological features necessitated suitable modifications of the existing techniques. While developing new techniques, as detailed below, the basic objective of measuring the pattern size (through ridge counts) was always taken into consideration, and in the case of two or three counts, the higher count was taken to represent the size of the pattern.

(1) Ridge counts of interdigital patterns

The patterns in the interdigital areas, when present, are mostly loops, and whorls which are invariably of small size and accompanied by accessory triradii occur only rarely (about 2%). The loops in these interdigital spaces are formed essentially by the curving of the main lines of the digital triradii towards the distal border of the palm. Sometimes, notably in the II and IV interdigital spaces, a loop is formed by an accessory triradius either independently or in conjuction with the main line A or B. The following situations in the interdigital spaces were encountered in the present series of 1498 palms, and the ridge counting was resolved as follows :

(a) Pattern formed independently by main lines A,B,C and D

Such patterns are always loops, and as in the case of digital loops, have only one count between the digital triradius and the core. For illustration see Fig. 1.

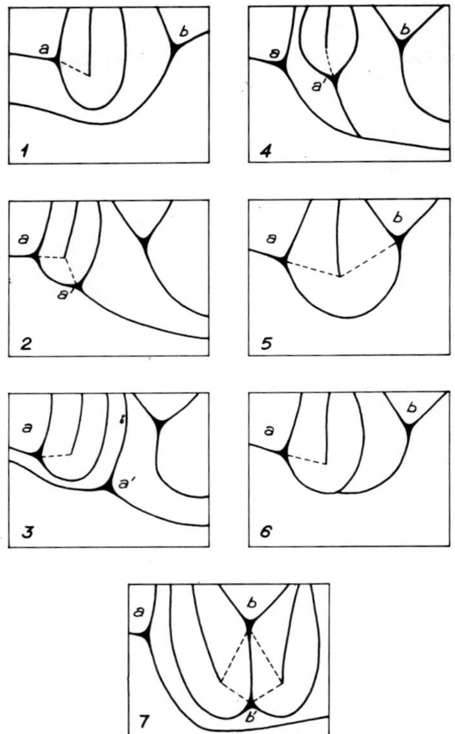

Figures 1-7. Details of methods followed in counting the ridges of the inter-digital patterns.

(b) <u>Pattern formed by the main line and proximal radiant of an accessory triradius, and the main line and one of the radiants of accessory triradii are fused</u>

Patterns formed this way are also always loops, and have two triradii and a common core. Consequently there are two ridge counts, one each from the triradius and the core (see Fig. 2). This situation is similar to digital whorls.

(c) <u>Pattern formed independently by the main line of a digital triradius but an accessory triradius is also present</u>

As illustrated in Fig. 3 only one count between the digital triradius and the core of the pattern was made, the pattern being treated as a loop. It may be noted here that ridge counts from the accessory triradius and the core were not taken since the latter triradius does not contribute in enclosing the pattern area.

(d) Pattern formed by the two distal radiants of an accessory triradius, and the main line and proximal radiant of an accessory triradius are fused

Such a situation is shown in Fig. 4. There is only one count from accessory triradius and the core, and for the reasons given in (c) above counts from the digital triradius and the core were not taken.

(e) Pattern formed by the fusion of main lines of two adjacent digital triradii

In such cases the pattern area is enclosed by the radiants of both the digital triradius and two counts, one each from the two triradius, are scored. Fig. 5 illustrates such a situation.

A variant of this situation is shown in Fig. 6; although the main lines of two digital triradii are fused but the pattern is enclosed by the continuation of one of the main lines. The counts are naturally done from the triradius whose main line encloses the pattern.

(f) Patterns formed by the fusion of main line of a digital triradius and a radiant of an accessory triradius

Such a case is illustrated in Fig, 7. Here for each of the patterns in the two adjacent interdigital spaces there are two counts, one from the digital triradius to the core and other from the accessory triradius to the core.

(2) Ridge counts of hypothenar patterns

This configurational area is characterized by the presence of a variety of patterns. Of these the true patterns are loops, whorls and tented arches; the last, however, does not have a ridge count as in the case of digital tented arches. The true patterns, in this area are formed by three different palmar elements : main line A, hypothenar triradii including extralimital triradius and axial triradii (Malhotra et al 1980). The patterns occur singularly or in duplex or triplex formations. The ridge counting of patterns in this area were resolved as follows :

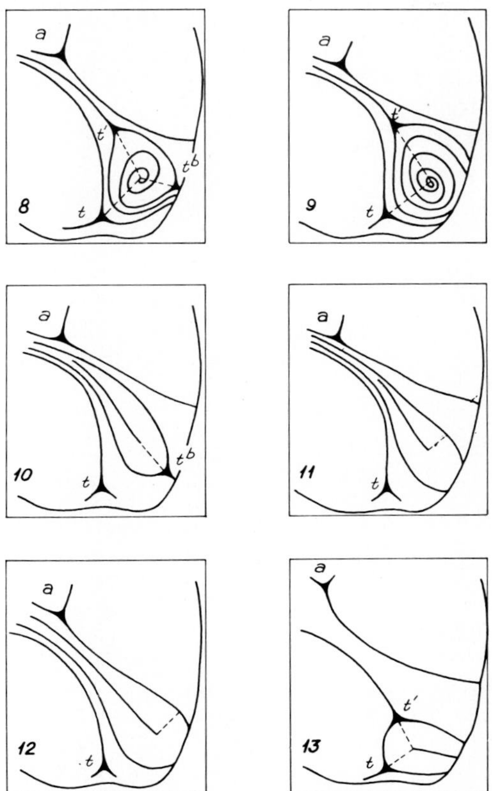

Figures 8-13. Details of methods followed in counting the ridges of the hypothenar patterns.

(a) Whorls

The whorls in the hypothenar area, as mentioned earlier, are formed by three triradii, and present usually two morphological situations : (i) when all the three triradii are present on the palm, and (ii) when only two triradii are present and the hypothenar triradius is extralimital.

In the first type of whorls with three triradii present on the palm, the highest of the three counts was used (see Fig. 8). In the second case also, infact we should have three counts, but because of the enormous subjectivity involved in descerning the expected position of extralimital triradius, only two counts from the triradii present on the palm were made, and the higher of the two counts was accepted (Fig. 9). It may be noted here that in similar type of digital situations, Holt (1958 : 159), in fact, counted ridges between the potential site of the extralimital triradius and the core.

(b) Loops

The loops in this area are rather complex and from the point of counting the ridges pose certain difficulties. In the case of single loops, the following four situations were encountered, and the ridge counting procedure adapted are as given below :

(i) Loop formed by hypothenar triradius t^u or t^b (border triradius; Penrose, 1968)

In such cases counts between the triradius and the core were made (see Fig. 10), and like the digital loops had only one count.

(ii) Loop formed by an extralimital triradius

In such cases the two radiants enclosing the pattern area were traced radialwards (such loops always open towards radial border). Then on the core line a perpendicular was drawn from the core on the distal radiant. The ridges along the perpendicular between the core and the distal radiant were counted (Fig. 11). For reasons mentioned earlier, while discussing hypothenar whorls, counts between the potential site of the extralimital triradius and the core were not attempted.

(iii) Loop formed by main line A

Such loops in fact are bounded by an extralimital triradius on the ulnar border of the palm. Thus the loop is formed by the two triradii, inter-digital 'a' and an extralimital. For reasons already given above counts between later triradius and core are not practical and counting between triradius 'a' and core presents technical difficulties, as the core line runs parallel through most of its course to the core. Hence procedures adopted in the case of (ii) above were followed (for illustration see Fig. 12).

(iv) Loop formed by two axial triradii

Such loops are bounded by the radiants of both the axial triradii, and, therefore, counts from each of the triradii to the core were made, the higher of the two counts was used (see Fig. 13).

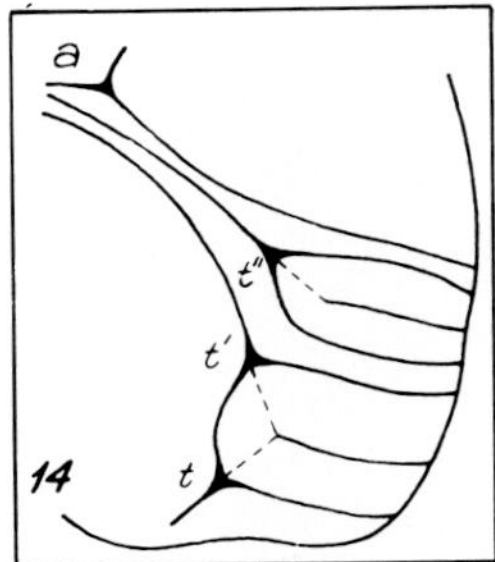

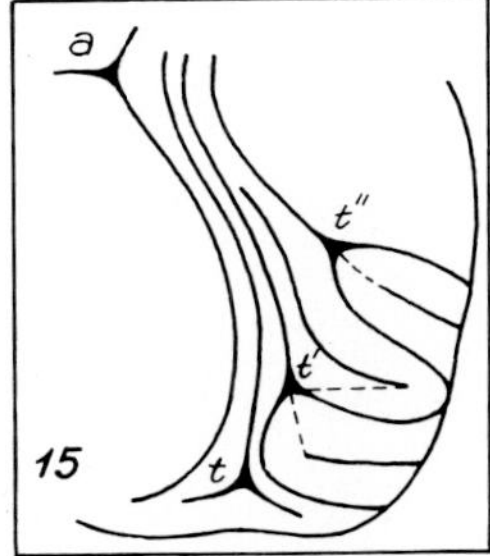

Figures 14-15. Details of methods followed in counting the ridges of the hypothenar patterns.

(c) Duplex and triplex patterns

Duplex patterns, in a majority of the cases, comprise of two loops, and very rarely a whorl and a loop; the procedure followed in ridge counting are detailed in Fig. 14.

Triplex formations involving three true patterns are extremely rare (approx. 1 in 3000 palms), and in the present series not even a single such pattern, was encountered. However, while analysing another series one such pattern was seen and the ridge counting in this case was resolved as shown in Fig. 15.

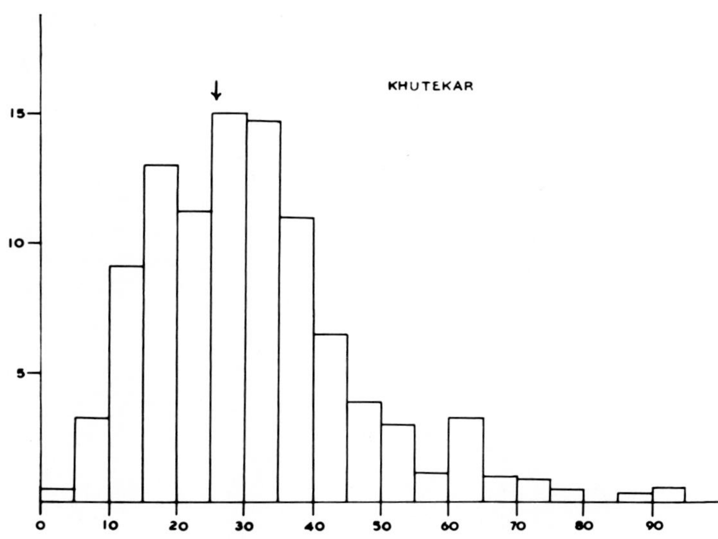

Fig. 16. Distribution of total palmar pattern ridge count among the Khutekar males (n=392).

Distribution of palmar pattern ridge counts

(i) The distribution of palmar pattern ridge counts in either sex and in either hand and combined total for right and left palms was found to be leptokurtic and positively skewed (see figures 16-17). The means of distributions of TPPRC among Khutekar males (n=392) is 26.2 ± 0.77 while among Nandiwalla males (n=202) and females (n=105) it is 26.73 ± 1.27 and 23.80 ± 1.32 respectively; sex difference, however, is non-significant (t=1.13, d.f.355).

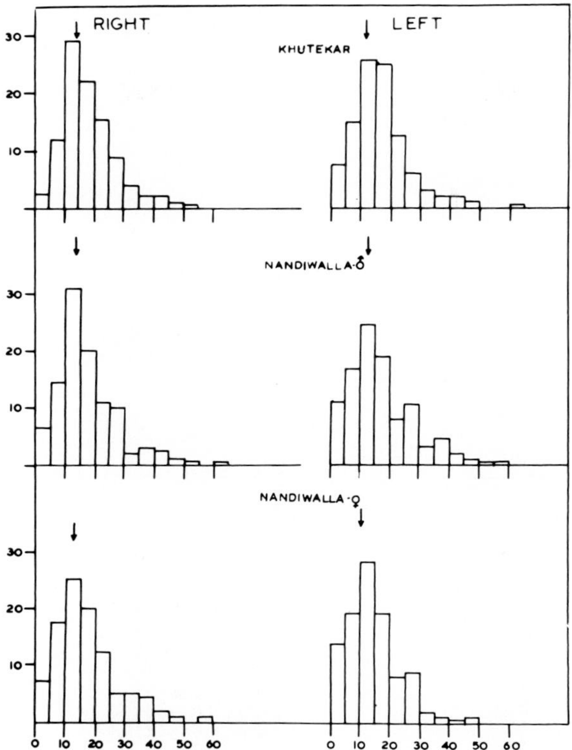

Fig. 17. Distribution of summed palmar pattern ridge counts on the right and left palms in three samples.

(ii) Distributions of ridge counts on interdigital areas III and IV are conspicuously bimodal while hypothenar area shows a tendency towards bimodality (figure 18). The highest mean ridge counts, in general, are those for IV interdigital followed by III, Hypothenar, II and Thenar/I interdigital. The hypothenar area shows greatest variability in ridge counts while Thenar/I interdigital the least (see figure 19 for details).

(iii) Except for interdigital areas Thenar/I interdigital and IV, the mean ridge counts are higher in other areas on the right palms; the only statistically significant differences were, however, observed between right and left interdigital areas Thenar/I and III.

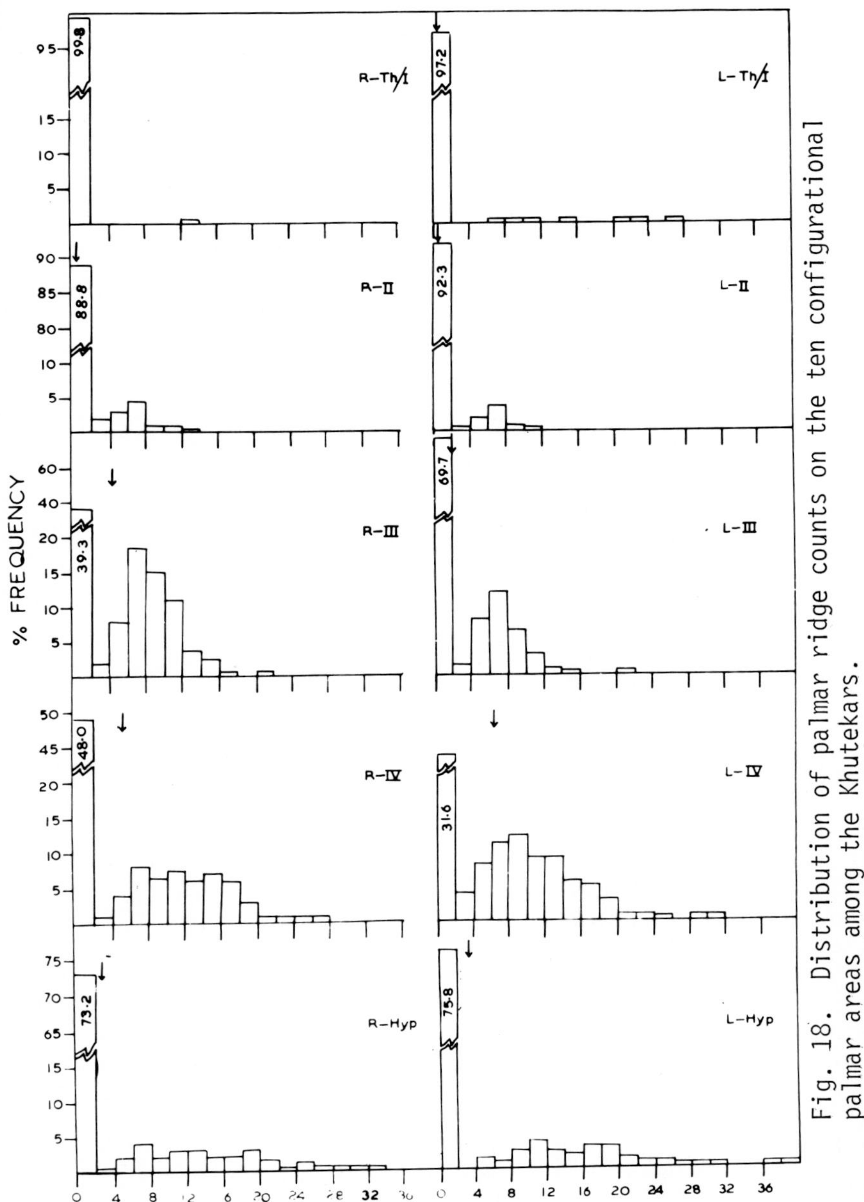

Fig. 18. Distribution of palmar ridge counts on the ten configurational palmar areas among the Khutekars.

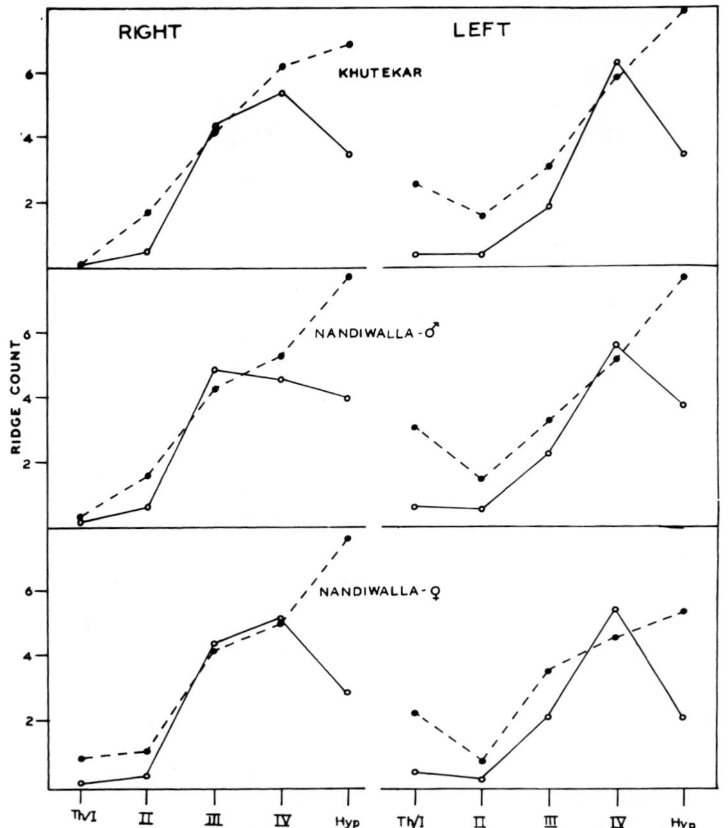

Fig. 19. Means (0-0) and standard deviation (0---0) on individual palmar areas.

Correlations

(i) Pattern ridge counts of all the five homologous areas are significantly correlated (correlations range between 0.31 to 0.64). The correlation values, however, fail to depict any systematic relationship between ridge counts of adjacent areas. The only consistent significant negative correlations between heterologous palmar areas is observed between interdigital areas III and IV (see table 1). Highly significant positive correlation occurs between the totals for right and left palms (range 0.38 to 0.58). The correlations between totals of each hand and combined totals for right and left hands are very high, positive and significant (all values are above 0.82). The character TPPRC is found to be highly positively correlated with number of triradii as well as with number of loops on the palm; average correlation between TPPRC and number of loops is 0.76 and between TPPRC and number of triradii is 0.7. Between TPPRC and total finger ridge count non-significant positive correlation has been observed (r=0.194).

Familial correlations

The genetics of the trait TPPRC was studied by examining the genetical correlations between pairs of relatives and between monozygotic twin-twin and dizygotic twin-twin pairs. Palmar prints of a sample of 110 families, comprising 513 persons, including 316 children (191 males and 125 females) and 102 twin pairs (MZ 52 and DZ 50) were analysed. The obtained correlation coefficients between pairs of relatives and between twin pairs are set out in table 2. Significant correlations between sib: sib, parent : child and MZ pairs (r=0.8) indicate that the TPPRC is strongly determined by heredity. The greater likeness between sibs than between parent and child, and the highly positively skewed distribution of TPPRC suggests a major influence of a dominant/recessive gene on the character.

The familial correlations, including twins were further analysed using the models and methods of path analysis (Malhotra and Rao 1981). It suggests that about one third variation in TPPRC is accounted for by additive genetic factors (h^2=0.37 ± .06). However, the observed MZ correlation (0.8) can not be explained in terms of h^2 alone, requiring either intra-uterine environment specific to MZ twins or dominance deviations. This second source of family resemblance can not be resolved in this material.

In view of the successful application of ridge counting technique to the palmar patterns, it should now be possible not only to extend it to sole patterns in Man, but could perhaps also be applied to the palmar patterns in non-human primates. Once these quantitative techniques are perfected we should be in a better position to understand the dermatoglyphic evolution. We have undertaken a series of investigations on these lines, and the preliminary results are indeed very encouraging.

Acknowledgements

We wish to express our deep appreciations to Dr. Anil P. Gore of Poona University, Pune, for his help in the statistical analysis of the data. This research was supported by the University Grants Commission, New Delhi and the Indian Statistical Institute, Calcutta.

Table 1. Correlation Coefficients between palmar configurational areas among the Khutekars.

Palmar areas	Th/I	II	III	IV	Hyp.
Th/I	-	-0.02	-0.05	+0.05	-0.03
II		-	+0.17*	-0.07	-0.04
III			-	-0.44*	-0.02
IV				-	-0.02
Hyp.					-

*Significant at 5% and below levels

Table 2. Correlation between relatives for total palmar pattern ridge count

Related pairs	Number of pairs	Observed Correlation coefficients ± S.E.
Parent-Parent	96	-0.13 ± 0.10
Mother-child	309	0.15*± 0.05
Father-child	306	0.15*± 0.05
Parent-child	617	0.14*± 0.04
Father-son	184	0.19*± 0.07
Mother-daughter	122	0.14 ± 0.09
Father-daughter	123	0.08 ± 0.09
Mother-son	186	0.13 ± 0.07
Daughter-daughter	95	0.13 ± 0.10
Son-son	190	0.18*± 0.07
Daughter-son	265	0.29*± 0.06
sib-sib	554	0.22*± 0.04
Midparent-child	299	0.20*± 0.05
Midparent-son	179	0.22*± 0.07
Midparent-daughter	112	0.19*± 0.09
Monozygotic twin-twin	52	0.80*± 0.05
Dizygotic twin-twin	50	0.29*± 0.13

* Significant at 5% and below levels

REFERENCES

Bonnevie K (1924). Studies on papillary patterns of human fingers. J Genet 15:1-111.

Dennis RLH (1977). "A study of dermatoglyphic variation in the human populations of the North Pennine Dales". University of Durham : Ph. D thesis.

Fang TC (1950). "The inheritance of the a-b ridge count on the human palm, with a note on its relation to Mongolism". University of London:Ph. D thesis.

Ford Walker N (1957). The use of dermal configurations in the diagnosis of mongolism. J Pediatrics 50 : 19-26.

Giepel G (1941) . Die Gesamtanzhl der fingerlristen alsneues merkmal zur Zwillings diagnose. Zeitscrift für Morphologie und Anthropologie 39 : 414-419.

Glanville EV (1965a). Heredity and line A in palmar dermatoglyphics. Am J Hum Genet 17 : 420-424.

Glanville EV (1965a). Heredity and dermal patterns in the interdigital areas of the palm. A Ge Me Ge 14 :295-304.

Henry ER (1901) . "Classification and uses of Finger-Prints." London : Routledge.

Holt SB (1952). Genetics of dermal ridges:inheritance of total finger ridge-count. Ann Hum Genet 17 : 140-161.

Holt SB(1956). Genetics of dermal ridges: parent-child correlations for finger ridge-count. Ann Hum Genet 20 :159-170.

Holt SB (1958). Genetics of dermal ridges: the relation between total ridge-count and the variability of counts from finger to finger. Ann Hum Genet 22:323-339.

Holt SB (1968). "The Genetics of Dermal Ridges". Springfield C.C. Thomas.

Karmakar B, Malhotra KC (1981). Genetics of palmar pattern ridge counts. IV. Correlation between total palmar pattern ridge count and total finger ridge count. Technical Report No. Anthrop./1/ 81, Indian Statistical Institute, Calcutta, India.

Loesch D (1971). Genetics of dermatoglyphic patterns on palms. Ann Hum Genet 34:277-293.

Loesch D (1974). Genetical studies of sole and palmar dermatoglyphics. Ann Hum Genet 37:405-420.

Malhotra KC, Reddy BM, Karmakar B, Vijayakumar M (1981). Relationship between types of axial triradii and true hypothenar patterns. In press- Dermatoglyphics.

Malhotra KC, Vijaykumar M, Karmakar B. (1981a). Genetics of palmar pattern ridge counts: I Frequency distribution of palmar pattern ridge counts. Technical Report No. Anthrop. /1/81, Indian Statistical Institute, Calcutta, India.

Malhotra KC, Karmakar B, Vijayakumar M. (1981b). Genetics of palmar pattern ridge counts. II. The correlation between ridge counts on different palmar configurational areas. Technical Report No. Anthrop./1/81, Indian Statistical Institute, Calcutta, India.

Malhotra KC, Karmakar B, Vijayakumar M. (1981c). Genetics of palmar pattern ridge counts. III. Correlation between total palmar pattern ridge count, number of palmar loops and number of palmar triradii. Technical Report No. Anthrop./1/81, Indian Statistical Institute, Calcutta, India.

Malhotra KC, Vijayakumar M, Karmakar B. (1981d). Genetics of palmar pattern ridge counts V. Familial correlations. Technical Report No. Anthrop./1/81, Indian Statistical Institute, Calcutta, India.

Malhotra KC, Reddy BM, Vijayakumar M, Karmakar B, Guha A, (1981e). Genetics of palmar pattern ridge counts. VI. Correlation analysis of some palmar dermatoglyphic characters in twins. Technical Report No. Anthrop./3/1981, Indian Statistical Institute, Calcutta, India.

Malhotra KC, Rao DC (1981). Path analysis of total palmar pattern ridge counts. Communicated to Am J Phys Anthrop.

Mukherjee DP (1966). Inheritance of total number of triradii on fingers, palms and soles. Ann Hum Genet 29: 349-352.

Newman HH (1931). Palm print patterns in twins. J Hered 22 : 41-49.

Pateria HN (1974). Genetic basis of a-b, b-c, and c-d ridge counts on human palms. Am J Phys Anthrop 40 : 171-172.

Penrose LS (1954). The distal triradius t on the hands of parents and sibs of mongol imbeciles. Ann Hum Genet 19 : 10-38.

Penrose LS (1968). Memorandum on dermatoglyphic nomenclature. Birth Defect Original Article Series 4 : 1-12.

Pons J (1954). Herencia de las lineas principales de la palma. Contribucion a la genetica de los caracteres dermapapilares. Trab Inst "Bernardino de Sahgun" de Anthropologia y Ethnologia del CSIC, Barcelona 14 : 35-50.

Pons J (1959). Quantitative genetics of palmar dermatoglyphics. Am J Hum Genet 11 : 252-256.

Pons J (1964). Genetics of a-b ridge count on the human palm. Ann Hum Genet 27 : 273-277.

Sciulli PW, Rao DC (1975). Path analysis of palmar ridge counts. Am J Phys Anthrop 43 : 291-294.

Smith GF (1964). Quantitative genetics of the patterns in the hallucal area of the sole. Ann Hum Genet 28 : 181-184.

Tiwari SC (1965). Genetical analysis of a-b ridge counts. Anthropologist 12 : 125-128.

Progress in Dermatoglyphic Research, pages 129–137

STUDY OF TOTAL PATTERN INTENSITY IN JAPANESE POPULATION WITH SPECIAL REFERENCE TO AUTOSOMAL ANEUPLOIDY

Ichiro Matsui, M.D.

Division of Research Promotion and Division of Medical Genetics, Kanagawa Children's Medical Center, Yokohama 232, Japan

An attempt has been made to evaluate the effects of autosomal aneuploidy on dermatoglyphics using total pattern intensity. The finger pattern intensity has been studied well in order to test the racial variation in physical anthropology, to determine the twin zygosity or to study the genetics of dermatoglyphics (Asaka 1975). However, the pattern intensity of the other dermatoglyphic areas, for example, palms, toes and soles has been investigated to a lesser extent. The pattern intensity refers to the complexity of ridge configurations and expressed by counting the number of triradii present. The total pattern intensity, the total number of triradii in all dermatoglyphic areas may offer a measure for the complexity of all ridge configurations in an individual.

Among the very large number of reports describing dermatoglyphics in chromosome aberrations, characteristic pecuriarities of ridge configurations have been demonstrated (Schaumann 1976, de Grouchy and Turleau 1977). In such hazzard condition as in autosomal aneuploidy which involves the severe disturbances of many organs and tissues, the dermatoglyphic changes compose the important part of the profound abnormal manifestations. However, the routine analysis of finger-, palm- and hallucal-prints for the diagnostic purpose of chromosome aberrations, has a limitation in assessing the total dermatoglyphic traits. Consequently, the evaluation and the comparison of total pattern intensity between the control population and the autosomal aneuploidy may provide the total exertion on dermatoglyphics in the latter condition.

METHODS AND CONTROL POPULATION

The " Dermatoglyphic Databanking System " using small-sized micro-computer has been developed for data processing in the present study. The micro-computer; SORD M-223, Mark V (Japan) with C.P.U. size of 64 K-Bite has been used appreciably. The data in the System are compatible with I.B.M. and standard computer by the minimal operations. The operations for data in-put, correction, erase, conditional search, retreaval, computation for statistical analysis, etc. are facile by the several steps of manipulation. For the Dermatoglyphic Databanking System a considerably large-size program of nearly 16,000 steps in Basic Language has been utilized (commercial software by Nippon Joho Kenkyu Center, Tokyo).

The stored data of control population in the Databanking System were composed of mentally and physically normal children in Nakada Primary School, Yokohama, aged six to twelve years old. The number of males, females and the total were 523, 503 and 1,026, respectively. However, the total 1,007 males and females were employed in the present tatal pattern intensity study. The rest 19 individuals were excluded for the reason of inappropriate dermatoglyphic information. No sibs were included in the control population.

The finger prints, palm prints and planta prints were examined, and toes by direct observations. The configurations of every dermatoglyphic area were analysed following the standards given by Cummins and Midlo (1961) and by Penrose (1968). The number of palmar triradii, plantar triradii and other informations were recorded. Each information was coded in numerical character and stored in the computer. Nearly 100 dermatoglyphic traits occupying 250 spaces in each individual, have been stored consecutively in the file.

The total pattern intensity (T.P.I.) designating the summation ofvalue 0 for arches, 1 for loops and 2 for whorls for ten fingers and toes, with the additional value of palmar and plantar triradii was calculated in each individual.

Area	Mean	S.D.	Skewness($\sqrt{b_1}$)	Kurtosis(b_2)	Fig.
Total Finger P.I.	14.129	3.525	1.358	2.170	(1)
Total Toe P.I.	9.984	3.299	-0.364	3.083	(2)
Total Finger and Palm (both hands) P.I.	24.714	3.790	0.556	2.627	(3)
Total Toe and Planta (both feet) P.I.	21.818	3.852	0.436	2.848	(4)
Left Hand and Foot P.I.	23.183	3.546	-0.265	3.008	(5)
Right Hand and Foot P.I.	23.353	3.234	0.246	2.868	(6)

Table 1. Pattern intensity of selected dermatoglyphic areas

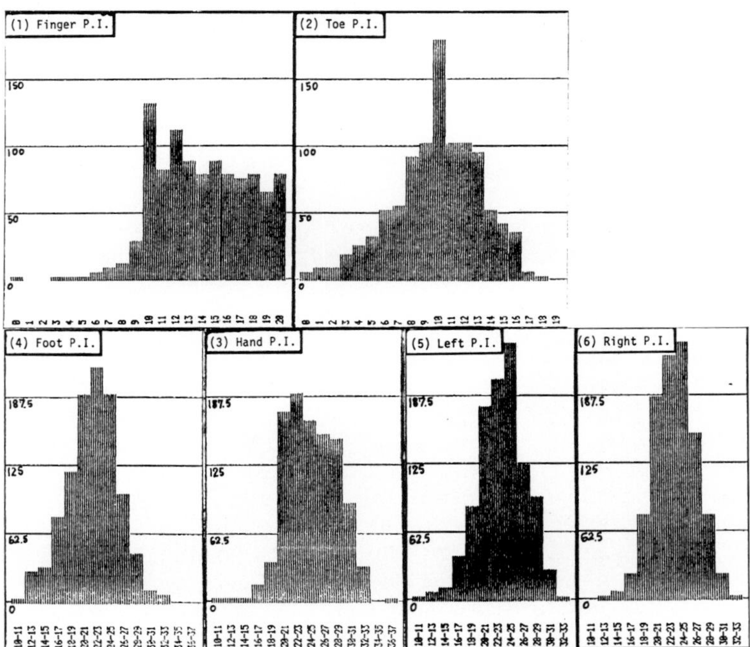

Figure 1. Distribution of pattern intensity of selected dermatoglyphic areas

DISTRIBUTION OF TOTAL PATTERN INTENSITY IN CONTROL POPULATION

The distribution of the pattern intensity (P.I.) of 1,007 males and females on some selected dermatoglyphic areas are presented in Figure 1. The ordinate and abscissa indicate the frequency and the value of P.I., respectively.

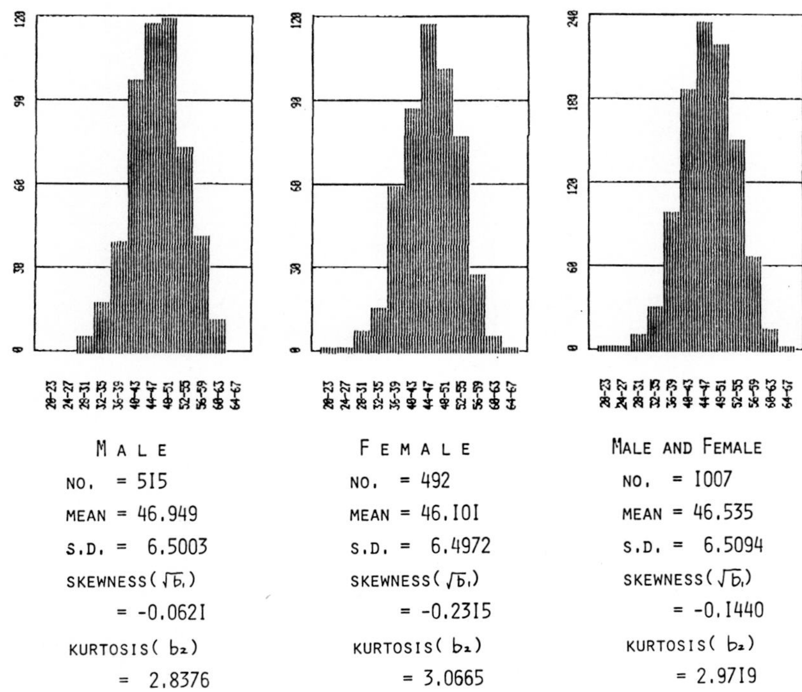

Figure 2. Distribution of T.P.I. in control population

The calculations of mean value, standard deviation, skewness and kurtosis given by Snedecor and Cochran (1967) for these groups are listed in Table 1. The distribution of total finger pattern intensity (F.P.I.) reveales marked positive skew and flatness (Fig. 1 - (1)).

The value for T.P.I. in the present control population range from 22 to 65. In Figure 2, the histograms for the distribution of T.P.I. for 515 males, 492 females and the total 1,007 are presented with the corresponding mean value, standard deviation, skewness and kurtosis below the histograms. In both sexes the distribution of T.P.I. skewed more or less negatively. In males mean value is 46.949 with S.D. 6.500, while in females mean value is 46.101 with S.D.6.497. The means between both sexes differ significantly(t=2.068). Deviations from normality, as measured by g_1(skewness) and g_2(kurtosis) have been calculated for the control population sample. For male distribution, g_1= - 0.062 (t =

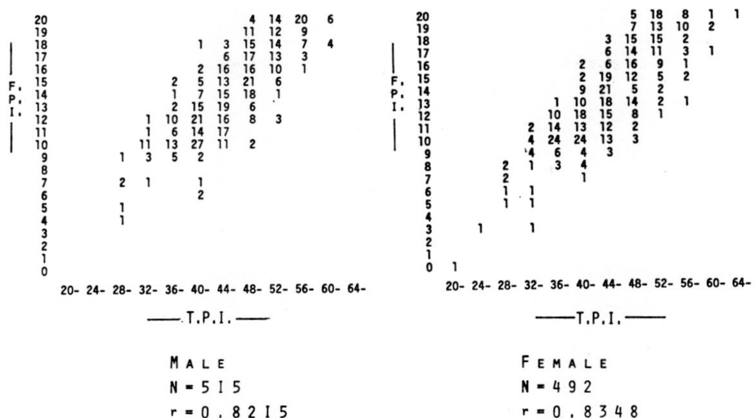

F.P.I. (rows) × T.P.I. (columns) — Male

F.P.I.	20-	24-	28-	32-	36-	40-	44-	48-	52-	56-	60-	64-
20								4	14	20	6	
19								11	12	9		
18						1	3	15	14	7	4	
17							6	17	13	3		
16						2	16	16	10	1		
15					2	5	13	21	6			
14					1	7	15	18	1			
13					2	15	19	6				
12				1	10	21	16	8	3			
11				1	6	14	17					
10				11	13	27	11	2				
9			1	3	5	2						
8												
7			2	1		1						
6						2						
5			1									
4			1									
3												
2												
1												
0												

—T.P.I.—

MALE
N = 515
r = 0.8215

F.P.I. (rows) × T.P.I. (columns) — Female

F.P.I.	20-	24-	28-	32-	36-	40-	44-	48-	52-	56-	60-	64-
20								5	18	8	1	1
19								7	13	10	2	
18							3	15	15	2		
17							6	14	11	3	1	
16						2	6	16	9	1		
15						2	19	12	5	2		
14						9	21	5	2			
13					1	10	18	14	2	1		
12					10	18	15	8	1			
11				2	14	13	12	2				
10				4	24	24	13	3				
9				4	6	4	3					
8			2	1	3	4						
7			2			1						
6			1	1								
5			1	1								
4												
3		1		1								
2												
1												
0	1											

—T.P.I.—

FEMALE
N = 492
r = 0.8348

Table 2. Correlation table between T.P.I.on F.P.I.

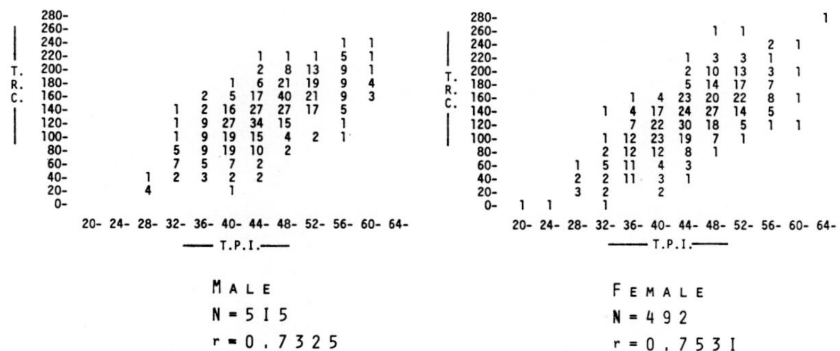

T.R.C. (rows) × T.P.I. (columns) — Male

T.R.C.	20-	24-	28-	32-	36-	40-	44-	48-	52-	56-	60-	64-
280-												
260-												
240-										1	1	
220-							1	1	1	5	1	
200-							2	8	13	9	1	
180-						1	6	21	19	9	4	
160-					2	5	17	40	21	9	3	
140-				1	2	16	27	27	17	5		
120-				1	9	27	34	15		1		
100-				1	9	19	15	4	2	1		
80-				5	9	19	10	2				
60-				7	5	7	2					
40-			1	2	3	2	2					
20-			4			1						
0-												

—T.P.I.—

MALE
N = 515
r = 0.7325

T.R.C. (rows) × T.P.I. (columns) — Female

T.R.C.	20-	24-	28-	32-	36-	40-	44-	48-	52-	56-	60-	64-
280-												1
260-								1	1			
240-										2	1	
220-							1	3	3	1		
200-							2	10	13	3	1	
180-							5	14	17	7		
160-					1	4	23	20	22	8	1	
140-				1	4	17	24	27	14	5		
120-					7	22	30	18	5	1	1	
100-				1	12	23	19	7	1			
80-				2	12	12	8	1				
60-			1	5	11	4	3					
40-			2	2	11	3	1					
20-			3	2		2						
0-	1	1		1								

—T.P.I.—

FEMALE
N = 492
r = 0.7531

Table 3. Correlation table between T.P.I. on T.R.C.

0.575) and g_2 = - 0.162 (t = 0.750),for female g_1 = - 0.232 (t = 2.109) and g_2 = 0.067 (t = 0.298), respectively. Three of these values are not significant for the deviation but that of g_1 in case of female distribution verges on significance. For the total male and female distribution, g_1 = - 0.144 (t = 1.87) and g_2 = - 0.028 (t = 0.182), being Gaussian distribution.

Table 2 demonstrates the correlation between T.P.I. on F.P.I. Observed correlation coefficients are 0.822 for males and 0.835 for females, respectively. Table 3 shows the correlation between T.P.I. on total finger ridge counts (

Unusual patterns			Controls	Syndromes [1]
Hypoplastic ridges			0 %	4p-(4/4), +18, +21,
FINGER	Radial loop	Digit I	0.5	+18(8/23),
		Digit IV	0.4	+18(6/23),5p-(2/11),+21(6%)
		Digit V	0.3	+18(4/23),+21(3%)
	7 or more arches		0.4	+18(14/23), 5p-(1/11)
PALM	Bilateral t''		1	+21(41%),+13(2/3),+18(12/23)
	Interdigital loop, II		0.5	18p-(1/2)
	Zygodactyly, II-III		0.05	8ptrisomy(1/1)
	Absent b or c triradius		7	5p-(3/11),4p-(1/3),18p-(1/2)
SOLE	Hallucal pattern	O	1.6	+18(3/16)
		A^t	8.3 [2]	+21(88%),+18(4/16),r(18)(1/1)
		A^f	0.8	4p-(1/3)
		L^t	8.6 [3]	4p-(2/3),+13(1/3),9ptris(1/1),5p-(1/7)
	Zygodactyly,II-III,others		7	+18(6/16),r(18)(1/1),5p-(4/11)
	Interdigital whorl,II III IV		1.1	+8(3/3)
TOE	Arches on all 10 toes		0.4	+8(2/3),+13(2/3),+18(6/16)
Flexion crease	Bilateral simian crease		4	+13(2/3),+21(40%),8ptris(1/1),9ptris(1/1),5p-(1/11)
	Single flexion crease, V		0	+18(6/16),+21(20%),8ptris(1/1),4p-(1/1),9ptris(1/1),5p-(1/11)

Remarks: 1) Frequency in each syndrome is expressed in (positive cases/ total cases examined)
2) A^t includes variations. Typical A^t is 3.1%. The rest 5.2% include patterns having seam, fan, ladder, very small pocket, or L-shaped right angle arch.
3) L^t also includes varations. Typical L^t is 5.9%

Table 4. Unusual dermatoglyphic findings in Japanese autosomal aneuploidy (Kanagawa Child. Med. CTR.)

F.R.C.) with correlation coefficients of 0.732 for males and 0.753 for females, respectively.

AUTOSOMAL ANEUPLOIDY AND T.P.I.

The unusual ridge configurations observed in autosomal aneuploidy in Kanagawa Children's Medical Center are itemized and listed in Table 4. The frequency of the corresponding dermatoglyphic traits in normal controls is determined by the out-put of our Dermatoglyphic Databanking

System (total 1,026 males and females). The abnormal dermatoglyphic trends in this series are consistent with those of Caucasian studied before (Schaumann and Alter 1976). The cases were confirmed by banding analysis.

The mean values of T.P.I. in autosomal aneuploidy are compared with the calculated normal standard curve of the control population (total 1,007 males and females) in Figure 3. The observation reveals that the T.P.I. means of all aneuploidy cases, except one case of 9p- syndrome, are situated in the left half of the normal standard distribution. However, the deviations from the normal mean in each

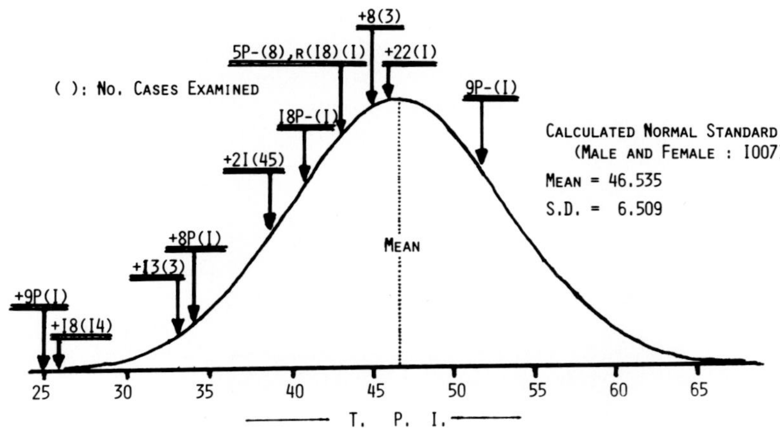

Figure 3. Mean T.P.I. values in autosomal aneuploidy, compared with the calculated normal standard curve of the control population

autsomal syndrome are considerably different. Marked decreases in T.P.I. means are observed in a case with +9p, +8p and cases with +18, +13 trisomic syndromes. It is of interest that the prominent contrast is present in T.P.I. values between +9p and 9p- syndrome, suggesting the relation of " le contre-type " manifestation in dermatoglyphics.

COMMENTS

The term " pattern intensity index " was first described by Cummins and Steggerda (1935) and defined as the average number of triradii occuring on fingers per individual. The studies of this trait have been, and still are, used to a considerable extent in physical anthropology. Later, the term " pattern intensity " was applied insted (Cummins and Midlo 1943, 1961). The pattern intensity had been used for the other dermatoglyphic areas such as palms and soles, and investigated mainly for comparative dermatoglyphics in primatology. In human dermatoglyphic research the pattern intensity has been substantially limited to F.P.I. untill nowadays.

The present investigation of T.P.I. in the Japanese control population revealed that the distribution of this trait was nearly consistent with the normal distribution with mean value of 46.949 for males and 46.101 for females. The significant negative skewness in female distribution could be explained in terms of the higher frequencies of arches on fingers and on toes in females than those in males (Matsui 1978). The values of T.P.I. highly correlate on F.P.I. and on F.R.C.

The appreciable decrease for the mean T.P.I. values in autosomal aneuploidy compared with the control population was demonstrated in this study. In the pediatric practice the quick diagnosis for chromosomal syndromes will be easily established with the aid of assessing finger, palm and hallucal configurations. However, total evaluations of every dermatoglyphic area may suggest the entire influences of serious distortions caused by autosomal aneuploidy. The evaluation of T.P.I. can be a useful trait for this purpose. In the present study, however, the precise trends of each autosomal trisomy or monosomy on T.P.I. has not been elucidated. Similar attempt has been performed by Penrose (1967), who demonstrated the clear effects of sex chromosome aneuploidy on T.R.C.

Furthermore, as the pattern intensity concerns the complexity of ridge configurations, the complexity of patterns increases in the order arch, loop, whorl and is accompanied by an increase in the number of triradii. The higher values indicate greater number and complexity of patterns. Conversely, a low value of pattern intensity or T.P.I. indicates lesscomplex, i.e. more simplified ridge configurations. The present observation of decreased mean T.P.I. values in autosomal aneuploidy permits the possibilities that the effects of autosomal aneuploidy on dermatoglyphics are indicative of a process of simplifying the ridge configurations in the embryonic dermatoglyphogenesis to some extent.

REFERENCES

Asaka A, Nakama T (1975). Pattern intensity of fingers in twins. Jpn J Human Genet 20:153.

Cummins H, Midlo C (1961). "Finger Prints, Palms and Soles." New York: Dover Publ.

Cummins H, Steggerda M (1935). Finger prints in a Dutsh family series. Amer J Phy Anthrop 20:19.

de Grouchy J, Turleau C (1977). "Clinical Atlas of Human Chromosomes." New York: John Willy & Sons.

Matsui I (1978). Dermatoglyphics and congenital abnormalities. Pediat Review 11:814 (JAPAN).

Penrose LS (1967). Finger print patterns and the sex chromosomes. Lancet 1:298.

Penrose LS (1968). Memorandum on dermatoglyphic nomenclature. Birth Defects 4(3):1.

Schaumann B, Alter M (1976). "Dermatoglyphics in Medical Genetics." New York: Springer-Verlag.

Snedecor GW, Cochran WG (1967). "Statistical Methods." Ames: Iowa State Univ Press.

Progress in Dermatoglyphic Research, pages 139–143

PALEODERMATOGLYPHICS

CHRISTOS S. BARTSOCAS, M.D.

Second Department of Pediatrics
University of Athens
P.O. Box 3064, Athens-617, Greece

INTRODUCTION

For most of us the study of dermatoglyphics for forensic, anthropological or genetic purposes is fairly modern. It is well known that the scientific classification of patterns used today was proposed by Galton (1892), who was the first to study dermal patterns in families and racial groups (Thompson and Thompson 1980). As we all know, Cummins was the first to use the term dermatoglyphics (Cummins and Midlo 1961). Nonetheless, the history of dermal pattern studies goes back into antiquity.
Purpose of this article is to present very briefly information on dermatoglyphics, dating back in Greek antiquity, to be used as a proof and justification for a new branch of our field to be called PALEODERMATOGLYPHICS.

MATERIALS AND METHODS

The material of this study should be divided into two categories:

a. archeological findings.
b. literature data.

Archeological findings include pottery, sculpture work, painting and building material on which finger prints may have been imprinted. Examples are shown in Fig. 1 and 2. Finger prints shown were sealed for identification purposes by the unknown potter who made amphoras found on the island of Amorgos 25 centuries ago. Finger prints were found in the interior of the bronze statue called Kouros of Piraeus,

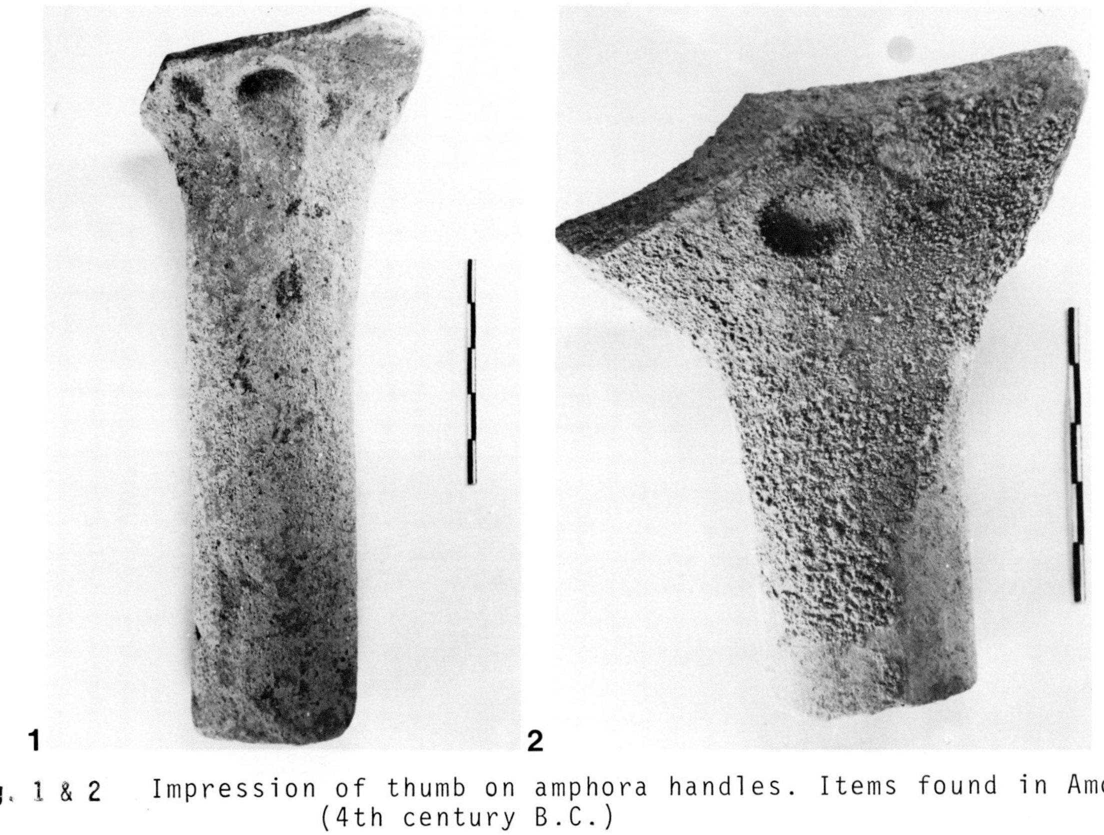

Fig. 1 & 2 Impression of thumb on amphora handles. Items found in Amorgos. (4th century B.C.)

as well as on tiles in Kassiopi, Epirus in Northern Greece, dating back to the 3rd century B.C. These are just a few examples, which may be of value to the study of dermatoglyphics on archeological material.

The ancient literature is also rich on information about knowledge of dermal and palmar patterns and their use in antiquity. The ancient Greeks believed that the stars were determining the future of every individual by contributing to the formation of his palmar creases at birth. Therefore, there was a widespread belief in "palamoscopy" (observation of the palms), in which 5 main and 5 secondary creases were used together with several creases of lesser importance. These lines or creases were studied for their length and depth, whether they were straight or bent, and what was their relationship to other regions of the hand. The hand was therefore considered as a map, where the future of the person was inscribed (Artemidoros 1805).

Artemidoros wrote a treatise entitled "Cheiroscopica", but considered the "cheiroscopes"(observers of the hands), as charlatans (Souidas 1705). Finger divination signs are written in code No. 3632 of the University Bologna library. Palamoscopes are mentioned by Nonnus in the 6th century and by Th. Valsamon in the 12th century. We don't know how the reading of palm patterns was performed, but we learn from Nonnus that the palmar creases were informative about what was destined to happen.

On an altar dedicated to Hermes Aristoteles found a treatise written with gold letters about "cheiromanty", which he gave as a present to Alexander the Great. This treatise was later translated into Latin by John the Spaniard, its use was wide-spread in Rome and formed the basis for the Roman cheiromanty.

According to Souidas (1705) Elenos had written a book on cheiroscopy. Belief in the importance of palmar creases as determining factors for the prognosis of the future was based on the ancient concepts that every part of our body is influenced by a star, which contributed to certain characteristic physical and emotional qualities (Maury 1857). Prognosis of the person's future from observing the palmar lines, finger creases or nail signs, continued through the Byzantine period (Koukoules 1948).

As recently as in the previous century the three main palmar creases were thought to tell how long someone was going to live. Happy was going to be the individual with more or less parallel palmar creases, as well as when the left hand creases would form the letter M.

DISCUSSION

Purpose of this brief article is to bring to our attention the importance of initiating a study of the prehistory of dermatoglyphics. It should be stressed to archeologists and anthropologists to observe carefully any dermatoglyphic material they may found as it may prove to be an important finding to our field.

Attention to dermatoglyphics in archeological material has been brought forward in the past by Cummins (1941), who reported ancient finger prints in clay and by Cummins and Midlo (1961) in their book on "Finger prints, palms and soles". They mention that favorable opportunities for impressing finger prints existed in clay workers and refer to aboriginal Indian carvings in Nova Scotia, as well as to a chinese clay seal of the 3rd century B.C. and a palestinian lamp dating to the 4th or 5th century A.D.

By studying dermatoglyphics on archeological findings one may establish racial evolutionary patterns at various periods, with implications to ethnology, physical anthropology and human genetics. The study of ancient texts of any nation is equally important to us. It will bring closer to modern scientists our professional ancestors the cheiroscopists and the palamoscopists.

Therefore, we propose the use of the term paleodermatoglyphics to be used for the study of dermatoglyphics through antiquity in archeological and anthropological material (mummies), as well as in the ancient texts.

Acknowledgement: The author is indebted to Prof. Lila Marangou and Mr. Petros Samsaris for archeological information and the photographs of figures 1 & 2.

REFERENCES

Artemidorus Daldianus (1805). Oneirocritica II, 69 ('Αρτεμιδώρου 'Ονειροκριτική) Sumtibus Siegfried Lebrecht Crusii, vol I, Lipsiae.

Bouché-Leclercq, A. (1879-1882). Histoire de la divination dans l' antiquité, Paris.

Cummins, H. (1941). Ancient finger prints in clay, Sci. Monthly 52 : 389-402.

Cummins, H. and Midlo, C. (1961). "Finger prints, palms and soles: an introduction to dermatoglyphics". Dover Publications, New York.

Galton, F. (1892). "Finger prints". Macmillan, London.

Koukoulés, Ph. (Κουκουλές, Φ.) (1948). "Life and civilization of the Byzantines . (Βυζαντινῶν Βίος καί Πολιτισμός)". Athens.

Maury, A. (1857). La magie et l' astrologie dans l' antiquité et au moyen-âge. Paris.

Souidae (1705). Lexicon Graece et Latine, vol I, Typis Academicis, Cantabrigiae (see Artemidorus and Elenus).

Thompson, J.S. and Thompson, M.W. (1980). "Genetics in Medicine", 3rd Edition, W.B.Saunders Company, New York.

Progress in Dermatoglyphic Research, pages 145-156

GRANDPARENTAL INFLUENCES IN THE EXPRESSION OF DERMATOGLYPHICS PATTERNS ON THE FINGERTIPS

Dr.Abdülbari BENER *

Istanbul Technical University,
Faculty of Engineering,
Dept. of Environmental Engineering,
Teknik Üniversite
Taksim, Taskısla
ISTANBUL - TURKEY

A B S T R A C T S

The study of the occurrance of like patterns in grandparents and grandchildren allows for eight different sequences of gametic involvement in the contribution to a specific phenotype. Correlation between paternal and maternal grandparents and their grandchildren of both sexes for the occurrence of the major dermatoglyphics patterns on specific fingertips have been calculated. Such correlations reflect the amount of hereditary likeness between clases of relatives and may provide clues to the number of loci involved and to degree of dominance that may exist for the specification of some patterns over other.

Using a synthetic index of pattern correlation, it was shown that patternal influence through two generations was least for the specification of whorls in males, and greatest for specification radial loops. In grandchildren of maternal grandmothers the influence on radial loops was least and greatest for specification of whorls, implying differential roles for chromosomal, oocytoplasmic and uterine environmental factors in patterns. A comparison of the pattern correlation indexes of the various grandparent - grandchild pairs might indicate whether this persumed difference in developmental influence is detectable.

* Present address:King Abdulaziz University,College of Engineering,Dept.of Industrial Engineering, P.O. Box 9027 , Jeddah , Kingdom of Saudi Arabia

INTRODUCTION

The nature of the primary genetic specification for pattern is not yet understood, although explanations for some patterns have been proposed (Slatis et al., 1976). To further this search, correlations for the occurrence of a given pattern on the same digit in grandparents and their grandchildren should be determined for each pattern from on each digit. Such correlations reflect the amount of hereditary likeness between classes of relatives, and may provide clues to the number of loci involved and to degree of dominance that may exist for the specification of some patterns over other.

The study of the occurrence of like patterns in grandparents and grandchildren allows for eight different sequences of gametic involvement in the contribution to a specific phenotype. Thus paternal grandfathers are linked to their grandsons through two sperm cells, whereas granddaughters trace their descent from their maternal grandmother through two egg cells (Fig. 1). Should either chromosomal or non-chromosomal influence be strong, a detectable relationship between certain grandparents and their grandchildren for pattern form should be demonstrable.

The study of grandparental influence on dermatoglyphic patterns requires the collection of prints from three generations of related persons. As part of the analysis of a large collection of fingerprints, data on grandparents and their grandchildren became available.

In the families collected in Poland by Dr.Danuta Z. Loesch Dermatoglyphic data were recorded. This data has kindly been put at my disposal by Dr.Loesch.

In theory a grandchild inherits one-fourth of its genome, on the average, from each grandparent. It is shown here that paternal and maternal grandparents exert quite different and identifiable chromosomal and oocytoplasmic influences on the specification of dermatoglyphic pattern form.

MATERIALS AND METHODS

The fingerprints data used and analysed in this study and investigation originally were collected by Dr.Loesch from villages in northeastern Poland, and have been used in her earlier studies (1971, 1974). The patterns were classified into the major categories of whorls, ulnar loops, and radial loops. Eight types of grandparent and grandchild pairs were examined for the occurrence of whorls, ulnar loops and radial loops on corresponding digits. For this study the prints from 516 grandparent and grandchild in 539 families are analysed.

Each grandparent and their grandchild pair (paternal and maternal) in which either member showed the fingertip pattern in question on a specific digit was examined for pair agreement on the same digit. Agreemenet for the pattern in question was valued one for each member of the pair, non-agreement was valued zero. Each value was standardized in the manner described previously (Bener, 1979 a-b, 1980). The variances and covariance were determined by the method detailed by Fisher (1970). The data were prepared for computer analysis by entering them on punched cards. Subs subsequently each pattern was analyzed for each digit.

The correlations between grandparents and grandchildren of both sexes in all combinations were determined. The calculations were done on the IBM 360/65 computer at the University College London Computer Centre, and employed a program prepared by the author.

RESULTS

The correlations obtained are presented in Tables 1, 2 and 3. In order to simplify fingertip nomenclature and to accord with the sequence of print-taking employed by Scotland Yard (U.K.) and the Federal Bureau of Investigation (USA) among others, the fingertips are designated from 1 to 10, ranging from the right thumb to the left little finger. The nomenclature employed here, equated with the other system commonly used, follows; Right hand: 1, thumb (R I); 2, fore finger (R II); 3, middle finger (R III); 4, ring finger (R IV); 5, little finger (R V). Left hand: 6, thumb (L I); 7, fore finger (L II); 8, middle finger (L III); 9, ring finger (L IV); 10, little finger (L V), (Erk and Bener,1980). Specific digits are identified according to the scheme originated by Henry (1900), whereby right-hand digits are designated 1 to 5, and left-hand digits 6 to 10. Confusion between the two hands is thereby minimised.

An estimate of the total digital correlation between a class of grandparents and a class of grandchildren can be obtained by summing arithmetically the separate correlations for the occurrence of a given pattern on each of the digits. This pattern correlation index (PCI) provides a convenient basis for comparing the eight types of grandparent-grandchild pairs. The PCI's are summarised in Table 4.

DISCUSSION

The dermatoglyphic patterns on fingertips are set several months before birth, and remain unchanged throughout life. On *a priori* considerations alone, paternal grandfather influence on both grandsons and granddaughters (Fig. 1 paths *a* and *b*) would be expected to be primarily chromosomal whereas maternal grandmother influence would reflect both the chromosomal and oocytoplasmic contributions from both the mother and grandmother (Fig. 1 path *g* and *h*). In addition, the *in utero* environments of both mother and grandmother could exert effects during embryogenesis. A comparison of the pattern correlation indexes of the various grandparent-grandchild pairs might indicate whether this persumed difference in developmental influence is detectable.

The PCI's for paternal grandfathers range from -0,23 (for Ulnar Loops in granddaughter) to -1,10 (for whorls in granddaughters) whereas maternal grandmaternal influence, as measured by PCI's, range from -1,16 (for Radial Loops in granddaughters), to -1,14 (for Whorls in grandsons). Even though the number of pairs available for analysis is limited, especially paternal grandmother-granddaughter and grandfather-granddaughter pairs, there is a precise inversion of values that occupy the extremes, and they relate to the same patterns in the same grandchildren. The implication is clear that chromosomal factors are much less important in specifying whorl patterns in grandsons than are oocytoplasmic or *in utero* environmental ones. On the other hand, Radial loops show positive PCI's with paternal grandparents and negative PCI's with maternal grandparents, suggesting that oocytoplasmic and maternal environmental factors are Stronger than chromosomal ones in Radial loop specification.

The other four classes of grandparent-grandchild pairs (Fig. 1, paths c, d, e, f) have mixed gametic sequences, and the PCI's are correspondingly intermediate in range and value: paternal grandmother PCI's range from -0.44 to -1.27, and maternal grandfather PCI's range from -1.16 to -0.19 (Fig. 2). When all grandparent-grandchild pairs are taken together, the PCI's are positive for each pattern except for the Ulnar loops, but highest for Radial loops.

The inadvisability of grouping all related pairs regardless of sex can be seen from Fig. 2. The diversity of maternal and paternal influence is obscured when grandparent grandchild correlations are calculated for the entire group. The diagram clearly shows that PCI's for Radial loops are always positive for paternal grandparents, and negative for maternal grandparents. Although Whorls also occupy extreme positions in some relationships, the range is much less than for Radial loops. Ulnar loops PCI's are negative.

This study suggest that observations taken over two generations are useful and perhaps necessary if the more subtle influences of male and female contributions to complex phenotypes are to be discovered. Larger samples of grandparent-grandchild pairs for various human traits under partial genetic control should be sought in order to explore further the potential of this kind of analysis.

SUMMARY

Correlations between paternal maternal grandparents and their grandchildren of both sexes for the occurrence of the major dermatoglyphic patterns on specific fingertips have been calculated. Using a synthetic index of pattern correlation, it was shown that paternal influence through two generations was least for the specification of whorls in males, and greatest for specification of radial loops. In grandchildren of maternal grandmothers the influence on Radial loops was least and greatest for specification of Whorls, implying differential roles for chromosomal, oocytoplasmic, and uterine environmental factors in pattern specification.

ACKNOWLEDGEMENTS

The author express his gratitude to Dr.Danuta, Z. Loesch, of the Department of Genetics, Psychoneurological Institute, Warsaw, for the use of data from Polish population dermatoglyphic study. He also express his appreciation to

Professors C.A.B. Smith and Frank C. Erk for the many courtesies extended to him while working at the Galton Laboratory, and to Dr.Sarah B. Holt for her most helpful comments on the manuscript.

R E F E R E N C E S

BENER, A., (1979a). Sex differences and bilateral asymmetry in Dermatoglyphic pattern elements on the fingertips. Annals of Human Genetics, 42, 333-342.

BENER, A., (1979b). Correlation between relatives, their theoretical values for autosomal and sex-linked characters with respect to Dermatoglyphic characters. Collegium Antropologicum, Vol. 3, No. 2. ,p.p.,211-223

BENER, A., and ERK, F.C., (1980). Correlation between relatives with respect to Dermatoglyphic patterns on specific fingertips. I. Sib-sib correlations. Human Biology, Vol 52, No 4, pp 765-772.

ERK, F.C., and BENER, A., (1980). Correlation between relatives with respect to Dermatoglyphic patterns on specific fingertips. II. Parent-Child correlations. Human Biology, Vol. 52, No. 4, pp 753-763.

FISHER, R.A., (1970). Statistical Methods for Research Workers. 14th Ed. Edinburgh: Oliver and Boyd.

HENRY, E.R., (1900). Classification and uses of Finger - Prints. London: Routledge.

LOESCH, D., (1971). Genetics of Dermatoglyphic patterns on palms. Annals of Human Genetics, 34, 277-293.

LOESCH, D., (1974). Genetical studies of sole and palmar Dermatoglyphics. Annals of Human Genetics, 37, 405-419.

SLATIS, H.M., KATZNELSON, M.B., and BONNE-TAMIR, B., (1976). The Inheritance of fingerprint patterns. American Journal of Human Genetics, 28, 280-289.

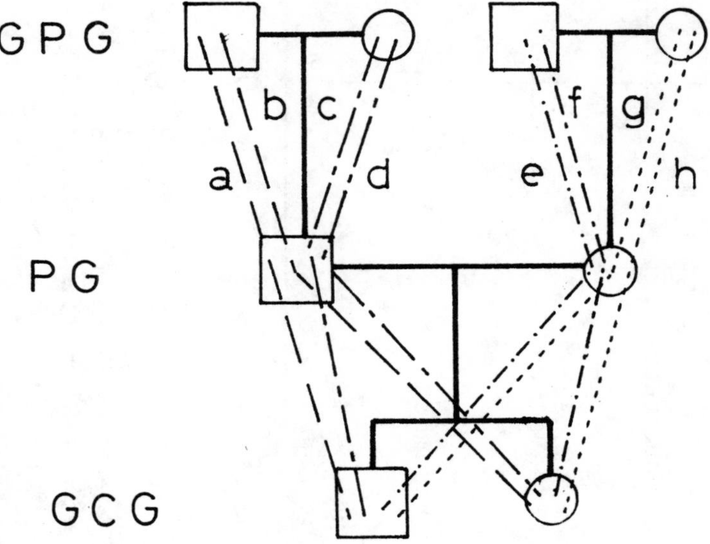

Figure: 1. The eight gametic sequences whereby grandparental influence is transmitted to grandchildren. (□= male, ○= female, GPG= grandparental generation, PG= parental generation, GGG= grandchild generation).

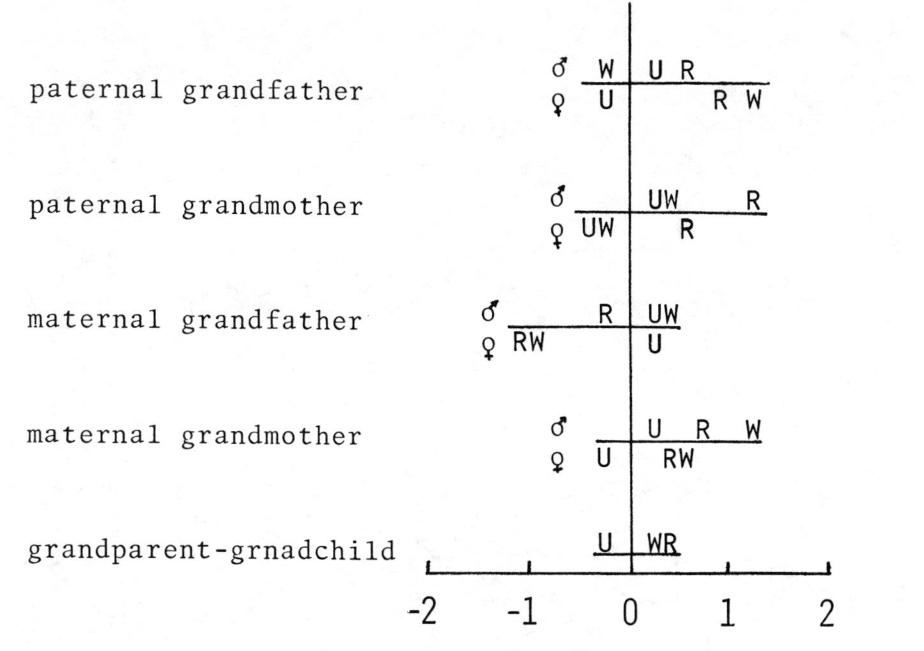

Figure: 2. Pattern correlation index ranges for the four grandparents of any child. (♂= grandson, ♀= granddaughter, W= whorls, U= ulnar loops, R= radial loops).

Table: 1. Correlations between grandparents and their grandchildren for the occurrence of whorls on specific fingertips.

	Paternal Grandfather-Grandson	Maternal Grandfather-Grandson	Paternal Grandfather-Granddaughter	Maternal Grandfather-Granddaughter	Paternal Grandmother-Grandson	Maternal Grandmother-Grandson	Paternal Grandmother-Granddaughter	Maternal Grandmother-Granddaughter	Grandparent-Grandchild
	N= 59	N= 53	N= 62	N= 55	N= 80	N= 74	N= 76	N= 56	N= 516
Right-Hand Fingertips									
1 (thumb)	0.02	0.11	0.09	0.02	-0.08	0.14	-0.14	0.21	0.03
2	-0.09	-0.12	-0.01	-0.02	0.14	0.06	0.01	-0.08	0.00
3	-0.01	0.11	0.00	-0.04	0.03	0.13	-0.26	-0.06	-0.02
4	0.09	-0.03	-0.14	-0.11	0.14	-0.06	0.08	-0.03	0.00
5	-0.06	0.28	0.23	-0.26	-0.07	0.13	0.20	-0.16	0.04
Left-Hand Fingertips									
6 (thumb)	0.13	0.03	0.02	0.09	0.04	0.18	-0.06	0.23	0.08
7	-0.13	0.06	0.20	0.11	0.05	0.00	0.02	0.13	0.05
8	0.04	-0.11	0.11	-0.16	0.17	0.18	0.09	0.12	0.07
9	-0.06	0.02	0.09	-0.14	0.22	0.23	-0.04	-0.09	0.04
10	0.07	-0.16	0.36	-0.20	0.13	0.15	0.34	0.01	0.11

Table: 2. Correlations between grandparents and their grandchildren for the occurrence of Ulnar Loops on specific fingertips.

	Paternal Grandfather-Grandson	Maternal Grandfather-Grandson	Paternal Grandfather-Granddaughter	Maternal Grandfather-Granddaughter	Paternal Grandmother-Grandson	Maternal Grandmother-Grandson	Paternal Grandmother-Granddaughter	Maternal Grandmother-Granddaughter	Grandparent-Grandchild
	N= 59	N= 53	N= 62	N= 55	N= 80	N= 74	N= 77	N= 56	N= 516
Right-Hand Fingertips									
1 (thumb)	0.01	0.01	0.00	0.01	-0.05	0.01	-0.04	0.02	-0.01
2	0.11	0.09	0.01	0.17	-0.04	0.14	-0.01	-0.01	0.05
3	-0.12	0.02	-0.37	-0.02	0.09	0.00	-0.08	-0.06	-0.06
4	-0.02	0.01	-0.02	0.01	0.00	-0.02	-0.01	-0.08	-0.01
5	0.01	-0.01	-0.01	-0.01	0.01	0.02	-0.05	0.02	0.00
Left-Hand Fingertips									
6 (thumb)	0.00	0.01	0.01	0.02	-0.07	-0.01	-0.07	0.03	-0.01
7	-0.14	0.05	0.17	0.00	0.06	-0.04	-0.16	-0.04	-0.05
8	0.20	0.01	-0.02	0.02	0.07	0.02	0.11	-0.04	0.05
9	0.00	-0.01	0.01	0.01	0.03	-0.00	0.07	-0.02	-0.01
10	0.00	0.00	-0.01	-0.02	-0.03	0.02	-0.06	0.02	-0.01

Table: 3. Correlations between grandparents and their grandchildren for the occurrence of Radial Loops on specific fingertips.

	Paternal Grandfather-Grandson	Maternal Grandfather-Grandson	Paternal Grandfather-Granddaughter	Maternal Grandfather-Granddaughter	Paternal Grandmother-Grandson	Maternal Grandmother Grandson	Paternal Grandmother Granddaughter	Maternal Grandmother-Granddaughter	Grandparent-Grandchild
	N= 59	N= 53	N= 62	N= 55	N= 80	N= 74	N= 77	N= 56	N= 516
Right-Hand Fingertips									
1 (thumb)	0.02	0.11	0.12	0.02	-0.07	0.15	-0.08	0.23	0.05
2	-0.08	-0.10	0.03	-0.12	0.33	-0.04	0.09	0.03	0.03
3	0.15	0.06	0.05	-0.16	-0.01	0.13	-0.17	-0.29	-0.03
4	0.15	-0.03	-0.04	-0.15	0.17	-0.05	0.12	0.10	0.04
5	-0.08	0.28	0.17	-0.33	-0.10	0.13	0.19	-0.21	0.01
Left-Hand fingertips									
6 (thumb)	0.16	0.01	-0.01	0.09	-0.02	0.15	0.11	0.31	0.10
7	0.06	0.07	-0.01	0.02	0.20	-0.19	0.09	0.11	0.04
8	0.11	-0.25	0.15	-0.08	0.40	0.21	-0.08	0.02	0.08
9	-0.03	-0.01	0.13	-0.18	0.19	0.22	-0.07	-0.08	0.03
10	0.16	-0.20	0.37	-0.27	0.18	0.16	0.31	0.01	0.11

Table: 4. Pattern correlation indexes for grandparents and their grandchildren indexes are arithmetic sum of coefficients of correlation calculated separately for each of ten digits (Tables 1, 2, 3).

	No. Pairs	WHORLS	ULNAR LOOPS	RADIAL LOOPS
PATERNAL GRANDPARENTS				
Grandfather-grandson	59	0.00	0.05	0.62
Grandfather-granddaughter	62	1.10	-0.23	0.96
Grandmother-grandson	80	0.67	0.01	1.27
Grandmother-granddaughter	77	-0.24	-0.44	0.51
MATERNAL GRANDPARENTS				
Grandfather-grandson	53	0.19	0.18	-0.06
Grandfather-granddaughter	55	-0.71	0.19	-1.16
Grandmother-grandson	74	1.14	0.14	0.87
Grandmother-granddaughter	56	0.28	-0.12	0.23
Grandparent-grandchild	516	0.40	-0.06	0.46

Progress in Dermatoglyphic Research, pages 157-173

FURTHER STUDIES ON DERMATOGLYPHIC ASSOCIATIONS

Virginia Inés FORTICH BACA.

Facultad de Filosofía y Letras, Departamento de Ciencias Antropológicas, Universidad de Buenos Aires, 25 de Mayo 217, 1002, Buenos Aires, ARGENTINA

In a previous study (Fortich Baca, 1978), it has been suggested that three dermatoglyphic variates: the axial triradius, the coefficient of Turpin and Lejeune and the hypothenar patterns, could be associated on acount of topographic reasons, that is, that the axial triradius would be a barrier for those palmar ridges running from the distal triradii and consequently modifying the coefficient of Turpin and Lejeune. At the same time and for similar reasons, the cited triradius would be an influence in the presence and type of hypothenar patterns.

This postulate has been analyzed here again, pointing out the statistical validity of the proposed association, in order to determine if these three variates can be taken altogether as a recurrent whole, for diagnostic purposes in racial and genetic studies.

If the proposed associations were really strong, it would be unnecessary to analyze separately each variate, for one would almost always involve the type of the other two.

MATERIAL AND METHODS

A group of 400 caucasian males and females (200 of each), from Buenos Aires city, all of them with a High school or University study was analyzed. Subject of analysis has been the hand and not the individual.

The coefficient of Turpin and Lejeune was divided into three categories: low, up to 19; medium from 20 up to 29; high, 30 or more. Axial triradius was classified into three categories too: t, t′ and t′′ . The index proposed by Norma Ford Walker (cf. Bartalos, M. and Baramki, Th., 1972: 286) for the classification of this triradius, has been applied. Cases of triradii off the end have been included in the t or low triradius group, because it could be assumed that this position is an exceedingly low one, that cannot alter the type of the other two variates.

There was only one hand with a t′′′ triradius and this was included in the t′′ group, because it represented a similar case, that is, a very high triradius.

Hypothenar patterns were divided into whorls and loops, this latter subdivided into four types: radial, ulnar, digital and carpal loops. Hypothenar arches were included in the "no pattern" category, for this configuration did not demand a triradius for its development.

Percentile distribution and statistical significance of percentile differences were tested. Sex and side differences were controled too, in order to establish if these variates had any influence in the results.

A X^2 test and a test of deviation from the normal curve have been applied here.

RESULTS

1.- Sex and side differences are non signigicant in relation with the distribution of hypothenar patterns. The coefficient of Turpin and Lejeune is influenced only by laterality, while axial triradius is conditioned only by sex.

2.- In relation with hypothenar patterns, predominate those hands without this kind of configurations. Digital and radial loops follow in order of absolute number, but percentile differences do not appear to be significant.

3.- Percentile differences in the triradius distribution are really significant, t being more frequent than t′ and this one more frequent than t′′.

4.- In relation with the coefficient of Turpin and Lejeune, a low coefficient is rather scarce, medium being the more frequent of the left hand, while on the right a high coefficient is more frequent.

5.- The coefficient of Turpin and Lejeune does not show any significant association with the other two variates.

6.- The position of axial triradius is significantly related to the hypothenar patterns.

7.- Axial triradius t''is more frequently associated with hypothenar whorls, than t or t'.

8.- A X^2 test applied ot prove the association among the three parameters denotes a significant relation in all cases, except for the left hand in the male group.

9.- The association among the axial triradius t, low coefficient and no hypothenar patterns, as well as that of axial triradius t, medium coefficient and no hypothenar patterns, is more frequent than t', medium coefficient and no configurations. At the same time,this latter is more frequent than a t'' triradius with medium coefficient and absence of patterns, independently of sex and side differences. On the other hand, there are no cases of axial triradius t, high coefficient and hypothenar whorls, and a t'' triradius with a high coefficient and hypothenar whorls is more occurrent than of t', high coefficient and palmar whorls.

DISCUSSION

The high percentage of absence of hypothenar patterns, no matter which position the corresponding axial triradius may have, is denoting that these patterns, although influenced by the palmar triradii, are not their necessary consequence.

Only two of the three variates analyzed here are really associated:they are the axial triradius and the hypothenar patterns. The coefficient of Turpin and Lejeune, on the contraty, shows to be independient of the position of the axial triradius or the presence and type of hypothenar patterns but, nevertheless, the association between these two variates is so strong that even when the three variates are correlated simultaneously, the X^2 test reveals still a positive significant association.

The variation of the coefficient of Turpin and Lejeune seems to be due to other conditions than the position of the axial triradius or the hypothenar configurations. These other conditions could be the existence of accessory distal triradii, interdigital patterns, etc. In a preliminary way, it could be said that this coefficient does not prove to be good for describing the general obliquity degree of palmar ridges.

Finally, it can be deduced from all the above that in a dermatoglyphic analysis, either one or the other of the associated variates can be taken on account as an index of diagnosis and classification, being unnecessary to use both.

REFERENCES

BANCROFT, H. (1968). "Introducción a la biostadística". Buenos Aires, EUDEBA.

BARTALOS, M. and BARAMKI, Th. (1972) "Citogenética Médica". Buenos Aires, EUDEBA.

CORTADA de KOHAN, N. and CARRO, J.M. (1975) "Estadística aplicada". Buenos Aires, EUDEBA.

FORTICH BACA, V.I. (1978). Acerca de la posible asociación entre los trirradios axiales, el coeficiente de Turpin-Lejeune y las figuras hipotenares. Rev. Biol. del Urug. 6 (2): p. 93.

SCHREIDER, E. (1966) "La Biometría". Buenos Aires, EUDEBA.

VESSEREAU, A. (1976) "La Estadística". Buenos Aires, EUDEBA.

VIDAL, O.R. (1966) Las crestas de las manos. Su importancia en citogenetica humana. Rev. Esp. de Ped. XXIII (133): p 1-22.

ABBREVIATIONS

M = Male
F = Female
L = Left Hand
R = Right hand
h = high coefficient
m = medium coefficient

l = low coefficient
u = ulnar hypothenar loop
r = radial hypothenar loop
d = digital hypothenar loop
c = carpal hypothenar loop
w = hypothenar whorl
0 = absence of hypothenar patterns
n.s. = non significant

TABLES

1

Percentile distribution of axial trirradius

	Males			Females		
	l	r	l+r	l	r	l+r
t	66.5	55.0	58.0	55.0	51.0	53.25
t'	33.0	39.0	36.0	29.5	36.5	33.0
t''	6.5	5.5	6.0	15.0	12.5	13.75
n^o	200	200	400	200	200	400

	Males+Females		
	l	r	l+r
t	58.0	53.25	43.12
t'	33.75	37.75	35.75
t''	10.75	9.0	9.87
n^o	400	400	800

2

Percentile distribution of the coefficient of Turpin and Lejeune

	Males			Females		
	l	r	l+r	l	r	l+r
h	23.5	49.5	36.5	25.0	42.5	33.75
m	69.5	47.5	58.5	67.0	54.0	60.5
l	7.0	3.0	5.0	8.0	3.5	5.75
n^o	200	200	400	200	200	400

	Males+Females		
	l	r	l+r
h	24.25	46.0	35.12
m	68.25	50.75	59.5
l	7.5	3.25	5.37
n^o	400	400	800

3

Percentile distribution of hypothenar patterns

	Males			Females		
	l	r	l+r	l	r	l+r
O	68.0	62.0	65.0	68.5	59.5	64.0
u	8.5	10.5	9.5	7.5	7.5	7.5
c	0.5	1.5	1.0	2.0	5.0	3.5
d	13.5	9.5	11.5	10.0	12.5	11.25
r	7.5	13.0	10.25	8.5	11.0	9.75
w	2.0	3.5	2.75	3.5	4.5	4.0
n^o	200	200	400	200	200	400

	Males+Females		
	l	r	l+r
O	68.25	60.75	64.5
u	8.0	9.0	8.5
c	1.25	3.25	2.25
d	11.75	11.0	11.37
r	8.0	12.0	8.0
w	2.75	4.0	3.37
n^o	400	400	800

4

PERCENTILE DIFFERENCES (Z test)

Axial triradius

	P_1	$\%P_1$	n^o	P_2	$\%P_2$	n^o	≠	Zc	Sign.
M.L.	t	66.5	200	t'	33.0	200	33.5	7.11	0.05
R.	t	55.0	200	t'	39.0	200	16.0	3.24	0.05
L.	t'	33.0	200	t''	6.5	200	26.5	2.05	0.05
R.	t'	39.0	200	t''	5.5	200	33.5	8.79	0.05
F.L.	t	55.0	200	t'	29.5	200	25.5	5.34	0.05
R.	t	51.0	200	t'	36.5	200	14.5	2.95	0.05
L.	t'	29.5	200	t''	15.0	200	14.5	3.54	0.05
R.	t'	36.5	200	t''	12.0	200	24.5	5.96	0.05
L+R	t M	58.0	400	F	51.0	400	7.0	1.99	0.05
	t'M	36.0	400	F	33.0	400	3.0	0.89	n.s.
	t''M	6.0	400	F	12.5	400	6.5	3.19	0.05
M t	L	66.5	200	R	55.0	200	11.5	2.37	0.05
t'	L	33.0	200	R	39.0	200	-6.0	0.37	n.s.
t''	L	6.5	200	R	5.5	200	1.0	0.42	n.s.
F.t	L	55.0	200	R	51.0	200	4.0	0.80	n.s.
t'	L	29.5	200	R	36.5	200	-7.0	1.48	n.s.
t''	L	15.0	200	R	12.5	200	2.5	0.72	n.s.

Coefficient of Turpin and Lejeune

	P_1	$\%P_1$	n^o	P_2	$\%P_2$	n^o	≠	Zc	Sign.
M.L.	m	69.5	200	h	23.5	200	46.0	8.37	0.05
R.	h	49.5	200	m	47.5	200	2.0	0.40	n.s.
L.	h	23.5	200	m	7.0	200	16.5	4.71	0.05
R.	m	47.5	200	l	3.0	200	44.5	11.91	0.05
F.L.	m	67.0	200	h	25.0	200	42.0	9.29	0.05
R.	m	54.0	200	h	42.5	200	11.5	2.31	0.05
L.	h	25.0	200	l	8.0	200	17.0	4.70	0.05
R.	h	42.5	200	l	3.5	200	39.0	2.44	0.05
L+R.h	M	36.5	400	F	33.75	400	2.75	0.81	n.s.
m	M	58.5	400	F	60.5	400	-2.0	0.57	n.s.
l	M	5.0	400	F	5.75	400	-0.75	0.47	n.s.

	P_1	$\%P_1$	n^o	P_2	$\%P_2$	n^o	≠	Zc	Sign.
M h	L	23.5	200	R	49.5	200	-26	5.6	0.05
m	L	69.5	200	R	47.5	200	22	4.58	0.05
l	L	7.0	200	R	3.0	200	4	1.84	n.s.
F h	L	25.0	200	R	42.5	200	27.5	5.91	0.05
m	L	67.0	200	R	54.0	200	13	2.68	0.05
l	L	8.0	200	R	3.5	200	4.5	1.94	n.s.

<u>Hypothenar patterns</u>

	P_1	$\%P_1$	n^o	P_2	$\%P_2$	n^o	≠	Zc	Sign.
M.L.	0	67.5	200	d	13.5	200	54.0	13.17	0.05
	d	13.5	200	u	8.5	200	5.0	1.60	n.s.
	u	8.5	200	r	7.5	200	1.0	0.36	n.s.
	r	7.5	200	w	2.0	200	5.5	2.60	0.05
	w	2.0	200	c	0.5	200	1.5	1.35	n.s.
M.R.	0	59.5	200	r	13.0	200	46.5	11.05	0.05
	r	13.0	200	u	10.5	200	2.5	0.77	n.s.
	u	10.5	200	d	9.5	200	1.0	0.12	n.s.
	d	9.5	200	w	3.5	200	6.0	2.45	0.05
	w	3.5	200	c	1.0	200	2.5	1.69	n.s.
F.L.	0	66.5	200	d	10.0	200	56.5	14.28	0.05
	d	10.0	200	u	7.5	200	2.5	0.34	n.s.
	u	7.5	200	r	8.5	200	-1.0	0.36	n.s.
	r	8.5	200	w	3.5	200	5.0	2.11	0.05
	w	5.0	200	c	2.0	200	1.5	0.91	n.s.
F.R.	0	55.5	200	d	12.5	200	43	10.18	0.05
	d	12.5	200	r	11.0	200	0.5	0.15	n.s.
	r	11.0	200	u	7.5	200	3.5	1.21	n.s.
	u	7.5	200	c	5.0	200	2.5	0.42	n.s.
	c	5.0	200	w	4.5	200	0.5	0.24	n.s.

	% left	n^o	% right	n^o	≠	Zc	Sign.
M.u	8.5	200	10.5	200	-2	0.68	n.s.
r	7.5	200	13.0	200	-5.5	1.82	n.s.
0	67.5	200	59.5	200	8.0	1.66	n.s.
d	13.5	200	9.5	200	4	1.25	n.s.
c	0.5	200	1.5	200	-1	0.80	n.s.
w	2.0	200	3.5	200	-1.5	0.57	n.s.
F u	7.5	200	7.5	200	no	difference	
r	8.5	200	11.0	200	-2.5	0.84	n.s.
0	66.5	200	55.5	200	11.0	2.26	0.05
d	10.0	200	12.5	200	-2.5	0.79	n.s.
c	2.0	200	5.0	200	-3.0	1.06	n.s.
w	3.5	200	4.5	200	=1	0.51	n.s.

Association of axial triradius with hypothenar patterns. Percentile differences.

	P_1	$\%P_1$	n^o	P_2	$\%P_2$	n^o	≠	Zc	Sign.
Males									
L+R	t'-w	20.27	143	t''-w	21.73	23	-17.54	2.0	0.05
L	t'-w	3.03	66	t''-w	15.38	13	12.35	1.2	n.s.
R	t'-w	5.19	77	t''-w	30.0	10	-24.81	1.68	n.s.
Females									
L+R	t'-w	3.03	132	t''-w	22.22	54	-19.19	3.28	0.05
L	t'-w	1.69	59	t''-w	20.68	29	-18.99	2.24	0.05
R	t'-w	4.10	73	t''-w	24.00	25	19.9	2.24	0.05
Males +Females									
L+R	t'-w	3.63	275	t''-w	22.07	77	18.44	3.80	0.05
L	t'-w	2.40	125	t''-w	19.04	42	16.64	2.67	0.05
R	t'-w	4.66	150	t''-w	25.71	35	21.05	2.77	0.05

Association of axial triradius, coefficient of Turpin and Lejeune and hypothenar patterns. Percentile difference.

	P_1	$\%P_1$	n^o	P_2	$\%P_2$	n^o	≠	Zc	Sign.
Males									
L+R	t-m-0	80.13	146	t'-m-0	58.9	73	21.23	3.19	0.05
	t'-m-0	58.90	73	t''-m-0	18.7	16	40.1	3.54	0.05
L	t-m-0	82.14	84	t'-m-0	58.13	43	24.0	2.78	0.05
	t'-m-0	58.13	43	t''-m-0	25.0	12	33.1	2.27	0.05
R	t-m-0	77.41	62	t'-m-0	60.0	30	17.4	1.67	n.s.
Females									
L+R	t-m-0	80.76	130	t'-m-0	52.56	78	28.2	4.25	0.05
	t'-m-0	52.56	78	t''-m-0	24.24	33	28.3	3.02	0.05
L	t-m-0	80.55	72	t'-m-0	59.52	42	21.0	2.36	0.05
	t'-m-0	59.52	42	t''-m-0	26.31	19	33.2	2.63	0.05
R	t-m-0	81.03	58	t'-m-0	44.44	36	36.5	3.75	0.05
Males +Females									
L+R	t-m-0	80.43	276	t'-m-0	55.62	151	24.8	5.28	0.05
	t'-m-0	55.62	151	t''-m-0	22.44	49	22.1	4.6	0.05
L	t-m-0	81.41	156	t'-m-0	58.82	85	22.59	3.62	0.05
	t'-m-0	58.82	85	t''-m-0	25.80	31	33.02	3.47	0.05
R	t-m-0	79.16	66	t'-m-0	51.51	66	27.65	3.85	0.05
Males									
L+R	t''-h-w	42.85	7	t'-h-w	4.73	63	38.09	2.01	0.05
R	t''-h-w	50.0	6	t'-h-w	4.44	30	45.56	2.19	0.05
Females									
L+R	t''-h-w	24.0	25	t'-h-w	2.63	114	21.3	2.46	0.05
R	t''-h-w	37.5	16	t'-h-w	2.46	81	35.0	2.86	0.05

5

Association between axial triradius and coefficient of Turpin and Lejeune. (Both hands).

	Males				Females				Males +Females			
	h	m	l	n^o	h	m	l	n^o	h	m	l	n^o
t	76	146	12	234	67	130	16	213	143	276	28	447
t'	63	73	7	143	51	78	3	132	114	151	10	275
t''	7	16	0	23	17	34	4	55	24	50	4	78
n^o	146	235	19	400	135	242	23	400	281	477	42	800

X^2 =6.955 =n.s. X^2 = 5.544 =n.s. X^2 = 7.789 =n.s.

6

Association between axial triradius and coefficient of Turpin and Lejeune. Males.

	Left				Right			
	h	m	l	n^o	h	m	l	n^o
t	28	84	9	121	48	62	3	113
t'	18	43	5	66	45	30	2	77
t''	1	12	0	13	6	4	0	10
n^o	47	139	14	200	99	96	5	200

X^2 = 4.575 = n.s. X^2 = 5.616 = n.s.

7

Association between axial triradius and coefficient of Turpin and Lejeune. Females.

	Left				Right			
	h	m	l	n^o	h	m	l	n^o
t	28	72	11	111	39	58	5	102
t'	15	42	2	59	36	36	1	73
t''	7	20	3	30	10	14	1	25
n^o	50	134	16	200	85	108	7	200

X^2 = 3.331 =n.s. X^2 = 4.678 = n.s.

8

Association between axial triradius and coefficient of Turpin and Lejeune. Males + Females.

	Left				Right			
	h	m	l	n^o	h	m	l	n^o
t	36	156	20	232	87	120	8	215
t'	33	85	7	125	81	66	3	150
t''	8	32	3	43	16	18	1	35
n^o	97	273	30	400	184	204	12	400

X^2 = 3.470 = n.s. X^2 =6.252 = n.s.

9

Association between axial triradius and hypothe patterns.

Males.

Left + Right

	u	r	c	d	w	0	n^o
t	2	27	0	23	0	182	234
t'	29	13	1	19	6	75	143
t''	7	2	2	4	5	3	23
n^o	38	42	3	46	11	260	400

$X^2 = 41.79 = 0.05$

Left

	u	r	c	d	w	0	n^o
t	1	9	0	12	0	99	121
t'	13	5	0	12	2	34	66
t''	3	1	1	3	2	3	13
n^o	17	15	1	27	4	136	200

$X^2 = 32.830 = 0.05$

Right

	u	r	c	d	w	0	n^o
t	1	18	0	11	0	83	113
t'	16	8	1	7	4	41	77
t''	4	1	1	1	3	0	10
n^o	21	27	2	19	7	124	200

$X^2 = 32.933 = 0.05$

10

Associataion between axial triradius and hypothenar patterns

Females.

Left + Right

	u	r	c	d	w	0	n^o
t	0	27	0	21	0	166	214
t'	18	12	2	23	4	73	132
t''	12	0	12	1	12	17	54
n^o	30	39	14	45	16	256	400

$X^2 = 72.813 = 0.05$

Left

	u	r	c	d	w	0	n^o
t	0	13	0	11	0	88	112
t'	8	4	1	8	1	37	59
t''	7	0	3	1	6	12	29
n^o	15	17	4	20	7	137	200

$X^2 = 39.385 = 0.05$

Right

	u	r	c	d	w	0	n^o
t	0	14	0	10	0	78	102
t'	10	8	1	15	3	36	73
t''	5	0	9	0	6	5	25
n^o	15	22	10	25	9	119	200

$X^2 = 49.963 = 0.05$

11

Association between axial triradius and hypothenar patterns. Males + Females.

Left + Right

	u	r	c	d	w	0	n^o
t	2	54	0	44	0	348	448
t'	47	25	3	42	10	148	275
t''	19	2	14	5	17	20	77
n^o	68	81	17	91	27	516	800

$X^2 = 82.963 = 0.05$

Left

	u	r	c	d	w	0	n^o
t	1	22	0	23	0	187	233
t'	21	9	1	20	3	71	125
t''	10	1	4	4	8	15	42
n^o	32	32	5	47	11	273	400

$X^2 = 43.694 = 0.05$

Right

	u	r	c	d	w	0	n^o
t	1	32	0	21	0	161	215
t'	26	16	2	22	7	77	150
t''	9	1	10	1	9	5	35
n^o	36	49	12	44	16	243	400

$X^2 = 55.440 = 0.05$

12

Association between coefficient of Turpin and Lejeune and Hypothenar patterns. Males.

Left + Right

	u	r	c	d	w	0	n^o
h	16	17	2	19	6	86	146
m	22	23	2	20	5	163	235
i	0	1	0	7	0	11	19
n^o	38	41	4	46	11	260	400

$X^2 = 13.180 =$ n.s.

Left

	u	r	c	d	w	0	n^o
h	3	3	0	10	1	30	47
m	14	12	1	12	3	97	139
l	0	0	0	5	0	9	14
n^o	17	15	1	27	4	136	200

X^2 = 11.323 =n.s.

Right

	u	r	c	d	w	0	n^o
h	13	14	2	9	5	56	99
m	8	11	1	8	2	66	96
l	0	1	0	2	0	2	5
n^o	21	26	3	19	7	124	200

X^2 = 10.619 =n.s.

13

Association between coefficient of Turpin and Lejeune and hypothenar patterns. Females.

Left + Right

	u	r	c	d	w	0	n^o
h	13	17	4	15	3	83	135
m	17	20	9	28	13	155	242
l	0	2	1	2	0	18	23
n^o	30	39	14	45	16	256	400

X^2 =10.395 = n.s.

Left

	u	r	c	d	w	0	n^o
h	3	8	1	4	0	34	50
m	12	9	3	14	7	89	134
l	0	0	0	2	0	14	16
n^o	15	17	4	20	7	137	200

X^2 = 12.157 = n.s.

Right

	u	r	c	d	w	0	n^o
h	10	9	3	11	3	49	85
m	5	11	3	14	6	66	108
l	0	2	1	0	0	4	7
n^o	15	22	10	25	9	119	200

X^2 = 9.457 = n.s.

14

Association between coefficient of Turpin and Lejeune and hypothenar patterns. Males + Females.

Left + Right

	u	r	c	d	w	0	n^o
h	29	34	6	34	9	169	281
m	39	43	11	48	18	318	477
l	0	3	1	9	0	29	42
n^o	68	80	18	91	27	516	800

$X^2 = 14.569$ = n.s.

Left

	u	r	c	d	w	0	n^o
h	6	11	1	14	1	64	97
m	26	21	4	26	10	186	273
l	0	0	0	7	0	23	30
n^o	32	32	5	47	11	273	400

$X^2 = 15.846$ = n.s.

Right

	u	r	c	d	w	0	n^o
h	23	23	5	20	8	105	184
m	13	33	7	22	8	132	204
l	0	3	1	2	0	6	12
n^o	36	48	13	44	16	243	400

$X^2 = 10.776$ = n.s.

15

Association among axial triradius, coefficient of Turpin and Lejeune and hypothenar patterns. Males.

Left + Right

		u	r	c	d	w	0	n^o
t	h	0	11	8	0	0	57	76
	m	2	16	11	0	0	117	146
	l	0	0	4	0	0	8	12
t'	h	15	6	10	0	3	29	63
	m	14	6	6	1	3	43	73
	l	0	1	3	0	0	3	7
t''	h	2	0	1	1	3	0	7
	m	5	2	3	1	2	3	16
n^o		38	42	46	3	11	260	400

$X^2 = 82.398 = 0.05$

Left

		u	r	c	d	w	0	n^o
t	h	0	1	3	0	0	24	28
	m	1	8	6	0	0	69	84
	l	0	0	3	0	0	6	9
t'	h	3	2	6	0	1	6	18
	m	10	3	4	0	1	25	43
	l	0	0	2	0	0	3	5

t''	h	0	0	1	0	0	0	1
	m	3	1	2	1	2	3	12
n^o		17	15	27	1	4	136	200

X^2 =45.935 = n.s.

Right

		u	r	c	d	w	0	n^o
t	h	0	10	5	0	0	33	48
	m	1	8	5	0	0	48	62
	1	1	0	0	1	0	2	3
t'	h	12	4	4	0	2	23	45
	m	4	3	2	1	2	18	30
	l	0	1	1	0	0	0	2
t''	h	2	0	0	1	3	0	6
	m	2	1	1	0	0	0	4
n^o		21	27	19	2	7	124	200

X^2 = 56.891 = 0.05

16

Association among axial triradius, coefficient of Turpin-Lejeune and hypothenar patterns. Females.

Left + Right

		u	r	c	d	w	0	n^o
t	h	0	14	7	0	0	46	67
	m	0	12	13	0	0	105	130
	l	0	1	1	0	0	14	16
t'	h	8	3	7	2	0	31	51
	m	10	8	15	0	4	41	78
	l	0	1	1	0	0	1	3
t''	h	5	0	1	2	3	7	18
	m	7	0	0	9	9	8	33
	l	0	0	0	1	0	3	4
n^o		30	39	45	14	16	256	400

X^2 = 97.687 = 0.05

Left

		u	r	c	d	w	0	n^o
t	h	0	7	2	0	0	19	28
	m	0	6	8	0	0	58	72
	l	0	0	1	0	0	10	11
t'	h	1	1	1	1	0	11	15
	m	7	3	6	0	1	25	42
	l	0	0	1	0	0	1	2
t''	h	2	0	1	0	0	5	8
	m	5	0	0	3	6	5	19
	l	0	0	0	0	0	3	3
n^o		15	17	20	4	7	137	200

X^2 = 79.920 = 0.05

Right

		u	r	c	d	w	0	n^o
t	h	0	7	5	0	0	27	39
	m	0	6	5	0	0	47	58
	1	0	1	0	0	0	4	5
t'	h	7	2	6	1	0	20	36
	m	3	5	9	0	3	16	36
	1	0	1	0	0	0	0	1
t"	h	3	0	0	2	3	2	10
	m	2	0	0	6	3	3	14
	1	0	0	0	1	0	0	1
n^o		15	22	25	10	9	119	200

X^2 =79.920= 0.05

17

Association among axial triradius, coefficient of Turpin and Lejeune and hypothenar patterns.

Males + Females.

Left + Right

		u	r	c	d	w	0	n°
t	h	0	25	15	0	0	103	143
	m	2	28	24	0	0	222	276
	1	0	1	5	0	0	22	28
t'	h	23	9	17	2	3	60	114
	m	24	14	21	1	7	84	151
	1	0	2	4	0	0	4	10
t''	h	7	0	2	3	6	7	25
	m	12	2	3	10	11	11	49
	1	0	0	0	1	0	3	4
n°		68	81	91	17	27	516	800

$X^2 = 126.004 = 0.05$

Left

		u	r	c	d	w	0	n°
t	h	0	8	5	0	0	43	56
	m	1	14	14	0	0	127	156
	1	0	0	4	0	0	16	20
t'	h	4	3	7	1	1	17	33
	m	17	6	10	0	2	50	85
	1	0	0	3	0	0	4	7
t''	h	2	0	2	0	0	5	9
	m	8	1	2	4	8	8	31
	1	0	0	0	0	0	3	3
n°		32	32	47	5	11	273	400

$X^2 = 70.148 = 0.05$

Right

		u	r	c	d	w	0	n°
t	h	0	17	10	0	0	60	87
	m	1	14	10	0	0	95	120
	1	0	1	1	0	0	6	8
t'	h	19	6	10	1	2	43	81
	m	7	8	11	1	5	34	66
	1	0	2	1	0	0	0	3
t''	h	5	0	0	3	6	2	16
	m	4	1	1	6	3	3	18
	1	0	0	0	1	0	0	1
n°		36	49	44	12	16	243	400

$X^2 = 98.198 = 0.05$

Progress in Dermatoglyphic Research, pages 175–188

A METHODOLOGICAL APPROACH TO THE DEVELOPMENT OF EPIDERMAL RIDGES VIEWED ON THE DERMAL SURFACE OF FETUSES

Michio OKAJIMA

Department of Forensic Medicine, Tokyo Medical and Dental University, Yushima, Bunkyo-ku Tokyo 113

The embryogenetic interest in dermatoglyphics is in two main areas: the first is the differentiation of epidermal ridges and the second is the formation of ridge patterns. Earlier studies on embryogenesis published by many workers were summarized by Schaumann and Alter(1976).

Bonnevie(1929) and other workers suggested the significance of peripheral nerves in initiating the differentiation of ridges. However, Hale(1952) stated that the presence of nerve filaments are not essential to the ridge differentiation, since ridges are seen to develop in regions where nerve twigs are not demonstrable. Hirsch and Schweichel(1973) confirmed that capillaries are distributed at regular intervals under the epidermal-mesenchyme border in the fetus from second to third month. They did not stress the significance of periphery nerves in the determination of epidermal ridges, although they reported that the neurite bundles are generally accompanied by capillaries or located near them and that vessel-nerve pairs are observed when the glandular folds are forming. Blechschmidt(1963) postulated that the glandular folds follow the main directions of blood vessels from which nourishment is supplied. Thus, the capillary vessels seem to influence the induction of epidermal ridges, but the detailed mechanism of ridge differentiation is still unknown.

The interaction between the dermis and epidermis, which has been widely studied in the morphogenesis of the integmental appendages(Spearman,1977), seems to be playing a great role in the differentiation of epidermal ridges as well. However, this basic process in the integmental development seems to have not yet been studied from the standpoint of dermatoglyphics because of the methodological limitation that experimental materials are not available in dermatoglyphic investigations. Similarly, the mechanisms in successive morphogenesis, i.e., furrow fold formation and dermal papilla differentiation, are not clear.

For the pattern formation, the hypothesis that the nature of volar pads is largely related to the ridge arrangement is generally accepted. It is also probable that the mechanical stresses in the skin growth that are induced by the volar curvature are involved in the mechanism(Mulvihill and Smith,1969). However, we have not sufficient data at present on the pattern formation of epidermal ridges.

OBSERVATION OF FETAL DERMATOGLYPHICS

For the dermatoglyphic study, the entire volar surface has to be observed. Though the undulations at the dermo-epidermal junction are occasionally observable through the half-transparent epidermis by the reflex of light in the earlier gestational stages, this is not applicable as a routine method for the entire volar skin.

Hale(1949) presented a new method of inspecting the ridge arrangement in fetus specimens that had been preserved in formalin, but this method has not yet been applied by other workers. According to this method, the cornified epithelial cells were rubbed away with a gauze pad. After this, the specimen was stained with hematoxylin solution, dehydrated, cleared, stored in oil and then inspected. Using specimens of this kind, he measured the breadth of epidermal ridges and counted minutiae per standard area in the earlier gestational stages.

Another surface examination of epidermal ridges was undertaken by Fleischhauer and Horstmann(1951/52), inspecting the undersurface of dried epidermis that was chemically abraded from fresh skin materials. Some other workers reconstructed dermatoglyphic configurations from serial histological sections(Bonnevie,1927; Schaeuble,1933; Babler,1978).

The present author developed a method to inspect dermatoglyphics on the exposed dermis of the fetus(Okajima,1975) and the human adult(Okajima,1979). This technique was

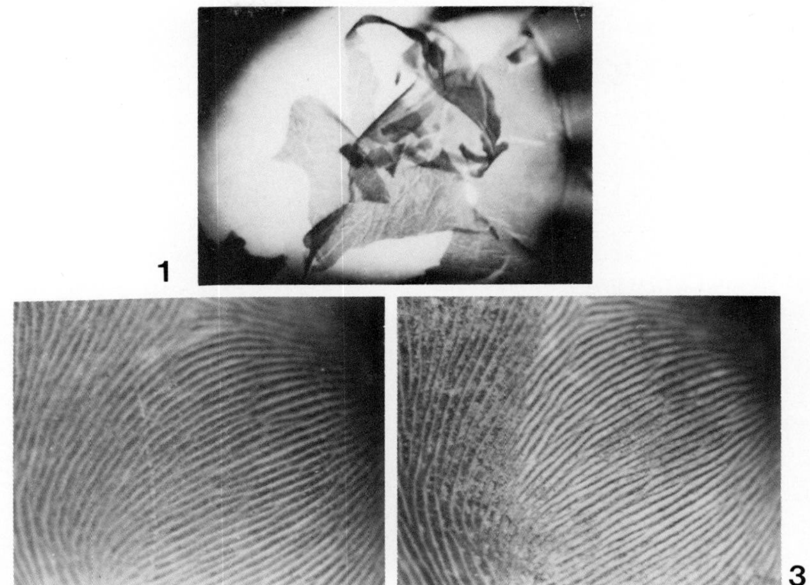

Fig.1 Peridermal layer, which is stained in a darker tone with toluidine blue(TB), is abrading from the subjacent intermediate layer.
Fig.2 Ridged structure displayed on the intermediate layer of the epidermis. (TB staining)
Fig.3 Ridged structure on the intermediate layer(left) and the mechanically abraded dermal surface. (TB staining)

recently applied to the dermatoglyphic examination of fetuses with chromosome anomalies(Suzumori,1980; Okajima et al.,1981) and technical revisions were made(Okajima et al.,1981). As the method is not yet widely used, details of the procedure and some findings accompanying the methodology are presented here.

METHODOLOGICAL PRESENTATION

The principle of our method is to remove all the epidermal layers and to observe undulations displayed on the dermal surface. For the examination, an entire hand or foot that was fixed in formalin prior to the preparation is used. For the convenience of subsequent chemical treatments and observations, it is first fixed on a rubber plate in an extended state with cotton thread.

The First Treatment with Alkaline Solution

As the first process, the specimen was incubated in 3% potassium hydroxide solution at 30°C for 15 to 20 hours. Then, it was washed in running water for several hours and left in 10% formalin for at least a few days. After this, the specimen was immersed in water and, under a stereomicroscope, the superficial layer of the epidermis was removed by brushing. The peridermal layer in younger fetuses(Fig.1) or the stratum corneum in older fetuses is easily separated, forming into large membranes, from the subjacent intermediate layer of the epidermis.

Ridged Structures on the Intermediate Layer

The exposed intermediate layer that is stained with toluidine blue represents a ridged structures whose arrangement is exactly consistent with that of the epidermal ridges (Fig.2).

If the intermediate layer is brushed vigorously, the dermal surface is exposed and the summit of the dermal projection is stained in a violet tone, while the groove where the sweat ducts are located remains unstained. Fig.3 demonstrates the anatomical relationship between the intermediate layer and the dermis. The intermediate layer is seen on the left side of the figure, while the dermal surface is shown in the central to right areas. The violet lines on the intermediate layer correspond anatomically to those on the dermal surface. The latter is represented more sharply. The pale ridges on the intermediate layer are located above the grooves of the dermis. Therefore, the arrangement of epidermal ridges can be examined and the ridge count performed on both surfaces. Thus, the intermediate layer provides dermatoglyphic information when the surface is intact.

Successive Treatments

Removing of the epidermal cells by vigorous brushing should be avoided, because intensive mechanical manipulation easily injures the dermal tissue, especially in younger fetuses. As the deeper layers of the epidermis remain firmly on the dermis after the first alkaline treatment, the second treatment, by which the specimen is incubated again in 3% potassium hydroxide solution at 30°C for 15 to 20 hours, is undertaken. Using the same procedure as described for the first treatment, the specimen is washed in running water and left in 10% formalin for more than a few days, preferably for a week or longer. The second treatment with the alkaline solution results in a lowering of the intercellular connections, and the epidermal cells are easily swept off by brushing.

When the effect of the treatment is sufficient, a gentle brushing is enough to remove the epidermal cells from the dermis. However, the cells of the basal layer tend to be attached more firmly to the dermis and they often remain even after the second treatment. In such cases, a third treatment with the alkaline solution is recommended. According to the author's experience, the epidermal cells separate more smoothly from the dermis when the specimen has been allowed to stand in formalin for a longer time after the treatment with alkaline solution. If the epidermal cells remain firmly attached, repeating the alkaline solution treatment for the same or a shorter time is more recommendable than intensifying the brushing. In general, repeated treatments as well as treatment for a longer time with alkaline solution do not give rise to unfavorable results.

The confirmation during the manipulation as to whether the epidermal cells still remain on the dermis can be made by staining the specimen with toluidine blue solution, since the epidermal cells and the dermis are stained differently.

Staining the Dermal Surface

The morphological features on the dermal surface are made visible by staining with toluidine blue. The specimen is immersed in 0.05% toluidine blue solution for about 30 seconds, with the length of immersion time varying depending upon the nature of the subject, and then rinsed in water. The inspection with a stereomicroscope is carried out with the specimen immersed in water.

Usually, the projected sites of the dermis, i.e., the terminal segments of the dermal papillae and the summit of the dermal ledges in younger fetuses, are stained in a violet tone by the reagent. On the contrary, the grooves and the basal segments of the dermal papillae remain unstained. The furrow presents a pale tone almost similar to the groove but, if inspected closely, it is slightly stained in a light blue tone.

When the examination is finished, the reagent on the dermis is removed by immersion in 70% alcohol. The specimen, thus decolorized, is preserved in 10% formalin and the examination can be repeated many times.

Comments on the Methodology

The revision of the preparation is the intensifying of the alkaline solution treatment. In our original report, alkaline solution was applied only once for 4 to 8 hours. However, in the revised one, the time of treatment is extended to 15 to 20 hours and the treatment is repeated at least twice.

What was the ridged structure that Hale(1949) viewed in his specimens, ridges on the dermal surface, on the intermediate layer, or both? I have not proved his original method. According to my experimental preparation, the epidermis could be removed by brushing with a cotton swab. In this procedure, the epidermis separates into two layers, the superficial layer and the deeper layer. By toluidine blue staining, the surface of the deeper layer usually did not display any clear ridged structure, contrary to the finding on the intermediate layer illustrated above. When the dermis was exposed, summits of the dermal projections were stained with toluidine blue. In this case, the dermis may be injured if the mechanical manipulation is not adequate. Therefore, I cannot answer the above question at present.

PRESENTATION OF SPECIMENS

In the present study, the growth of fetuses was indicated by the length of the foot for all the specimens. As is well known, the fetal age provided by obstetricians' records is occasionally not consistent with the fetal growth. This was also true in the present materials. Besides, the crown-rump

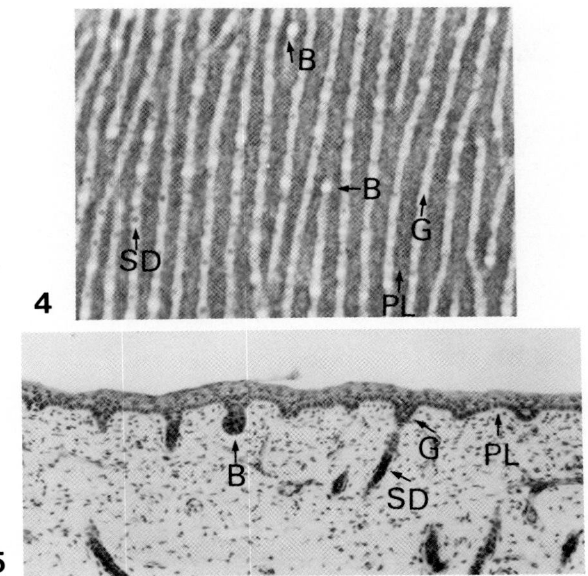

Fig.4 Dermal ridges of the foot from a fetus whose foot length(FL) was 31mm. The estimated fertilization age is about 17 weeks. The summit of the dermal projection(primary ledge, PL, primary dermal ridge) is stained in a violet tone. The groove(G) remains unstained. Sweat ducts(SD) are represented as dark spots in the groove. White holes in the groove are dermal depressions caused by the bud(B) formation, the initial form of sweat duct differentiation. (TB staining)
Fig.5 Histological section from the opposite foot of the same fetus as in Fig.4. Undulations at the dermo-epidermal junction are arranged at regular intervals. (HE staining)

length(CRL), which is widely used for estimating the fetal age, was not available in some of our samples. It has been revealed by previous studies that the foot length is very consistent with the CRL. Therefore, I used the foot length (FL) as the main indicator of the fetal growth(Moore,1973).

Fig.4 shows the hypothenar area of a foot from a fetus whose FL was 31mm. The CRL was not available, but it was estimated from the foot length to be about 150mm. Similarly, the

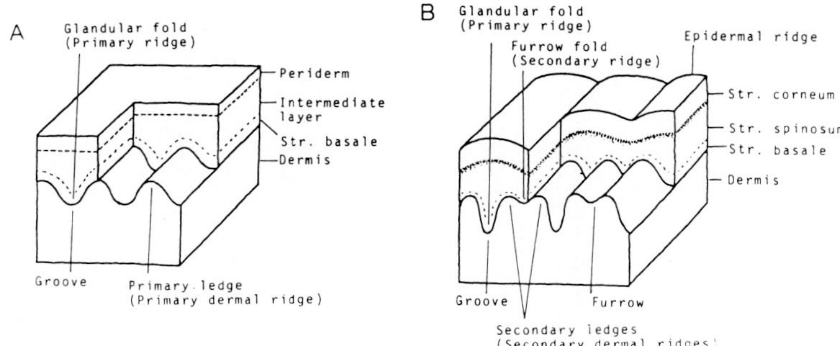

Fig.6 Diagrams of ridge differentiation.

fertilization age was estimated to be about 17 weeks. The dermal surface displays a ridged structure where the summit of the lineal dermal projection is stained in a violet tone but the grooves are not stained. Sweat ducts in the dermis are represented as blue spots in the grooves, since the cells of the ducts are stained intensively with the reagent. Besides these blue spots, round white impressions are observable scattered in the grooves. These are dermal depressions caused by the bud formation that is the initial developmental form of the sweat duct.

A histological section(Fig.5) from the foot of the opposite side of the same fetus shows that the surface is covered with flat periderm. The undulations at the dermo-epidermal junction are arranged at regular intervals. Sweat ducts are developing from the basis of the groove. The bud formation is recognized as a condensation of proliferated epidermal cells projecting into the dermis. Thus, new sweat ducts differentiate between the existing ones for a fairly long fetal period.

The dermal projection that is represented as a violet line in the surface view is morphologically a temporal structure observed only in an earlier fetal period. In successive stages, it is transformed into different appearances by the formation of furrows and dermal papillae(Penrose,1968). This dermal projection was termed the "primary dermal ridge" in the previous paper(Okajima,1975). However, the author

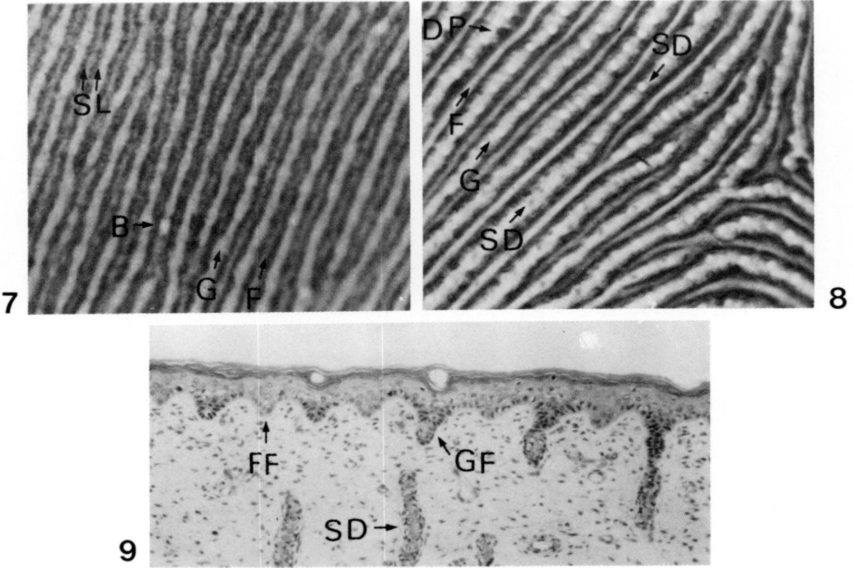

Fig.7 Dermal ridges of the foot from a fetus whose FL was 44mm and CRL 190mm. Estimated fertilization age is about 21 weeks. Dermal furrow(F) and secondary ledges(SL, secondary dermal ridges) are formed. Sweat ducts and formation of a few buds are observed. (TB staining)

Fig.8 Histological section from the opposite foot of the same fetus as in Fig.7. The dermo-epidermal junction presents contours of the groove, furrow and secondary ledges. Glandular fold(GF). Furrow fold(FF). (HE staining)

Fig.9 Dermal ridges of the foot from a fetus whose FL was 56mm. Estimated fertilization age is about 26 weeks. Dermal papillae(DP) are developing on the secondary ledges. (TB staining)

proposes here that this characteristic be named the "primary ledge" of the dermis for the convenience of embryological description and to avoid terminological confusion(Fig.6).

Fig.7 shows the hypothenar area of a foot from a fetus whose FL was 44mm and CRL 190mm. The fertilization age was estimated to be about 21 weeks. In the surface view, the summit of the primary ledge is subdivided on the midline into two lineal daughter projections by the formation of a furrow. The summits of the daughter projections are stained in a violet tone, while the furrow remains in a light tone.

The differentiation of the furrow occurs chronologically differently between the hands and feet of the same fetus and between varying sites in the same hand or foot. The hand antedates the foot in the differentiation. In the core area of the dermatoglyphic patterns, where the ridges are densely arranged, the furrow formation tends to be delayed or the width remains narrower. Orifices of the sweat ducts are viewed as blue spots. Formation of new buds still continues in this stage, though the number is extremely reduced.

The author again proposes terming the daughter projections "secondary ledges" of the dermis, as illustrated in Fig.6. These were called the "secondary dermal ridges" in the last paper.

Fig.8 shows a histological section of the opposite foot of the same fetus. The dermo-epidermal junction illustrates the contour of the furrow and the secondary ledges. The glandular and furrow folds of the epidermis are arranged alternately and can be distinguished by the contours as well as by the different reactions to the staining. The epidermal cells in the basal layer are stained less intensively by basic dyes in the furrow fold than in the glandular fold.

Fig.9 shows the palmar interdigital area of a fetus whose FL was 56mm. The fertilization age was estimated to be about 26 weeks. Bulge-like projections on the secondary ledges are dermal papillae that are now developing. In this specimen, formation of the bud is not recognized. Differentiation of the sweat ducts usually ends before the differentiation of dermal papillae begins. In this figure, some of the orifices of the sweat ducts are recognized as blue spots, while others are represented as small white holes in the groove. This difference in the reaction of the sweat ducts depends where the cells remain in the ducts. If the cells remain in the upper part of the ducts, orifices of the sweat ducts are marked as blue spots. On the contrary, if the cells are discharged by the treatment from the upper part of the ducts, they appear as empty white holes.

However, blue spots do not appear promptly after the

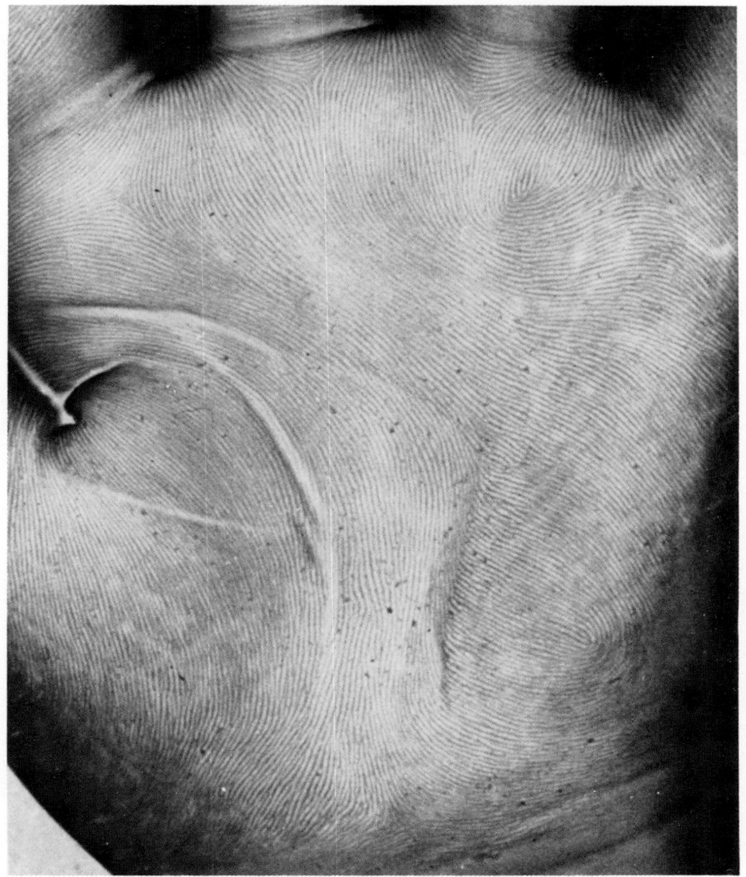

Fig.10 Palm of a fetus whose FL was 20mm. Differentiation of dermal ridges has just extended over the whole palm. (TB staining)

toluidine blue staining, but a few minutes later at least. The reagent infiltrates slowly through the cells of the sweat duct. Therefore, if a specimen is observed immediately after the staining, blue spots cannot be detected. A few minutes later, blue spots become gradually visible under the microscope.

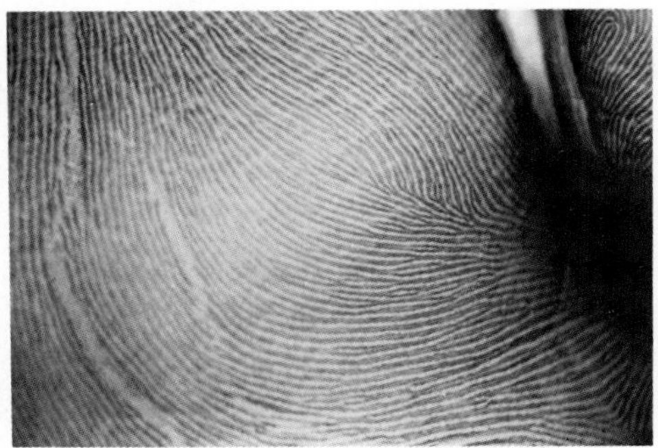

Fig.11 Hallucal pattern (arch tibial) of a fetus diagnosed as trisomy 21. (TB staining)

On the other hand, if the epidermal cells remain on the groove, the sweat ducts are not stained. Therefore, care must be taken in the examination of the sweat ducts, as their reaction varies according to the conditions of the sweat ducts themselves and to the time after the staining.

An entire palm surface of a fetus is presented in Fig.10. The FL was 20mm. The fertilization age was estimated to be about 14 weeks. The differentiation of the grooves extended over the entire palm surface just before this fetal stage. The ridges are sharp enough to be classified and counted.

CHROMOSOME ANOMALIES

Recently, the author published dermatoglyphic data of two fetuses with trisomy 21. These fetuses were diagnosed by amniocentesis, and abortion was induced in the 20th and 22nd week, respectively, from the last menstrual period. Dermatoglyphic diagrams and ridge counts were presented (Okajima et al., 1981). Fig.11 shows the hallucal area of the first fetus and the arch tibial pattern was observed. Suzumori (1980) described unusual dermatoglyphic features in hands of five fetuses--three with Down syndrome, one with 5p- and one with 18 trisomy--using this technique. I have not heard of further studies in which this methodology was applied.

CONCLUSION

The main points presented above and the advantages of the author's technique are as follows.

1. The original method presented by the author in 1975 was recently revised by the introduction of repeated alkaline solution treatments and extending the treatment time. The technique is not difficult.
2. Specimens fixed in formalin can be used.
3. The examination can be repeated many times.
4. The ridged structure can be observed on the dermal surface as well as on the intermediate layer of the epidermis.
5. The author proposed the terms "primary and secondary ledges" for the convenience of embryological description.
6. Orifices of the sweat ducts may appear differently according to the conditions of the specimen and staining.
7. Dermatoglyphic classification as well as ridge counts can be made in normal and chromosomally abnormal fetuses.

The new methodology presented here has just started to be used. If many specimens of good quality are prepared from various fetuses, normal and abnormal, it is expected that new findings will be obtained and contribute to better understanding of the embryogenesis of dermal ridges and pattern formation.

ACKNOWLEDGMENTS

This research was supported by grant No.357194 of the Japan Ministry of Education.

REFERENCES

Babler WJ (1978). Prenatal selection and dermatoglyphic patterns. Am J Phys Anthrop 48:21.

Blechschmidt E (1963). Die embryonalen Gestaltungsfunktionen der menschlichen Oberhaut. II. Mitteilung: Die Entstehung des Papillarkörpers in den proximalen und distalen Abschnitten der Fingerbeere. Z Morph Anthrop 54:163.

Bonnevie K (1927). Die ersten Entwicklungsstadien der Papillarmuster der menschlichen Fingerballen. NYT Magazin for Naturvidenskaberne B. 65:19.

Bonnevie K (1929). Was lehrt die Embryologie der Papillarmuster über ihre Bedeutung als Rassen- und Familien-charakter? Z indukt Abstam Vererb L 50:219.

Fleischhauer K, Horstmann E (1951). Untersuchungen über die Entwicklung des Papillarkörpers der menschlichen Palma und Planta. Z Zellforsch 36:298.

Hale AR (1949). Breadth of epidermal ridges in the human fetus and its relation to the growth of the hand and foot. Anat Rec 105:763.

Hale AR (1952). Morphogenesis of volar skin in the human fetus. Am J Anat 91:147.

Hirsch W, Schweichel JU (1973). Morphological evidence concerning the problem of skin ridge formation J ment Defic Res 17:58.

Moore KL (1973). "The Developing Human. Clinically Oriented Embryology." Philadelphia: Saunders, p78.

Mulvihill JJ, Smith DW (1969). The genesis of dermatoglyphics. J Pediat 75:579.

Okajima M (1975). Development of dermal ridges in the fetus. J Med Genet 12:243.

Okajima M (1979). Dermal and epidermal structures of the volar skin. In Wertelecki W, Plato CC (eds): "Dermatoglyphics--Fifty Years Later," Birth Defects: Orig Art Ser 15(6), New York: Alan R Liss, p 179.

Okajima M, Ikeuchi H, Tonomura A (1981). Dermatoglyphics of two fetuses with trisomy 21 diagnosed by amniocentesis. Jpn J Hum Genet 26:61.

Penrose LS (1968). Memorandum on dermatoglyphic nomenclature. Birth Defects: Orig Art Ser 4(3):1.

Schaeuble J (1933). Die Entstehung der palmaren digitalen Triradien. Z Morph Anthrop 31:403.

Schaumann B, Alter M (1976). "Dermatoglyphics in Medical Disorders." New York: Springer-Verlag, p 1.

Spearman RIC (1977). Hair follicle development, cyclical changes and hair form. In Jarrett (ed): "The Physiology and Pathophysiology of the Skin," Vol 4, London: Academic Press, p 1255.

Suzumori K (1980). Dermatoglyphic analysis of fetuses with chromosomal abnormalities. Am J Hum Genet 32:859.

Progress in Dermatoglyphic Research, pages 189–202

NONHUMAN PRIMATE DERMATOGLYPHICS: IMPLICATIONS FOR HUMAN BIOMEDICAL RESEARCH

Laura Newell-Morris, Carol E. Fahrenbruch
and Cynthia Yost
Depts. Anthropology and Orthodontics and Regional
Primate Research Center, University of Washington
Seattle, Washington 98195

The title of this paper is in actuality far too general for the topics I shall be discussing here, for two reasons. First, for the term "primates," substitute macaque monkey. This substitution is not meant to imply that macaque monkeys necessarily present us with the best models for research relevant to human dermatoglyphics. Rather, the choice is dictated by the traditional use of the macaque in biomedical research, the vast amount of data already available for the genus and the relatively greater availability of these primates compared to that of other species. Finally, my own research has focused on one species of the genus, viz., the pigtail macaque (*Macaca nemestrina*).

The second part of the title "Implications for Human Biomedical Research" could refer to almost anything, although in this case, almost nothing might be more descriptive. Research that addresses the relevance of nonhuman primate dermatoglyphics to problems of human development is almost totally lacking, especially as to the manifestation of these problems in the clinical setting. Thus, an almost infinite number of topics could be discussed with relative impunity, given the absence of results to counter even the wildest speculation. Yet fascinating as speculation may be, I shall confine myself here to two areas of research that I view as eminently feasible, given the data presently available on macaque monkeys in breeding colonies or research laboratories. The areas which will be considered are:

1. The genetics of dermatoglyphics
2. Fluctuating dermatoglyphic asymmetry

NONHUMAN PRIMATE DERMATOGLYPHICS - INTRODUCTION

Before I address these topics, however, a few general remarks about the dermatoglyphics of the nonhuman primates might be helpful in providing some background information. (For more detail the reader is referred to Midlo and Cummins, 1942; Biegert, 1961; Newell-Morris, 1979.) The human species, together with monkeys, apes and the less familiar prosimiians, comprise the taxonomic order Primates. Some years ago a prominent physical anthropologist commented on how fortunate we are in being the only species capable of studying its own evolutionary history, and at the same time to be surrounded by about 200 nonhuman primate species that very generally represent the evolutionary steps we have taken on our way to becoming the genus Homo. More importantly, from the perspective of this symposium we are fortunate in yet one more respect, viz., that all of our nonhuman relatives possess a system of dermal ridges covering to a greater or lesser extent the volar surfaces of their hands and feet. The dermal ridge system is ancient to the order, and its appearance undoubtedly is related to the arboreal mode of life which was the successful evolutionary strategy "seized upon" by the earliest ancestors of the primate lineage (Cartmill, 1974). A greatly elaborated tactile sense in combination with a non-slip surface, both provided by the dermal ridges and grooves, laid the groundwork for a myriad of primate life styles. Various selective forces related to life style have operated on the basic pentadactyl limb and its system of dermal ridges to produce a marvelous array of hands and feet within the primate order. For example, Figure 1 shows the hands of two prosimiians (representative of a very early stage of primate evolution), a galago from Africa and a lemur from Madagascar. Yet, as aberrant as the gross morphology of these species may appear, they show the same type of dermal ridge patterning that characterizes our own species.

Here, let me set forth one basic assumption that at least to date seems to be a sound one. Although the hands and feet of the various primate species may differ widely in their gross morphology, the dermal ridges are arranged in the basic pattern types familiar to anyone who works with human dermatoglyphics, i.e., open fields, arches, loops and whorls. This universality of pattern supports the idea set forth by Mulvihill and Smith (1969) that the developmental problem posed by an elevated surface to be covered with a system of parallel ridges is basically a mechanical one with limited solutions. Thus it is, that nonhuman primate species differ for the most part, as do human populations, quantitatively, rather than qualitatively in their dermatoglyphic patterns.

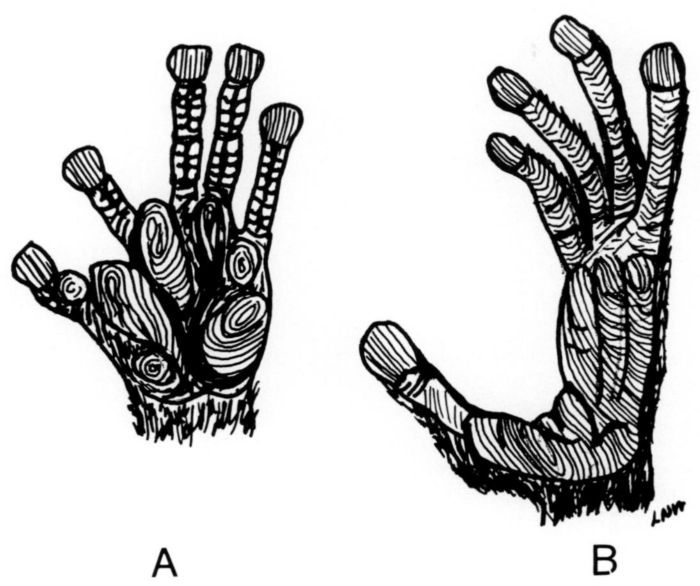

Fig. 1. Hands of a galago (A) and a lemur (B). Modified from Biegert (1961).

Perhaps more interesting from the point of view of this symposium is the finding that certain pattern types cluster normally in particular nonhuman primate species, yet in humans these same pattern clusterings are associated with specific chromosomal diseases and serve to separate an abnormal sample from a normal one. I have referred to this phenomenon elsewhere as the primate normal-abnormal continuum (Newell-Morris, 1979). A case in point is the occurrence in chimpanzee samples of a high frequency (47%) of the ulnar loop pattern on the second digit, a tibial arch in the hallucal area, and of course the aptly named "simian" crease - all of which are viewed as diagnostic features of trisomy 21 in human patients. Certainly it would seem worthwhile to begin looking for dermatoglyphic features that may normally cluster within particular nonhuman primate species to better understand their clustering in human disease states.

THE GENETICS OF DERMATOGLYPHICS

Pedigree Analysis

Just as the dermal ridges of all primate species share in a universality of pattern types, the genetic mechanisms controlling the conformation of the patterns are probably also universal. In other words, there are presently no data indicating that the genetic mechanisms differ interspecifically. In fact, to the contrary, the little genetic analysis that has been done (at least among macaques) yields heritability estimates for ridge counts equivalent to those obtained in human familial studies (Kerr, 1969). However, as several investigators have pointed out, the genetic study of polygenic characters such as dermatoglyphics is fraught with difficulties (Froehlich, 1976). Yet possibly some of the difficulties encountered by human studies, confined as they are to small pedigrees and very limited generational depth, might be overcome with nonhuman primate pedigree data.

Nonhuman primates raised in breeding colonies such as the one maintained by the Regional Primate Research Center of the University of Washington are bred in harem groups of one male and 6-12 females. At the present there are approximately 600 female and 70 male *M. nemestrina* adult breeders and four generations represented in our colony. The results of this type of breeding system are obvious, viz., the production of large numbers of offspring related through the father, i.e., paternal half-sibs; maternal half-sibs and full sibs are also available, but in fewer numbers. In any event, after three generations several of our best male breeders have transmitted their genes either directly or indirectly to large numbers of colony members. As shown in Table 1 breeding male No. 57199 is related to 312 individuals in the colony.

Degree of relatedness refers to the percent of genes the male and the individual in question share in common, for example, the degree of relatedness of the male's offspring is 0.50. There are 70 of these, and some will be full sibs, but the vast majority will be paternal half-sibs, produced by different mothers. Reported studies on human half-sibs are few, yet they offer interesting possibilities for genetic research. The genetic relationship between half-sibs is as close as that between grandparents and grandchildren and between uncles and nephews, but the former have the distinct advantage of belonging to the same generation. In addition, investigation of the various types of half-sibs enables us to partition out the father's and mother's effects on offspring more easily than the study of full sibs.

TABLE 1. Degree of Relatedness of Male No. 57199 to Colony Members

Relatedness	No.	Percent
0.75	9	0.03
0.62	1	0.00
0.50	70	0.22
0.38	9	0.03
0.25	205	0.66
0.12	18	0.06
Total	312	

It is obvious from this one example, and No. 57199 is no exception in our colony, that the potentiality for genetic analysis is rich. The sheer amount of available data subjected to new statistical techniques such as factor analysis may quickly yield the type of information that Holt (1968) calls for in more and larger human pedigree studies.

Genetic Marker Studies

One of the more exciting possibilities offered by the pedigrees available in breeding colonies is that of linkage studies. In defining the direction that human genetic research should take Thoday (1967) has urged the search for major genes with large effects on continuous variables. To accomplish this goal, the analysis must maximize effective heritability and limit the number of genes studied. Dermal ridge counts show high heritability, and therefore satisfy the first criterion. For the isolation of a limited number of genes Thoday recommends the identification of suitable single locus markers through studies of genetic association. Some human studies have already yielded the promising possibility of association between digital patterns and the Lewis blood group and the haptoglobin loci (Froehlich, 1976). Given the identity of large numbers of structural proteins and serological components already described in the human and macaque the search for marker loci for dermatoglyphic variation might be a profitable one, especially as the identification is best accomplished in segregating sib pairs. The identification of pleiotropic markers would be a major step forward in the delineation of the genetic controls over dermatoglyphics. In fact, it has been suggested (Froehlich, 1976) that with the delineation of only two pleiotropic markers, it should be possible to demonstrate the additive inheritance of fingerprints in man. Perhaps these markers will be provided by macaques.

FLUCTUATING ASYMMETRY

Bilateral structures rarely exhibit the developmental ideal of perfect symmetry. It has been suggested that fluctuating asymmetry, i.e., the random non-directional differences between sides, may be an indication of the developing organism's inability to buffer environmental disturbances (Van Valen, 1962). In fact, some investigators have proposed that the degree of fluctuating asymmetry may be positively correlated to the magnitude of local developmental disturbances (Townsend and Brown, 1980). The interpretation of asymmetry as related to differential developmental homeostasis, or in Waddington's term "canalization" (Waddington, 1957), is supported by three lines of evidence based primarily on dental asymmetry, i.e., i) the greater asymmetry in males as opposed to females (Tanner, 1978), ii) the increase of asymmetry associated with inbreeding (Bader, 1965; Doyle and Johnston, 1977), and iii) the increase of asymmetry in individuals with genetic disorders such as cleft lip (Woolf and Gianis, 1976; Morton and Niswander, 1967; and Sofaer, 1979) and Down's Syndrome (Garn et al., 1970).

To date, the majority of studies dealing with asymmetry have been carried out on human populations where the exact relationships between asymmetry, genotype and environmental stress are unclear (c.f., Bailit et al., 1970). However, a number of results confirming the conclusions drawn from human data have been obtained from experimental studies on mice and rats (e.g., Sciulli et al., 1979). All these results suggest that fluctuating asymmetry may provide an important measure of developmental decanalization in response to environmental stress. But experimental studies are needed to identify the nature and interaction of specific environmental stresses and the implications of observed asymmetry for the total organism.

Experimental Asymmetry in Macaques

Two studies are presently being conducted at the Regional Primate Research Center at the University of Washington that provide the ideal opportunity to examine the relationship between experimental environmental insult to the pregnant female during the first trimester and dermatoglyphic asymmetry in her offspring. The first experimental protocol involves the application of psychological stress (Sackett et al., in prep.) and the second, administration of a teratogenic agent in the form of ethanol (Bowden et al., 1981).

Casts were made of the right and left hand on each animal with Dow Corning Silastic. Intercore ridge counts were done in three areas, A, B and C, of the palm (Figure 2). A thread was extended between pins inserted in the pattern cores of adjacent areas and all ridges (excluding the core itself) intersecting the lines were counted. Counting was done under a dissecting microscope by one person (C.Y.). The mean error was one ridge which is well below the mean normal asymmetry figure.

The number of ridges were recorded for each intercore area, right and left hands; the count of the right hand was then subtracted from the count of the left hand for each animal to yield a residual asymmetry value for each intercore area. The three areal residuals were then added (sign ignored) to yield a total asymmetry value. Statistical testing showed that there were no significant differences by side, and that we were in fact dealing with a case of fluctuating asymmetry.

Prenatal Psychological Stress Protocol. Dermatoglyphics were available on eight stressed animals (four females, four males) and ten controls (six females, four males) bred under the same conditions within a five year-period. The stress condition involved catching the pregnant female, holding her in gloved hands, and then returning her to the cage. Capture occurred once a day, five days per week between 30 - 130 days of gestation. (Mean length of gestation in this species is 173 days.) In contrast, the individually caged unstressed females were handled as little as possible throughout their pregnancies. All pregnancies were monitored and found to be normal, and the fetuses were delivered vaginally between 164 to 187 days of gestation at normal birth weights.

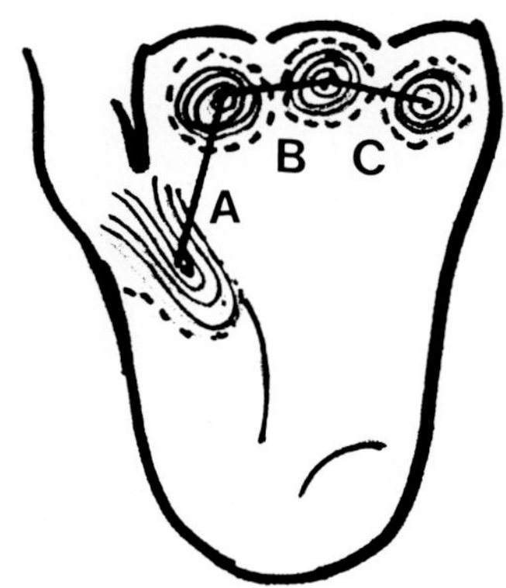

Fig. 2. Location of intercore areas A, B and C. All ridges intersecting the intercore connection lines between adjacent core areas are counted.

Ethanol Protocol. Three animals identified as fetal alcohol syndrome (FAS) were the offspring of females who had received ethanol nasogastrically, weekly from 40 days gestation. Two females received moderate doses of 2.5 g/kg (offspring MDA), one received high doses of 4.1 g/kg (offspring HDA). Peak blood ethanol levels were 200 - 300 mg % 2h for the moderate dose females, whereas those for the high dose female were 300 - 450 mg %. Pregnancies were normal and the infants delivered at term with normal APGAR scores. However, subsequent growth and developmental assessment revealed that the MDA male infant was hyperkinetic and retarded in facial expression and cognitive performance. The female MDA had retarded reflex development for ten days, but was normal thereafter. The HDA infant showed craniofacial abnormalities and severely retarded behavioral development. For example, walking, normally present at seven days did not occur until 80 days, cognitive performance appropriate for 22 days did not appear until 116 days (Bowden et al., 1981).

Results. Although the samples are too small to permit meaningful statistical testing, the results shown in Table 2 indicate that stress both of a psychological nature and through the administration of a known teratogenic agent has increased dermatoglyphic asymmetry in the developing embryo when compared to non-stressed controls.

TABLE 2. Total Asymmetry of Stressed and Fetal Alcohol Syndrome (FAS) Infants Compared to Unstressed Controls

Females	Mean	S.D.	N	Range
Control	6.83	3.55	6	3 - 13
Stressed	9.50	2.65	4	7 - 13
FAS (MDA)*	6.00	-	1	-
FAS (HDA)*	10.00	-	1	-
Males				
Control	5.00	2.00	7	2 - 7
Stressed	8.00	3.56	4	3 - 11
FAS (MDA)*	8.00	-	1	-

* see text for explanation.

In fact, only two animals, stressed male 2800 (Table 3) and female FAS (MDA) (Table 2) have asymmetry counts less than the control sample's mean.

Table 3. Areal Intercore Ridge Count Residuals, Stressed Group

Animal	Sex	A	B	C	Total
276	F	3	4	3	10
280	F	3	0	4	7
380	F	7	2	4	13
177	F	4	1	3	8
277	M	5	1	5	11
280	M	4	1	5	10
2800	M	2	0	1	3
279	M	4	2	2	8

Two of the FAS animals fall in the high asymmetry range, whereas one is well within the normal range. Again, although the sample numbers are too small to allow for any definitive conclusions, the results are in the direction expected for the environmental insult administered to the embryo via a known teratogenic agent. Interestingly, the degree of asymmetry seems to correlate with the severity of the other phenotypic defects, with the HDA infant showing the highest asymmetry. The response of the developing dermal ridge system to ethanol has also been noted in human clinical studies showing that FAS patients differed in pattern frequencies from a matched control sample (Qazi et al., 1980). However, the latter study did not look at asymmetry, and our sample is too small to allow for pattern comparisons. On the basis of our results we conclude that ethanol administered to the pregnant macaque during the first trimester of pregnancy can disrupt normal fetal pad development, and leave a lasting imprint in the form of increased ridge count asymmetry.

The areal intercore residuals show that the greatest contribution to the total asymmetry is made by areas A and C.

Table 4. Total Areal Intercore Ridge Counts, Stressed

Female	No.	A	B	C
Left	4	45.5	29.5	32.0
Right	4	44.8	28.3	28.5
Male				
Left	4	47.5	33.3	35.8
Right	4	44.8	34.3	32.5

Although the argument might be made that the higher contribution by area A is expected, given its higher total ridge count (Table 4), the argument does not hold for area C. Areas B and C show approximately the same ridge count, whereas the mean residual for area B is 1.4 and that of area C is more than two times greater, 3.4. Both areas B and C include one-half the total ridge count of interdigital pad III which tends to have a whorl pattern. Although the ridges were not analyzed with a developmental field concept in mind, it is interesting to note that the significantly lesser asymmetry noted for area B (between Interdigital pad cores II and III) when compared to area C (between Interdigital pad cores III and IV) is consistent with the data on human fingerprint patterns and ridge counts. It has been shown that digits II and III of the radial side are developmentally grouped, as are digits IV and V of the ulnar side. Furthermore, digit II on the radial side of the hand shows the least bilateral asymmetry of all the digits (Siervogel et al., 1979). Area B of our study falls within the radial compartment of the hand and seems to exhibit the most canalized development least easily deflected by environmental insult, as adjudged by degree of asymmetry.

If our results are biologically meaningful, albeit the small sample sizes dictate caution in interpretation, then several interesting questions can be raised. First, we have in the macaque (or perhaps in any other primate) a model in which the questions of why? how? and what does it mean? as they relate to asymmetry in general, and dermatoglyphic asymmetry, in particular, can be subjected to experimental testing. The facts that asymmetry exists and that frequently increased asymmetry is associated with environmental or genetic insult to the embryo do not in themselves resolve the paramount question of what asymmetry means in terms of total developmental outcome. Is there for example, correlation between increased asymmetry and lowered individual fitness? Is there a threshold effect, i.e., a level of asymmetry that cannot be violated without significantly increasing the chance of *in utero* or neonatal death? Do aborted and stillbirth populations show greater asymmetry than normal samples, and do they differ between themselves? To what extent is asymmetry a component of the human syndromes? These and many other questions remain, and we hope that our continued studies on the breeding colony of macaques at the University of Washington will contribute to their answers.

ACKNOWLEDGEMENTS

This work was supported by NIH grants HD08633 and HD02774 from NICHHD Mental Retardation Branch; RR 00166 from Animal Resources Branch; USPH grants NS10804 and NS15017; and RSA grant 16P56818.

REFERENCES

Bader RS (1965). Fluctuating asymmetry in the dentition of the house mouse. Growth 29:291.

Bailit HL, Workman PL, Niswander JD, MacLean CJ. Dental asymmetry as an indicator of genetic and environmental conditions in human populations. Hum Biol 42:626.

Biegert J (1961). Volarhaut der Hände und Füsse. Primatologia, Handbuch der Primatenkunde," Vol. 2. Basel: Karger.

Bowden DM, Weathersbee PS, Clarren S, Fahrenbruch CE, Goodlin B, Caffery S (1981). A binge model of fetal alcohol syndrome in the pig-tailed macaque. Am J Primatol 1:341.

Cartmill M (1974). Pads and claws in arboreal locomotion. In Jenkins FA (ed): "Primate Locomotion," New York Academic Press, p. 45.

Doyle WJ, Johnston O (1977). On the meaning of increased fluctuating dental asymmetry: A cross-population study. Am J Phys Anthrop 46:127.

Froehlich JW (1976). The quantitative genetics of fingerprints. In Giles E, Friedlaender JS (eds): "The Measures of Man," Boston: Peabody Museum Press, p. 260.

Garn SM, Cohen MM and Gecianskas MA (1970). Increased crown-size asymmetry in trisomy G. J Dent Res 49:465.

Holt SB (1968). "The Genetics of Dermal Ridges." Springfield: Charles C. Thomas.

Kerr BA (1969). "Digital and Palmar Dermatoglyphics in Macaca nemestrina." Unpublished MA thesis, University of Washington, Seattle.

Midlo C, Cummins H (1942). "Palmar and Plantar Dermatoglyphics in Primates." American Anatomical Memoirs No. 20, Philadelphia: Wistar Institute of Anatomy and Biology.

Morton SA, Niswander JD (1967). Developmental "noise" and a congenital malformation. Gen Res 10:313.

Mulvihill JJ, Smith DW (1969). The genesis of dermatoglyphics. J Pediatr 75:579.

Newell-Morris L (1979). Midlo and Cummins updated: Primate dermatoglyphics today and tomorrow. In Wertelecki W, Plato C (eds): "Dermatoglyphics - Fifty Years Later," New York: Alan R. Liss, p. 135.

Qazi QH, Masakawa A, McGann B, Woods J (1980). Dermatoglyphic abnormalities in the fetal alcohol syndrome. Teratology 21:157.

Sackett GP, Frederickson WT, Erwin J (n.d.). Sires and stress affect pregnancy outcomes of pigtail macaques. In preparation.

Sciulli PW, Doyle K, Siegel P, Siegel M (1979). The interaction of stressors in the induction of increased levels of fluctuating asymmetry in the laboratory rat. Am J Phys Anthrop 50:274.

Siervogel RM, Roche AF, Roche EM (1979). The identification of developmental fields using digital distributions of fingerprint patterns and ridge counts. In Wertelecki W, Plato C (eds): "Dermatoglyphics-Fifty Years Later," New York: Alan R. Liss, p. 135.

Sofaer JA (1979). Human tooth-size asymmetry in cleft lip with or without cleft palate. Arch Oral Biol 24:141.

Tanner JM (1978). "Foetus into Man: Physical Growth from Conception to Maturity." London: Open Books.

Thoday JM (1967). New insights into continuous variation. In Crow JF, Neel JV (eds): "Proceedings Third International Congress of Human Genetics," Baltimore: Johns Hopkins University Press.

Townsend GC, Brown T (1980). Dental asymmetry in Australian aboriginals. Hum Biol 52:661.

Van Valen L (1962). A study of fluctuating asymmetry. Evolution 16:125.

Waddington CH (1957). "The Strategy of the Genes." London: George Allen.

Woolf CM, Gianis HD (1976). Congenital cleft lip and fluctuating dermatoglyphic asymmetry. Am J Hum Gen 26:400.

Progress in Dermatoglyphic Research, pages 203-246

PALMAR HYPOTHENAR TRIRADII IN PRIMATES: SOME METHODOLOGICAL AND EVOLUTIONARY CONSIDERATIONS

K.C. MALHOTRA

Anthropometry and Human Genetics Unit, Indian Statistical Institute,
203, B.T. Road, Calcutta-700035, INDIA

INTRODUCTION

The palmar hypothenar area in primates, in general, and in Man in particular, is characterized by several distinguishing features not met with in other palmar configurational areas. Some of the features, among several others, are: (a) presence of a variety of both true and vestigial patterns, (b) occurence of highest frequency of duplex, triplex patterns and whorls, (c) hypothenar loops open towards all the four borders of the palm-radial, ulnar, proximal and distal, (d) hypothenar patterns unlike in other areas, are formed by three palmar elements - proximal radiant of digital triradius a, hypothenar triradius h (notation after Malhotra et al 1980a) and axial triradii t (Malhotra et al 1980b), and (e) the topography of ridge alignment (transverse/oblique), and the size of the patterns in this area occasionally force the hypothenar triradii to be situated out side the area of the ridged skin. Cummins and Midlo (1943) termed these triradii as <u>extralimital</u>(p.59).

It is thus obvious that the hypothenar area morphologically is very complex (Mavalwala 1978), and of special interest. It is, therefore, not surprising that considerable attention in the past has been paid to this area.

The frequency distribution of hypothenar patterns among several population groups has been documented (see Mavalwala 1977). The genetics of hypothenar patterns have been investigated by several workers (among others see, Weninger 1947; Vrydagh-Laoureux 1971; Holt 1975; Sognier et al 1979; Pons 1979). Loesch (1971) using the topological classification of Penrose and Loesch (1970) investigated the inheritance of hypothenar loops - peripheral (H), central ($\hat{H}$) and radial (H^r) - as well as hypothenar triradii t^b (border triradius including extralimital triradii). Loesch concluded that loops H and $\hat{H}$ and triradius t^b are strongly influenced by heredity and are 'mainly determined by single loci'(p. 289).

It is, however, quite surprising that till recently not much work has been done on hypothenar triradii themselves, and, despite a few methodological attempts, considerable confusion persists in terms of nomenclature and types of hypothenar triradii. Recently Malhotra et al (1980a, 1981) and Karmakar and Malhotra (1981) investigated a number of aspects of hypothenar triradii in man.

Among the non-human primates although a great deal of data on the frequency of hypothenar patterns and pattern intensities are now available (among others see, Midlo and Cummins 1942; Biegert 1961; Iwamoto 1964, 1967; Brehme

1967, 1975; Newell-Morris 1979a, 1979b), data on type of hypothenar triradii are conspicous by their absence.

The purpose of this paper, therefore, is fourfold: (i) to synthesize and further analyse results of previous studies on hypothenar triradii in humans, (ii) to examine the extent and nature of variation of hypothenar triradii in 14 non-human primates, hetherto unknown (iii) to compare the incidence of hypothenar triradii among human and non-human primates, and (iv) to discuss probable evolutionary implications of hypothenar triradii, in general, and extra-limital in particular.

The materials, for the sake of convenience, are presented under the following five heads:

(i) Methodological issues.
(ii) Hypothenar triradii in humans.
(iii) Hypothenar triradii in non-human primates.
(iv) Comparative analysis.
(v) Evolutionary implications.

METHODOLOGICAL ISSUES

Four studies (Cummins and Midlo 1943; Penrose and Loesch 1970; Schauman and Alter 1976; Malhotra et al 1980a) have so far considered the methodological issues involved in respect of the hypothenar triradii.

Cummins and Midlo (1943) devised a very powerful method of encapsuling most of the information conveyed by various palmar elements into a formula designated as 'palmar formula'. Unfortunately no provision was made to record types of hypothenar triradii, through information about the hypothenar patterns was documented. These authors, however, must be credited for noting the existance of hypothenar triradii including the extralimital ones. In the elaborate topographic scheme they designated separately all the palmar triradii (digital, accessory, axial) except for the hypothenar triradii, and surprisingly no reason was given for this glaring omission. However, label H was used to designate the hypothenar area.

Penrose and Loesch (1970) proposed a new scheme of classification of the palmar elements based on topological principles. In the scheme these authors did recognize the importance of the hypothenar triradii and categorized them into: (i) t^u (a triradius near the center of the hypothenar eminence), (ii) t^r (a very rare triradius deviating to the radial side of the palm), and (iii) t^b (a triradius either found in the hypothenar region very near the ulnar border of the palm, or is extralimital).

The scheme proposed by Penrose and Loesch suffers on account of atleast four reasons, namely (a) there is no justification in labelling hypothenar triradii as t, which is a label for axial triradii; the implied meaning is that hypothenar triradii are a variant of axial triradii and are therefore nothing but accessory to t, (b) no explanation has been offered for clubbing hypothenar border triradius and extralimital triradius in to one category t^b, (c) often the hypothenar triradii when present on palm may not be located exactly in the center, and in the existing scheme there is no provision for inclusion of such triradii, and (d) if a hypothenar triradii shifts towards the radial side, beyond the axis of the axial triradii, then, in terms of the basic plan of configurational fields, it should be called thenar triradius rather than t^r.

The scheme proposed by Schaumann and Alter (1976) is almost similar to the one proposed by Penrose and Loesch except for two significant departures: (a) that because "there is no definite anatomical landmark to allow a distinction between the ulnar and border triradii, all triradii shifted towards the ulnar side of the palm can be termed t^u." (p. 53), and (b) that information about these triradii should be incorporated in the palmar formula soon after the axial triradii. For example, presence of a triradius t^u will be recorded as D.C.B.A.-tt" t^u-.... (see fig. 3. 15, p. 46) and presence of a border triradius will be recorded as D.C.B.A.-tt't"t^b-..... (see fig. 3. 16, p. 47).

In short, the methodological improvements suggested by Schumann and Alter in respect of hypothenar triradii leave much to be desired. The fundamental error being that they also considered hypothenar triradii as variants of triradius t.

Recently Malhotra et al (1980a) critically examined the above three schemes and demonstrated their inadequacies. They proposed the following scheme which is more meaningful morphologically, eliminates subjectivity and provides maximum information: (a) all triradii situated towards the ulnar side in the hypothenar area (whether present on the palm or extralimital) in relation to the "narrow field aligned with the axis of the fourth digit" (Cummins and

Midlo 1943, p. 99) should be designated as hypothenar triradii and labelled h (following the general principle of designating other palmar triradii) to distinguish it from axial triradii t, (b) all triradii present on the hypothenar eminence irrespective of their location - center, border etc - as designated as h^p (superscript p stands for present on the palm), and those triradii which lie out side the ridged skin be designated as h^{ext} (superscript ext stands for extralimital), (c) all triradii placed towards radial side (cf. triradius t^r of Penrose and Loesch, 1970) beyond the axis of the axial triradii should not be treated as hypothenar triradii, instead to considered as thenar triradii, and (d) details about hypothenar triradii (h) be entered in the palmar formula soon after the axial triradii -.e., D.C.B.A. t.h. Th/I. II. III. IV. Hyp. It may be noted that after the axial triradius t, period has been used to emphasize the independent status of triradius h.

HYPOTHENAR TRIRADII IN HUMANS

In a series of three articles Malhotra et al (1980a, 1981) and Karmakar and Malhotra (1981) studied the nature and extent of variation in types of hypothenar triradii, using the methods of Malhotra et al (1980a), among 5,004 persons (10,008 palms) belonging to 34 different population groups from the Indian sub-continent. Of the total subjects studies 4838 were males and 166 females. Except for the Nepali sample from Nepal, the remaining 33 samples belonged to four north-Western states of India: Himachal Pradesh(N=4), Punjab(N=3), Rajasthan (N=5), and Maharashtra (N=21). The geographical location of the groups studied is shown in Fig. 1. The sample sizes vary between 48 and 631, the series average being 147. The distribution of the sample, separately for each group, is shown in table 1.

In terms of ethnic affiliation, except for the Bhils, a tribal population of Rajasthan and Nepalis, the remaining 32 groups belong to the Hindu caste system. The studied Hindu castes represent various social hierarchies.

Further details about sampling techniques and other ethnographic details about the groups studied could be found in Malhotra (1974, 1979); Malhotra et al (1978, 1980a, 1981); and Karmakar and Malhotra (1981).

From the three studies mentioned above and further analysis attempted here the following main points emerge:

(i) <u>Hypothenar triradii h^p</u>

An inspection of table 1 shows that the variation in perecent frequencies of triradius h^p among 34 groups is wide and statistically highly heterogeneous for either right (range 0 - 23.0, $p<0.001$) or left palms (range 0 - 21.0, $p<0.001$) or average of the two (range 0.5 - 20.0, $p<0.001$). There is a marked tendency for the right plams to show higher frequency of h^p (20/35, 57.1%). However, the bilateral differences in all the groups and in both sexes, except for the Nepalis ($p<0.001$) were non-significant. The only population for which data on both sexes were available, show statistically higher incidence of h^p on left palm ($p<0.001$) and totals of both palms ($p<0.01$) among females. This is consistent with the fact that females invariably show higher frequencies of hypothenar patterns than males (Cummins and Midlo 1943, p. 274.)

It may be noted that usually only one triradius h^p occurs on a single palm. Malhotra et al (1981), however reported 4 (0.16%) palms (1 left, 3 right), in a series of 2486 palms having 2 h^p each.

(ii) Hypothenar triradii h^{ext}

A statistically highly significant inter-group diversity is also observed in respect of percent frequency of triradius h^{ext} for right (range 2.1 - 20.4, $p<0.001$) or left palm (range 2.0 - 25.0, $p<0.001$) and average of both palms (range 4.0 - 21.0, $p<0.001$). There appears to be a notable tendency for the left palms to show higher incidence of h^{ext} (L>R 51.4%; R>L 31.4%; R=L 17.2%). The bilateral differences however, attain significance level at 5% only among the Agarwals.

(iii) Hypothenar triradii h (h^p+h^{ext})

The percent frequency of h, as expected, also depicts significant inter-group diversity for either right (range 8.8 - 29.0, $p<0.001$) or left palms (range 10.9 - 31.0, $p<0.001$) or average of both palms (11.7 - 30.0, $p<0.001$). The bimanual differences in both sexes and in all the groups are non-significant.

(iv) Bilateral symmetry

Malhotra et al (1981) studied bilateral asymmetry

among 13 populations. The results are presented in table 4. The degree of bilateral symmetry is high in all the groups ranging from 74% to 85% with a series average of 78.5%. The differences between population were found to be non-significant ($p < 0.90$).

(v) Relative incidence of h^p and h^{ext}

The frequencies of triradius h^{ext} show higher frequencies than triradius h^p in a majority of the groups on either right (25/35, $p < 0.001$) or left palm (26/35, $p < 0.001$) or both palms (24/35, $p < 0.001$). For the pooled series the average percent frequencies of triradius h^{ext} on right, left and average of both palms are 11.5, 12.2 and 11.8, respectively; the corresponding frequencies of h^p are 7.7. 6.6, and 7.2, respectively. These differences are highly significant for either right or left palm or average of both palms: in all cases p is < 0.001.

Generally on a given palm either h^p or h^{ext} occurs. However, Malhotra et al (1981) reported 11 (0.44%) out of 2486 palms - 5 right, 4 left of different persons and both palms of one person having both h^p and h^{ext} triradii.

(vi) Variation within different states

As noted earlier, except in the case of Nepal which is represented only by one group, from the remaining each of the Indian states at least 3 populations were sampled. It would therefore, be of interest to examine whether various groups sampled in a state show any differences in types of hypothenar triradii. For each of the states the homogeneity between groups was tested separately for triradius h^p or h^{ext} and for either right or left palms or totals of both palms. The frequencies of triradius h^p on both palms as well as totals of both palms show homogenous distribution within each state: the only exception being the 21 populations of Maharashtra state; they differ for right ($p < 0.01$) or left palm ($p < 0.001$) or totals of both ($p < 0.001$). In respect of triradius h^{ext}, the populations of Himachal Pradesh alone show homogeneous distribution. The populations within each of the remaining three states show varying degree of variation: the frequencies of h^{ext} on left palm show significant differences ($p < 0.05$) among the 3 groups of Punjab; the frequencies of h^{ext} differ significantly on right, left and totals of both palms among 5 groups of Rajasthan and 21 groups of Maharashtra.

It is highly noteworthy that when the frequencies of sum totals of triradius h^p and h^{ext} were considered either for right or left palm or totals of both, only groups in Rajasthan state showed significant differences for sum totals of both palms ($p < 0.005$). It is evident, therefore, that the power of discrimination between groups within a state, or between groups of different states, decreases enormously when sum totals of h^p and h^{ext} are considered than each of these treated separately.

A comparison of variances in respect of triradius h^p and h^{ext} within states reveal interesting results. In the case of triradius h^p the populations of Himachal Pradesh depict highest variability followed by states of Punjab, Maharashtra and Rajasthan. In respect of triradius h^{ext} the highest variability is observed in the populations of

Rajasthan followed by Maharashtra, Punjab, and Himachal Pradesh. The sum totals of h^p plus h^{ext} show highest variability in Rajasthan followed by Himachal Pradesh, Maharashtra and Punjab.

(vii) Variation between states

The summary means and standard errors for populations within each state are presented in table 2 for each of the 9 variables. For examining inter-state differences, t-values were computed for all possible state-pairs for each of the 9 variables. The results are presented in table 3. The highest degree of variation is observed between population groups of Himachal Pradesh and Maharashtra (they differ in 8 variables out of 9) followed by Maharashtra and Punjab (differ in 5 variables out of 9). The populations of Punjab and Himachal Pradesh show least differences: they differ in only one variable.

It is noteworthy that of the two types of hypothenar triradii maximum differences between populations of different states are observed in triradius h^p (12/18 instances) followed by h^{ext} (7/18 instances). The sum totals of h^p plus h^{ext} display least differences (3/18 instances).

(viii)North south cline

An examination of data presented in table 2 and plotted in Fig. 2, reveal striking north-south cline in the frequency distribution of either triradius h^p or h^{ext}. The summary means of frequencies for h^p are highest for

Himachal Pradesh and lowest for Maharashtra: there is a consistent decrease in the frequency of h^p from north to south. The frequency distribution of triradius h^{ext} on the contrary shows highest mean frequency among the sampled populations of Maharashtra and lowest in Himachal Pradesh; a consistent and gradual decrease from south to north is evident. However, when means of sum of h^p plus h^{ext} are considered Maharashtra shows the lowest mean, while in the other three states the incidence is more or less of the same order.

(ix) Variation within castes of the same social rank

In the 34 populations considered here there were five instances in which more than one population belonging to the same social status was sampled either within a state or from different states. In order to examine whether castes of the same social status showed homogeneous distribution among themselves, chi-square statistics was applied separately for each of the 9 variables. It is observed that (a) the three scheduled castes - Ramdasis of Punjab, Harijan Chammars of Himachal Pradesh and Meghwals of Rajasthan - who enjoy the lowest social status in the Hindu caste system show significant differences in the incidence of h^p ($p < 0.025$) and h^{ext} ($p < 0.025$) on the right palms, (b) the two Brahmin populations sampled from Rajasthan and Himachal Pradesh having the highest social status depict significant differences for totals of h^p on right plus left palms ($p < 0.001$) and sum of h^p plus h^{ext} on both palms ($p < 0.01$), (c) the two Rajput castes sampled from Rajasthan and Hmiachal Pradesh belong to middle social order. They differ only for sum of h^{ext} on both palms

($p < 0.05$), (d) the two trading castes, namely, Agarwals and Oswals, sampled from Punjab and Rajasthan differ for totals of both palms for h^p ($p < 0.025$) and h^{ext} ($p < 0.001$), (e) except for the Nandiwallas the remaining 21 populations sampled from Maharashtra belong to one caste-cluster of pastoral castes called Dhangars. They differ significantly in the frequency distribution of both h^p or h^{ext} either on left or right palms or total of both.

(x) Variation between ethnic groups

Malhotra et al (1981) attempted inter-ethnic variation in hypothenar triradii among 13 populations of four states: Himachal Pradesh, Punjab and Rajasthan in India and Nepalis.Of these the Bhils are Australoid, the Nepalis are Mongoloid and the remaining 11 groups are representatives of Caucasoids. Due to only one sample each of Australoid and Mongoloid the present materials are clearly insufficient for any detailed inter-ethnic analysis. The limited data, however, shows that the frequency of hypothenar triradii tends to be low in Mongoloids, and high in the Australoids, while the Caucasoids, though variable among themselves, occupy an intermediate position. The Australoid Bhils differ significantly from the Mongoloid Nepalis in the incidence of h^{ext} on right, left as well as sum of both palms. Bhils also differ from the pooled Caucasoid averages for h^{ext} on either right or left palms or sum of both, and for totals of h^p plus h^{ext} on left palm and sum of both palms. The Nepalis also differ from Caucasoids for h^p on right palm and h^{ext} on right palm.

The limited inter-ethnic comparisons attempted here indicate the possibility of existence of wide diversity in the frequency distribution of hypothenar triradii among major ethnic groups.

HYPOTHENAR TRIRADII IN NON-HUMAN PRIMATES

A review of the dermatoglyphic literature on non-human primates reveal that while several studies have reported frequencies of types of hypothenar patterns and pattern intensities (among several others see, Midlo and Cummins 1942; Biegert 1961; Brehme 1967, 1968, 1975; Iwamoto 1964, 1967; Newell - Morris 1979a, 1979b) among a number of non-human primates, surprisingly not even a single attempt has been made in the past to furnish data on hypothenar triradii. In fact, even the frequency distribution of hypothenar triradii or for that matter of any other configurational area, or total palm, are yet to be documented in non-human primates.

The present study, therefore, could be regarded as the first contribution aimed at understanding the nature and extent of diversity in types of hypothenar triradii among non-human primates. In fact, there is an urgent need to document the frequencies of triradial points in each of the configurational areas to permit more rigorous comparisons between various primates including man.

METHODOLOGICAL ISSUES

The hypothenar area among non-human primates morphologically is far more complex than in human. Unlike in humans, this area among non-human primates, in general, comprises of two distinct elements, hypothenar distal (H^d) and hypothenar proximal (H^p). In humans the hypothenar and thenar eminences are differentiated by depressed surface where in the proximal and central portions of the palm axial triradii occur. Among non-human primates also these areas are clearly differentiated by a definite parathenar configuration (P-th). This configuration provides a useful landmark for locating hypothenar triradii. Thus, all triradii occuring on the ulnar side of the axis of configuration P-th on the hypothenar eminence be designated as hypothenar triradii(h). Those present on the palm be designated as h^p and those lying outside the ridged skin be labelled as h^{ext}. Both h^p and h^{ext} then be scored separately for distal (h^{dp} or $h^{d\ ext}$) and proximal (h^{pp} or $h^{p\ ext}$) hypothenar areas. This procedure thus permits a direct comparison of types of hypothenar triradii in primates including humans.

SOURCE OF DATA

The data presented here were generated by inspecting illustrations of palmar prints of non-human primates provided by Midlo and Cummins (1942) in their monumental work entitled "Palmar and Plantar Dermatoglyphics in Primates". Besides, 8 illustrations of palms of Pygmy Chimpanzee (_Pan paniscus_) provided by Brehme (1975) were also used.

This procedure, though not the ideal, had to be adopted due to non-availability of palmar prints of non-human primates. It is appropriate that relevant details are provided about the nature of the data used here. In regard to the illustrations Midlo and Cummins (1942) write: "The first step in study of the actual hand or foot was to locate triradii (emphasis mine) and to trace the radiants extended from them. With these landmarks inserted in the outline, the courses of ridges were then traced in accord with direct observation. The tracing aimed to show only the general morphological characteristics of the configurations, distinguishing open fields, vestiges and the various pattern types without attention to the details of individual ridges". (p. 23). They further state that the prints chosen for illustrations were selected to secure comprehensiveness of these graphic records' (p. 23), and that 'the left hands are reversed in drawings, to obviate the difficulty of comparing the mirrored relationships of right and left members' (p. 23).

It is thus evident that the illustrations of palms provided are highly reliable especially in terms of location of triradial points. However, since only select and not random illustrations are provided our estimates of frequency distributions among non-human primates will not be very reliable, although qualitative inferences will still be highly valid. Further, because the left hands are reversed in drawings, bilateral comparisons can not be attempted.

Using the methodology of Malhotra et al (1980a) and as extended here for application to non-human primates, altogether drawings of 254 palms (right, left undifferentiated) of 14 non-human primates were analysed for types of hypothenar triradii. In fact Midlo and Cummins (1942) provided illustrations of hands of 35 species of the order primate comparising prosimians, Old and New World monkeys, apes, and human species. Owing to rather small number of illustrations, 20 species could not be utilized in the present study. The 14 species dealt in here belonged to five different families: Callitrichanae (N=1), Cebidae (N=5), Cercopithecine (N=4), Hylobatidae (N=1) and Pongidae (N=3). The names of the 14 primates investigated together with number of palms examined are given in table 5.

DISTRIBUTION OF HYPOTHENAR TRIRADII IN NON-HUMAN PRIMATES

For the sake of convenience distal and proximal hypothenar areas have been considered separately.

Distal hypothenar areas: In table 5 are given the frequencies of triradii h^p and h^{ext} in the distal hypothenar areas among 14 non-human primates. An inspection of this table reveals the following main observations: (a) a wide and significant range of variation in the frequencies of both triradii h^p and h^{ext} exists among the studied non-human primates, (b) strikingly both these triradii are absent among Aotus and Hylobates - these species usually lack true patterns in the distal area, and (c) Cebus and all the three species of family Pongidae lack triradius h^{ext}.

Due to rather small sample sizes rigorous analysis of variation within and between families in respect of hypothenar triradii could not be attempted. It appears, however, that considerable variation exists within and between families for both h^p and h^{ext}. In respect of h^p no systematic, decreasing or increasing, trend is decernible. Triradius h^{ext}, however, shows a decreasing trend, and while among all the 4 species of family Cercopithecinae h^{ext} is present, strikingly it is absent in Pongidae. This observation is in confirmity with the earlier observation of Midlo and Cummins (1942, p. 121) that pattern intensities in distal hypothenar area among Pongo (0.00), Gorilla (0.35) and Pan (0.04) occur in rather low frequencies.

Proximal hypothenar area: In table 5 the frequency distribution of hypothenar triradii in the proxiamal hypothenar area, separately for each of the 14 non-human primate, is presented. Since on a single palm often both h^p and h^{ext} triradii occur, the data were further analysed as given in table 6. From table 5 and 6 three main points emerge: (a) a wide diversity exists among the studied non-human primates in the frequencies of triradii h^p and h^{ext}, (b) among several species both h^p and h^{ext} occur in varying frequencies on a single palm, and (c) in terms of sum total of palms having either h^p or h^{ext} although no systematic trend is seen upto Hylobates, after Hylobates, however, there is a consistent decrease in the following order: Hylobates (100%) $>$ Pongo (91.7%) $>$ Gorilla (45.5%) $>$ Pan (45.5%).

Relative occurence of triradii h^p and h^{ext}

From the data presented in table 7 and plotted in figure 3 it is observed that among 12 out of 14 non-human primates the frequency of triradius h^p exceeds that of

h^{ext}, and in many cases these differences are significant; the reverse is true only among Oedipomidas and Aotus. In terms of relationship between triradius h^p and h^{ext} although no consistent pattern emerges, two types of negative relationships are noticeable: (i) an increase in h^p results in decrease in h^{ext} (Oedipomidas, Aotus, Atles, Papio, Lasiopyga, Pygathrix, and Hylobates); the other type of negative relationship i.e., decrease in h^p and increase in h^{ext}, is observed among all the three members of family Pongidae.

Relationship between triradius h^{ext} and pattern intensities

In figure 4 are presented data on the frequencies of h^{ext} and pattern intensities (after Midlo and Cummins, table 4, p. 121) in the proximal hypothenar area. Almost similar negative relationship, as observed between h^p and h^{ext} exists between h^{ext} and pattern intensities among a majority of the primates; some, however, show positive relationship. We shall say more about it a bit later.

COMPARATIVE ANALYSIS

In the preceding pages an analysis of the distribution of frequencies of types of hypothenar triradii among 34 human populations and 14 non-human primates have been presented. We shall now attempt a comparison between human and studied non-human primates, in general, and apes in particular. As noted earlier, the analysis among non-human primates is based on a rather small number of palmar prints and therefore, conclusions drawn should be viewed with due caution. The salient features emerging out of comparative analysis are given below: (i) as noted earlier, the hypothenar area among the non-human primates, in general, consists of two distinct elements, distal and proximal, which often bear true patterns. In humans the distal area, for all practical purposes, is pattern less (in a series of 1176 palms, Midlo and Cummins (1942) did not find even a single palm with pattern in distal area), and consequently lacks a triradius. The zero incidence of triradius h^p among humans is also observed among Aotus, Hylobates and Pongo. In general, the incidence shows progressive increase from Callitrichinae to Cebidae to Cercopithecinae, and progressive decrease from Hylobatidae to Pongidae to humans; (ii) it is noteworthy that triradius h^{ext} in the distal area is present among several non-human primates but is absent among the three great apes and humans; the only other three primates having zero incidence are Aotus, Cebus and Hylobates; (iii) the total number of hypothenar triradii (h^p+h^{ext}) in the proximal area show no consistent trend: however, except for Saimiri and Aotus the remaining members of families Cebidae and Cercopithecinae exhibit consistengly high values ranging between 81.8% to 100%. Strikingly from Hylobates onwards there is a progressive decrease, the order being: Hylobates (100%) $>$ Pongo (91.7%) $>$ Gorilla (55.6%) $>$ Pan (45.5%) $>$ Homo (22.2%). Midlo and Cummins (1942) observed similar situation in respect of pattern intensities: Pongo (0.96) $>$ Hylobates (0.84) $>$ Gorilla (0.49) $>$ Pan (0.31) $>$ Homo (0.21); (IV) the above relationship is also true in the case of triradius h^p: Hylobates (90.9%) $>$ Pongo (78.6%) $>$ Gorilla (71.4%) $>$ Pan (66.7%) $>$ Homo (57.1%); (v) it is highly noteworthy that hypothenar extralimital triradius (h^{ext}) is not a unique feature found among humans but is also present among all the 14 non-human primates except among Aotus. However, quantitatively humans possess the highest incidence (42.9%). Although no systematic trend is exhibited by members of Cebidae and Cercopithecinae families, a consistent progressive pattern emerges Hylobates onwards: Hylobates (9.1%) > Pongo (21.4%) > Gorilla (28.6%) > Pan (33.3%) > Homo (42.9%); (vi) on several individual palms both triradius h^p and h^{ext} occur. This situation occurs in the case of a hypothenar whorl or duplex pattern. It is noteworthy that high frequency of such palms are seen among several members of both Cebidae and Cercopithecinae families - the highest value is observed among Cebus (53.3%). There is a progressive decrease from apes to humans: Pongo (25%) > Gorilla (22.2%) > Pan (9.1%) > Homo (0.4%); (vii) in general, the frequency of triradius h^p exceeds that of h^{ext} both among humans and non-human primates, and the relationship between h^p and h^{ext} appears to be negative in most of the primates (Fig. 3), and (vii) the incidence of triradius h^{ext} among a majority of the primates shows negative relationship with pattern intensities (Fig. 4). That occurence of h^{ext} is not a direct function of pattern intensities is clearly demonstrable among Gorilla, Pan and Human; in these primates although the values of pattern intensities are quite low compared to several other primates, the incidence of triradius h^{ext} is considerably higher. Infact, this is most forcefully seen among humans who have the lowest pattern intensities (0.21) but have the highest frequency of h^{ext}; the only exception being Aotus, pattern intensity being 0.18 but have zero incidence of h^{ext}.

It is, therefore, evident that although unless a pattern exists, topologically it is impossible to get an extralimital triradius, but presence of a pattern per se does not guarantee occurence of h^{ext}. Instead the occurence of h^{ext} depends upon perhaps the type and size of the pattern and the general palmar ridge alignment.

EVOLUTIONARY IMPLICATIONS

From the preceding analysis it is evident that enormous diversity exists in humans and non-human primates in respect of hypothenar triradii h^p and h^{ext}. It is noteworthy that triradius h^{ext} occurs not only among humans but also among several non-human primates. It is highly significant that despite the considerable reduction in pattern intensities among apes and humans the frequency of h^{ext} shows a pattern of consistent increase from Pongo to Gorilla to Chimpanzee to humans. The obvious question to ask then is how do we explain the increasing number of extralimital triradii? The answer certainly does not lie in the number of patterns or degree of pattern intensities, as has been shown earlier in Fig. 4. It seems most likely that the following three developments during the evolution of palmar dermatoglyphics have led to progressive increase in extralimital triradii: (i) the distinction between distal and proximal hypothenar elements have progressively become less apparent, and infact in man it has nearly completely desappeared. The obvious result has been that the total hypothenar area has substantially increased and it can now accommodate relatively larger patterns than before, (ii) the general course of ridge alignment has also undergone substantial changes, and (iii) the changes that have occured in the length and breadth proportions of hands.

It may be mentioned here that infact extralimital triradii also frequently occur in the hallucal area of the distal sole (the frequencies have, however, yet to be empirically documented) and much less frequently on finger and toe patterns (Cummins and Midlo 1943). Holt (1968) reported occurence of extralimital triradii among Britishers in about 0.7 per cent of females and 1.4 per cent of males.

Cummins and Midlo (1943, p. 58-59) in respect of the occurence of extralimital triradii wrote: "A pattern may be so expanded that its margins encroach into the zone of junction of ridged skin and the generalized skin of the dorsum of the finger." As is evident this is rather a morphological description than an explanation.

The general courses of palmar ridges in great apes range from strictly longitudinal to oblique while in man the palm presents a combination of longitudianl and diagonal alignment (Midlo and Cummins 1942).

Thus it appears that it is the oblique and diagonal ridge alignment coupled with enhanced total hypothenar configurational area that has created morphological opportunities for the occurence of extralimital triradii. This is fully substantiated by an examination of the palms in man where the main line A (proximal radiant of triradius a) travels diagonally to position 3, recurves back and forms a large hypothenar radial loop. Such loops often are associated with extralimital hypothenar triradii. If, however, the main line travelled strictly longitudinal it will exist at position 1, and if its course is nearly transverse it will exist in the distal palmar area(positions

5' and 5"). In both these situations the main line A has hardly any possibility of recurving back and forming a loop. All the evidence at our disposal strongly suggests that it is primarily the evolution of diagonal ridge alignment in human palm in general, and in hypothenar area in particular, that has provided morphological opportunities for the occurence of extralimital triradii.

It is also probable that changes in the length and breadth proportions of hand, in general, and palm in particular among primates is associated with absence or presence of extralimital triradii. In the present study this could not be examined for want of relevant data.

In conclusion, it may be emphasized that our understanting of the causes of occurence of extralimital triradii is far from complete and more work is essential especially among the non-human primates. We are currently persuing a number of projects directed towords unravelling the evolutionary history of extralimital triradii in man and non-human primates.

Acknowledgements

I thank Mr. M. Vijayakumar, my student, for inking the four text figures. I also thank MS B. Karmakar for rendering various kinds of help.

REFERENCES

Biegert J (1961). "Volarhaut der Hände und Füsse. Primatologia, Handbuch der Primatenkunde", Vol. 2. Basel: S. Karger.

Brehme H (1967). Untersuchungen am Haytleistensystem der Palma and Planta Von Colobus polykomos, Colobus badius, Colobus verus, und Nasalis larvatus. Folia Primatologica 6: 243-283.

Brehme H (1968). The variability of the epidermal palm and sole patterns in the genera Cercopithecus and Erythrocebus patas. Folia Primatologica 9: 41-67.

Brehme H (1975). Epidermal patterns of the hands and feet of the pygmy chimpazee (Pan paniscus). Am J Phys Anthrop 45: 255-262.

Cummins H, Midlo C (1943). "Finger prints, palms, and soles. An introduction to dermatoglyphics". Philadelphia: Blakiston.

Holt S B (1968). "The Genetics of Dermal Ridges". Spring field: C.C. Thomas.

Holt S B (1975). The hypothenar radial arch, a genetically determined epidermal ridge configuration. Am J Phys Anthrop 42: 211-214.

Iwamoto M (1964). Morphological studies of Macaca fuscata. I. Dermatoglyphics of the hand. Primates 5: 53-73.

Iwamoto M (1967). Morphological study of Macaca fuscata.V. Dermatoglyphics of the foot. Primates 8: 155-180.

Karmakar B, Malhotra K C (1981). Ethnic variation in hypothenar triradii, h. South Asian Anthrop(in press)

Loesch D (1971). Genetics of dermatoglyphic patterns on palms, Ann Hum Genet 34: 277-293.

Malhotra K C (1974). Socio-biological investigations among the Nandiwallas of Maharashtra. Bull Urgt Anthrop Ethnol Sci 16: 63-102.

Malhotra K C (1979). Inbreeding among Dhangar castes of Maharashtra. J Biosoc Sci 11: 397-410.

Malhotra K C, Chakraborty R, Chakravartti A (1978). Gene differentiation among the Dhangar caste-cluster of Maharashtra, India. Hum Hered 28: 26-36.

Malhotra K C, Karmakar B, Reddy B M, Vijayakumar M (1980a). Ulnar triradius (t^u), border triradius (t^b) and extralimital triradius (t^{ext}), the neglected triradii on human palm. Technical Report No. Anthrop./7/1980, Indian Statistical Institute, Calcutta, India.

Malhotra K C, Reddy B M, Karmakar B, Vijayakumar M (1980b). Relationship between types of axial triradii and true hypothenar patterns. Technical Report No. Anthrop. 5/1980, Indian Statistical Institute, Calcutta, India.

Malhotra K C, Karmakar B, Vijayakumar M (1981). Diversity in hypothenar triradii among some population groups from the Indian sub-continent. Communicated to Am J Phys Anthrop.

Mavalwala J (1977). "Dermatoglyphics An International Bibliography". The Hague: Mouton.

Mavalwala J (1978). A methodology for dermatoglyphics - fingers and palms. In: "Dermatoglyphics An International Perspective", ed J Mavalwala. The Hague: Mouton, pp. 19-54.

Midlo C, Cummins H (1942). Palmar and plantar dermatoglyphics in primates. An Ant Mem 20: 1-198.

Newell - Morris L (1979a). Midlo and Cummins Updated: Primate Dermatoglyphics Today and Tomorrow. In: "Dermatoglyphics Fifty Years Later", eds W Wertelecki, C C Plato. New York: Alan R. Liss, Inc., pp 739-764.

Newell - Morris L (1979b). Functional considerations of interspecific variation in dermatoglyphic pattern intensity in Old World Monkeys. In: "Dermatoglyphics Fifty Years Later", eds W Wertelecki, C C Plato. New York: Alan R Liss Inc. pp 765-789.

Penrose L S, Loesch D (1970). Topological classification of palmar dermatoglyphics. J Ment Def Res 14: 111-128.

Pons J (1979). Genetics of dermal ridges: pattern inheritance in the hypothenar area. In: "Dermatoglyphics Fifty Years Later", eds W Wertelecki, C C Plato, New York: Alan R Lies Inc., pp. 539-542.

Schaumann B, Alter M (1976). "Dermatoglyphics in Mental Disorders." New York: Springer - Verlag.

Sognier M A, Kloepfer H W, Cummins H (1979). The Inheritance of hypothenar whorl. In: "Dermatoglyphics Fifty Years Later", eds W Wertelecki, C C Plato, New York: Alan R Liss Inc., pp 543-556.

Vrydegh - Laoureux S (1971). Heredite des dermatoglyphes. II. Dermatoglyphes des paumee et des pieds. Bull et Mem de la Soc d Anthrop Paris 7: 281-305.

Weninger M (1947). Zur vererburg der hautleistenmuster am hypothenar der menschlichen hand. Mitteilungen der Anthropologischen Gesellschaft in Wien 73-77: 55-82.

Table 1. Percent frequencies of types of hypothenar triradii among 34 groups from the Indian sub-continent.

Pupulations	Side	No.of palms	h^p	h^{ext}	h	Source
INDIA						
HIMACHAL	R	100	23.0	6.0	29.0	MALHOTRA et al
PRADESH	L	100	17.0	6.0	23.0	" " '81
1. Brahmins	R & L	100	20.0	6.0	26.0	
2. Choudhury	R	100	17.0	5.0	22.0	" " "
	L	100	21.0	7.0	28.0	
	R & L	100	19.0	6.0	25.0	
3. Harijian-	R	48	22.9	2.1	25.0	" " "
Chammar	L	48	8.3	10.4	18.7	
	R & L	48	15.6	6.2	21.8	
4. Gaddi	R	100	12.0	5.0	17.0	" " "
Rajput	L	100	12.0	3.0	15.0	
	R & L	100	12.0	4.0	16.0	
MAHARASHTRA						
5. Ahir	R	323	4.0	13.3	17.3	KARMAKAR &
	L	323	3.0	13.9	16.9	MALHOTRA 1981
	R & L	323	3.5	13.6	17.1	
6. Dange	R	201	5.5	13.4	18.9	" " "
	L	201	2.5	17.9	20.4	
	R & L	201	4.0	15.6	19.6	
7. Gadhari-	R	110	6.4	7.3	13.7	" " "
Dhengar	L	110	4.5	13.6	18.1	
	R & L	110	5.4	10.4	15.8	
8. Gadhari-	R	87	4.6	21.8	26.4	" " "
Nikhar	L	87	0	17.2	17.2	
	R & L	87	2.3	19.5	21.8	
9. Hande	R	98	6.1	6.1	12.2	" " "
	L	98	5.1	8.2	13.3	
	R & L	98	5.6	7.1	12.7	
10. Hatkar	R	631	7.5	10.6	18.1	MALHOTRA et al
	L	631	7.3	10.9	18.2	1980a
	R & L	631	7.4	10.7	18.1	
11. Kannade	R	92	1.1	17.4	18.5	KARMAKAR &
	L	92	0	17.4	17.4	MALHOTRA '81
	R & L	92	0.5	17.4	17.9	

Cont.....

12. Khatik	R	167	3.0	19.8	22.8	KARMAKAR &
	L	167	4.2	17.4	21.6	MALHOTRA '81
	R & L	167	3.6	18.7	22.2	
13. Khutekar	R	509	6.3	10.2	16.5	MALHOTRA et
	L	509	7.1	11.2	18.3	al 1980a
	R & L	509	6.7	10.7	17.4	
14. Kurmar	R	103	8.7	17.5	26.2	KARMAKAR &
	L	103	2.9	20.4	23.3	MALHOTRA '81
	R & L	103	5.8	18.9	24.7	
15. Ladshe	R	120	2.5	10.0	12.5	" " "
	L	120	2.5	8.4	10.9	
	R & L	120	2.5	9.2	11.7	
16. Mendhe	R	183	3.8	12.6	16.4	" " "
	L	183	1.6	13.1	14.7	
	R & L	183	2.7	12.8	15.5	
17. Sangar	R	89	7.9	10.1	18.0	" " "
	L	89	4.5	10.1	14.6	
	R & L	89	6.2	10.1	16.3	
18. Shegar	R	83	1.2	15.7	16.9	" " "
	L	83	0	14.5	14.5	
	R & L	83	0.6	15.1	15.7	
19. Telangi	R	91	2.2	13.2	15.4	" " "
	L	91	3.3	13.2	16.5	
	R & L	91	2.7	13.2	15.9	
20. Thellari	R	117	0	15.4	15.4	" " "
	L	117	3.4	19.6	23.0	
	R & L	117	1.7	17.5	19.2	
21. Unni-kankan	R	67	1.5	14.9	16.4	" " "
	L	67	3.0	14.9	17.9	
	R & L	67	2.2	14.9	17.1	
22. Varhade	R	76	2.6	17.1	19.7	" " "
	L	76	1.3	25.0	26.3	
	R & L	76	1.9	21.0	23.0	
23. Zende	R	160	4.4	10.6	15.0	" " "
	L	160	1.2	15.6	16.8	
	R & L	160	2.8	13.1	15.9	
24. Zade	R	79	2.5	6.3	8.8	" " "
	L	79	7.6	10.1	17.7	
	R & L	79	5.0	8.2	13.2	

Cont.......

25. Nandiwalla (males)	R	209	6.2	11.5	17.7	MALHOTRA et al 1980a
	L	209	2.4	11.5	13.9	
	R & L	209	4.3	11.5	15.8	
Nandiwalla (females)	R	166	9.0	5.4	14.5	
	L	166	9.0	4.8	13.9	
	R & L	166	9.0	5.1	14.2	
PUNJAB						
26. Agarwal Bania	R	100	18.0	8.0	26.0	MALHOTRA et al 1981
	L	100	16.0	2.0	18.0	
	R & L	100	17.0	5.0	22.0	
27. Jat Sikh	R	100	10.0	14.0	24.0	" " "
	L	100	13.0	8.0	21.0	
	R & L	100	11.5	11.0	22.5	
28. Ramdasis	R	100	15.0	9.0	24.0	" " "
	L	100	7.0	12.0	19.0	
	R & L	100	11.0	10.5	21.5	
RAJASTHAN						
29. Bhil	R	100	11.0	18.0	29.0	" " "
	L	100	9.0	22.0	31.0	
	R & L	100	10.0	20.0	30.0	
30. Brahmin Palival	R	100	7.0	6.0	13.0	" " "
	L	100	10.0	8.0	18.0	
	R & L	100	8.5	7.0	15.5	
31. Meghwals (Chammar)	R	100	7.0	16.0	23.0	" " "
	L	100	9.0	8.0	17.0	
	R & L	100	8.0	12.0	20.0	
32. Rajput	R	100	7.0	11.0	18.0	" " "
	L	100	15.0	7.0	22.0	
	R & L	100	11.0	9.0	20.0	
33. Oswal Bania	R	101	5.9	19.8	25.7	" " "
	L	101	11.9	15.8	27.7	
	R & L	101	8.9	17.8	26.7	
NEPAL						
34. Nepalis	R	94	18.1	2.1	20.2	" " "
	L	94	4.2	7.4	11.6	
	R & L	94	11.1	4.7	15.8	
ALL POPULATIONS	R	5004	7.7	11.5	19.2	
	L	5004	6.6	12.2	18.7	
	R & L	5004	7.2	11.7	18.9	

Table 2. Summary of Means and Standard Error within groups of each state.

STATE / VARIABLE	Himachal Pradesh (N=4) Mean±S.E.	Maharashtra (N = 21) Mean±S.E.	Punjab (N = 3) Mean±S.E.	Rajasthan (N = 5) Mean±S.E.
Triradius h^p				
Right	18.72±2.64	4.41±0.57	14.33±2.33	7.58±0.88
Left	14.57±2.78	3.47±0.55	12.00±2.64	10.98±1.13
Both palms	16.65±1.81	4.01±0.47	13.17±1.96	8.07±1.41
Triradius h^{ext}				
Right	4.52±0.84	12.74±0.97	10.33±1.85	14.16±2.51
Left	6.60±1.52	14.04±1.01	7.33±2.90	12.16±2.92
Both palms	5.55±0.52	14.73±0.87	8.83±1.92	13.16±2.50
Triradius h^p+h^{ext}				
Right	23.25±2.53	17.15±0.90	24.67±0.66	21.74±2.83
Left	21.17±2.80	17.52±0.80	19.33±0.88	23.14±2.72
Both Palms	22.20±2.25	17.31±0.73	22.00±0.29	22.44±2.60

Table 3. Obtained t-values for inter-state comparisons.

Pairs of states	h^p			h^{ext}			$h^p + h^{ext}$		
	R	L	R & L	R	L	R & L	R	L	R & L
1. Himachal Pradesh x Maharashtra	5.29*	3.91*	6.74*	6.39*	2.97*	9.09*	2.27*	1.25	2.07*
2. " " x Punjab	1.24	0.67	1.30	2.85*	0.22	1.65	0.38	0.62	0.09
3. " " x Rajasthan	3.99*	1.19	3.73*	3.64*	1.22	2.98*	0.40	0.50	0.07
4. Maharashtra x Punjab	4.13*	3.16*	4.55*	1.15	1.53	2.80*	6.71*	1.52	0.78
5. " " x Rajasthan	3.02*	5.95*	2.72*	0.53*	0.04	0.59	1.54	1.99	1.90
6. Punjab x Rajasthan	2.71*	0.35	2.12	1.23	1.17	1.37	1.01	1.33	0.17

* Significant at 5% and below levels.

Table 4. Percent bilateral symmetry among 13 groups of Himachal Pradesh, Punjab, Rajasthan and Nepal[1].

Groups	Absent on both palms	h^p present on both palms	h^{ext} present on both palms	Palmar symmetry[2]	Palmar asymmetry
1. Brahmin	64.2	10.0	2.0	76.0	24.0
2. Choudhury	69.0	8.0	4.0	81.0	19.0
3. Harijan-Chammar	72.9	8.3	2.1	83.3	16.7
4. Gaddi Rajput	72.0	2.0	1.0	75.0	25.0
5. Agarwal Bania	68.0	6.0	1.0	75.0	25.0
6. Jat Sikh	72.0	7.0	6.0	85.0	15.0
7. Ramdasis	69.0	3.0	6.0	78.0	22.0
8. Bhils	62.0	2.0	10.0	74.0	26.0
9. Brahmin Palival	76.0	2.0	1.0	79.0	21.0
10. Meghwal	70.0	1.0	6.0	77.0	23.0
11. Rajput	71.0	4.0	4.0	79.0	21.0
12. Oswal	63.4	2.0	10.9	76.2	23.8
13. Nepalis	77.7	2.1	2.1	81.9	18.1
Pooled 13 groups	69.8	4.4	4.3	78.5	21.5

1. Source: Malhotra et al 1981, 2. Frequencies of the same type of hypothenar triradii plus absent from both palms.

Table 5. Incidence of hypothenar triradii in non-human primates and man.

Primates[1]	No. of palms	Hypothenar triradii: Hd h^p	Hd h^{ext}	Hp h^p	Hp h^{ext}
Anthropoidea Callitrichanae					
1. Oedipomidas geoffroyi	10	2 (20.0)	2 (20.0)	2 (20.0)	1 (10.0)
2. Cebidae Aloutta[4]	16	1 (6.2)	13 (81.2)	7 (43.7)	10 (62.5)
3. Saimiri	12	8 (66.7)	2 (16.7)	1 (8.3)	2 (16.7)
4. Aotus Zonalis	12	0 (0.0)	0 (0.0)	1 (8.3)	0 (0.0)
5. Ateles[4]	20	8 (40.0)	1 (5.0)	20 (100.0)	2 (10.0)
6. Cebus[4]	15	8 (53.3)	0 (0.0)	14 (93.3)	9 (60.0)
Cercopithecinae					
7. Papio[4]	11	6 (54.5)	5 (45.5)	9 (81.8)	4 (36.4)
8. Pithecus (Maccaca[4])	59	41 (69.5)	19 (32.2)	57 (96.6)	32 (54.2)
9. Lasiopyga[4]	15	1 (6.7)	1 (6.7)	12 (80.0)	5 (33.3)
10. Pygathrix[4]	12	9 (75.0)	1 (8.3)	11 (91.7)	2 (16.7)
Hylobatidae					
11. Hylobates[4]	40	0 (0.0)	0 (0.0)	40 (100.0)	4 (10.0)
Pongidae					
12. Pongo pygmaeus[4]	12	0 (0.0)	0 (0.0)	11 (91.7)	3 (25.0)

13. Gorilla	9	3 (33.3)	0 (0.0)	11 (55.6)	3 (25.0)
14. Pan	11	2 (18.2)	0 (0.0)	4 (36.4)	2 (18.2)
Hominidae					
15. Homo[2]	10,008	0 (0.0)	0 (0.0)	716 (7.15)	1186 (11.85)

1. Except for data on Pan paniscus which have been inferred from the illustrations provided by Brehme (1975), data pertaining to other primates have been generated by examining the manus illustrations given by Midlo and Cummins (1942).
2. Data after Malhotra et al (1980a, 1981) and Karmakar and Malhotra (1981).
3. Figures in parenthesis are percentages.
4. On a single palm more than one triraddii h^p or h^{ext} occure.

Table 6. Incidence of types of hypothenar proximal triradii among primates.

Primates	No. of palms	Hypothenar triradii(proximal region)				
			Present			
		Absent	h^p	h^{ext}	$h^p + h^{ext}$	Total present
1. Oedipomidas geoffroyi	10	7 (70.0)[1]	2 (20.0)	1 (10.0)	0 (0.0)	3 (30.0)
2. Aloutta	16	0 (0.0)	6 (37.5)	9 (56.2)	1 (6.2)	16 (100.0)
3. Saimiri	12	9 (75.0)	1 (8.3)	2 (18.7)	0 (0.0)	3 (25.0)
4. Aotus Zonalis	12	11 (91.7)	1 (8.3)	0 (0.0)	0 (0.0)	1 (8.3)
5. Ateles	20	0 (0.0)	18 (90.0)	0 (0.0)	2 (10.0)	20 (100.0)
6. Cebus	15	0 (0.0)	6 (40.0)	1 (6.7)	8 (53.3)	15 (100.0)
7. Papio	11	2 (18.2)	5 (45.4)	0 (0.0)	4 (36.4)	9 (81.8)
8. Pithecus (Maccaca)	59	3 (5.1)	25 (42.4)	0 (0.0)	31 (52.5)	36 (94.9)
9. Lasiopyga	15	2 (13.3)	8 (53.3)	1 (6.7)	4 (26.7)	13 (86.7)
10. Pygathrix	12	1 (8.3)	9 (75.0)	0 (0.0)	2 (16.7)	11 (91.7)
11. Hylobates	40	0 (0.0)	36 (90.0)	0 (0.0)	4 (10.0)	40 (100.0)
12. Pongo	12	1 (8.3)	8 (66.7)	0 (0.0)	3 (25.0)	11 (91.7)
13. Gorilla	9	4 (44.4)	3 (33.3)	0 (0.0)	2 (22.2)	5 (55.6)

14. Pan	11	6 (54.5)	3 (27.3)	1 (9.1)	1 (9.1)	5 (45.5)
15. Homo	2486	1933 (78.8)	311 (12.5)	231 (9.3)	11 (0.4)	553 (22.2)

1. Figures in parenthesis are percentages.

Table 7. Relative occurence of hypothenar triradii h^p and h^{ext} in the proximal hypothenar area among primates.

Primates	Hypothenar triradii		
	h^p	h^{ext}	Total h
1. Oedipomidas geoffroyi	2 (66.7)*	1 (33.3)	3
2. Aloutta	7 (41.2)	10 (58.8)	17
3. Saimiri	1 (33.3)	2 (66.7)	3
4. Actus Zonalis	1 (100.0)	0 (0.0)	1
5. Atles	20 (90.9)	2 (9.1)	22
6. Cebus	14 (60.9)	9 (39.1)	23
7. Papio	9 (69.2)	4 (30.8)	13
8. Pithecus (Maccaca)	56 (64.4)	31 (35.6)	87
9. Lasiopyga	12 (70.6)	5 (29.4)	17
10. Pygathrix	11 (84.6)	2 (15.4)	13
11. Hylobates	40 (90.9)	4 (9.1)	44
12. Fongo	11 (78.6)	3 (21.4)	14
13. Gorilla	5 (71.4)	2 (28.6)	7
14. Pan	4 (66.7)	2 (33.3)	6

15. Homo (based on 2486 palms)[1]	322 (57.1)	242 (42.9)	564

* Figures in parenthesis are percentages
1 After Malhotra et al (1981).

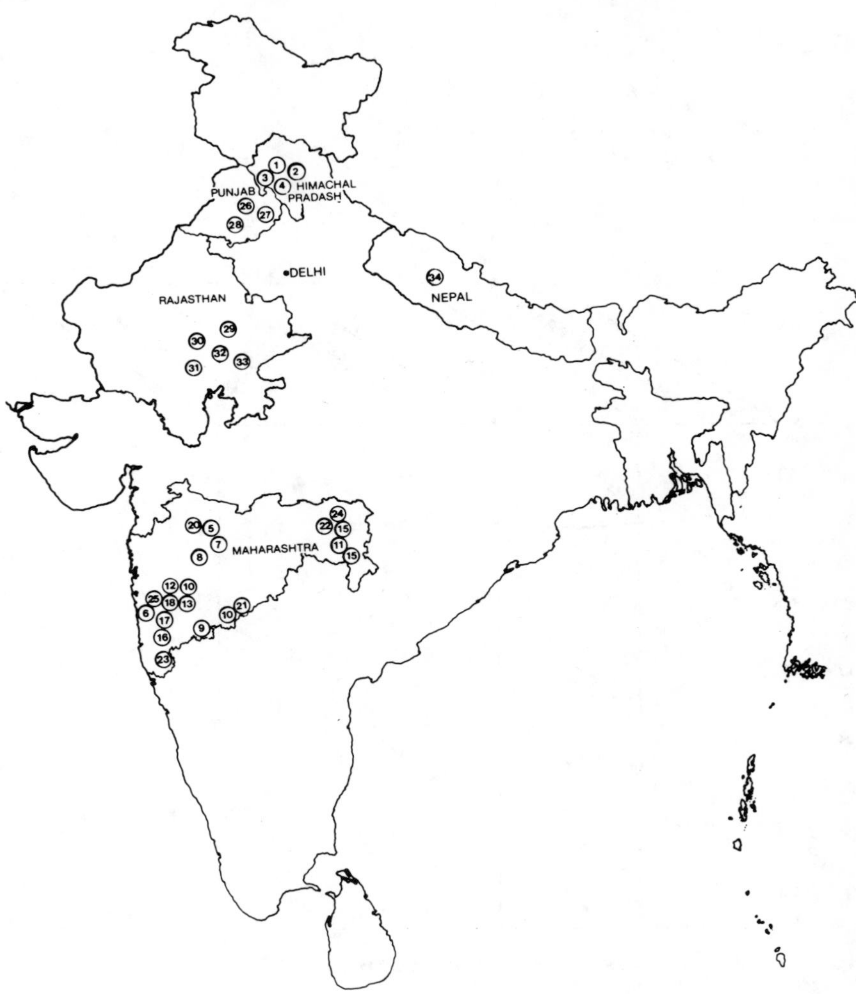

Fig. 1. Geographical location of the 34 human populations in the Indian sub-continent. The number within the circles correspond to the population numbers given in table 1.

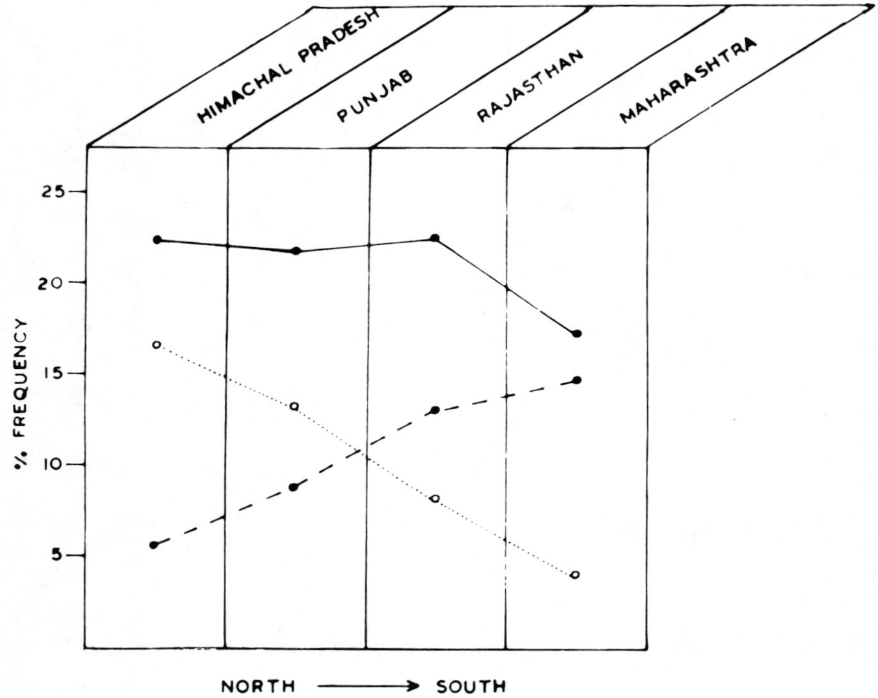

Fig. 2. Distribution of average frequencies of hypothenar triradii h^p (0....0) and h^{ext} (0---0) in four Indian states, arranged in the north-south axis. Note the progressive decrease in the frequency of h^p from north to south, and progressive increase in h^{ext} from north to south.

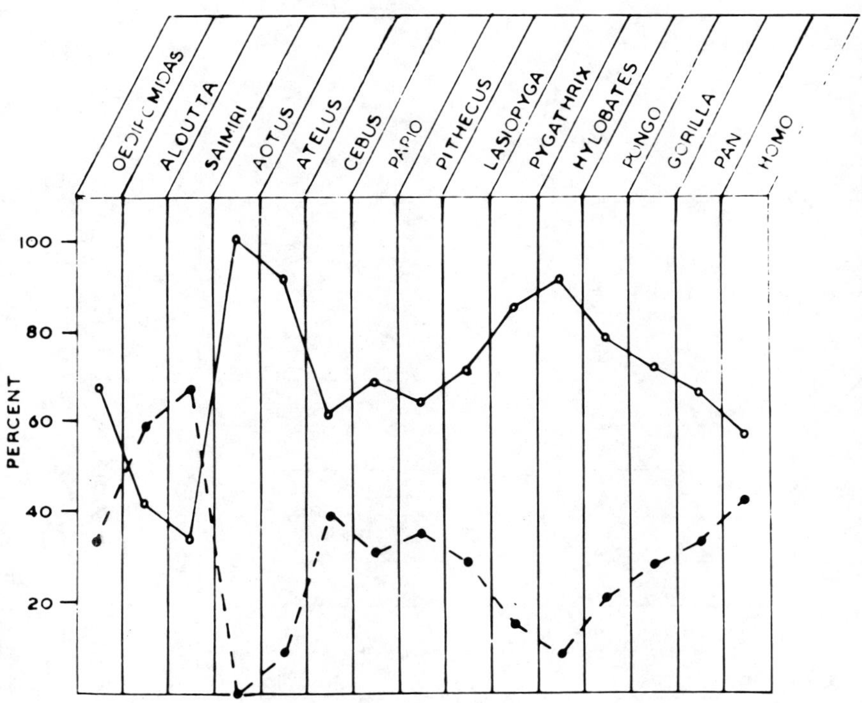

Fig. 3. Relative frequencies of hypothenar triradii h^p (0——0) and h^{ext} (0---0) among 14 non-human primates and man.

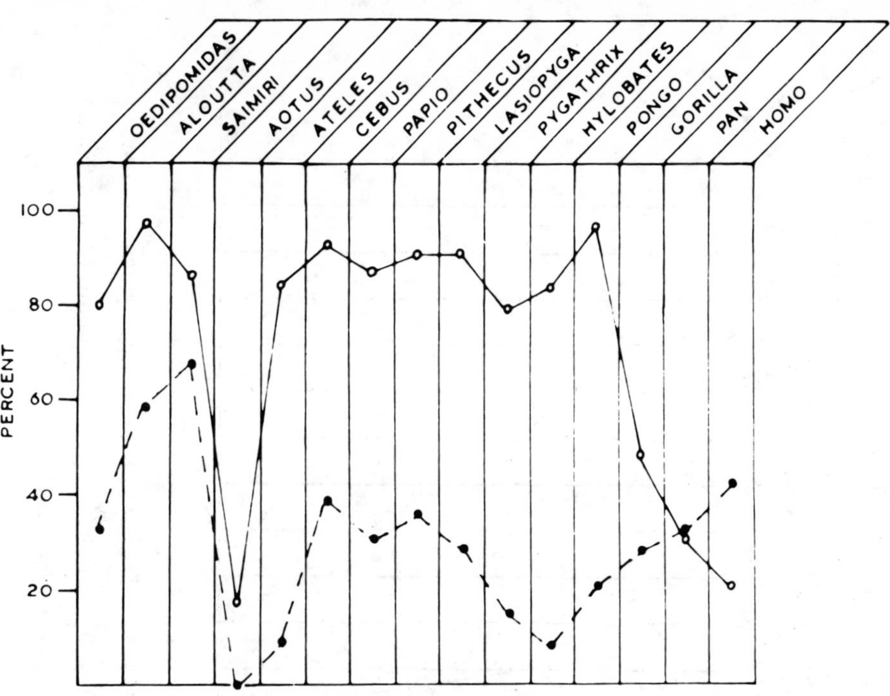

Fig. 4. Joint distribution of pattern intensities (0——0) after Midlo and Cummins, (1942), and hypothenar triradius h^{ext} (0----0) among 14 non-human primates and man.

Progress in Dermatoglyphic Research, pages 247-267

DIGITAL AND PALMAR DERMATOGLYPHICS IN GREEKS

C.S. BARTSOCAS[1], TH. PANAYOTOU[2], S. VARONOS[3], S. KRITSIKIS[2], C.C. PLATO[4] and C.J. PAPADATOS[1]

[1]2nd Department of Pediatrics, University of Athens, "P. & A. Kyriakou" Children's Hospital, Athens, Greece

[2]Department of Cardiology, University of Athens

[3]Athens Naval Hospital

[4]Gerontology Research Center, NIA, NIH, Baltimore City Hospitals, Baltimore, Maryland 21224, U.S.A.

INTRODUCTION

Information on dermatoglyphic frequencies among Greeks is minimal. It is composed of four studies. One by Margarite Weninger (1974), the other by D. F. Roberts (1965) on the island of Tinos, the third by C. C. Plato (1970) among Greeks of Cyprus. The fourth study deals with the frequencies of the Greeks of the Soviet Union (Heet 1982). In the present study we provide additional data by studying the dermatoglyphic frequencies of two Greek samples which differ in terms of region as well as age composition.

MATERIAL AND METHODS

The present study reports on the dermatoglyphics of two Greek samples. The first sample is composed of bilateral digital and palmar prints from 201 students (117 boys and 84 girls) under the age of 17 years. They were all military dependents born in various parts of Greece. The second sample was collected from 210 adults (93 men and 117 women) all residents of the island of Salamis. Only prints with bilaterally readable dermatoglyphic features were included in the analysis. The prints were evaluated for 1) digital pattern frequencies, 2) modal types of the C and D lines, 3) presence of palmar patterns in the hypothenar, thenar/I and the II, III, and IV interdigital areas of the palm, 4) presence of palmar accessory triradii, and 5) presence of simian or sydney palmar creases. We also studied the degree of bilateral symmetry in each of these traits. Male and female frequencies were done separately and separate comparisons were made for each sex and hand.

Dermatoglyphic prints were evaluated utilizing the standard methodology of Cummins and Midlo (1943). However, the classification of modal types of the C line and palmar pattern subtypes were those of Plato (1970) and Plato and Wertelecki (1972), respectively. Frequencies for all dermatoglyphic traits studied were calculated and presented separately by sex, hand, and bilateral symmetry. In this paper, we followed the same table format as that presented in our earlier publications (Plato et al., 1975 and Steinberg et al., 1975) allowing easier comparisons of the dermatoglyphics of Greeks with those of other populations. Statistical comparisons were carried out using chi-square contingency tables and Student's t-test.

RESULTS

In general the dermatoglyphic frequencies of the two regions are similar (table 1). Dermatoglyphic comparisons of the two male samples showed no significant differences in any of the variables studied. Comparisons of the female samples resulted in significant differences in digital pattern frequencies ($P < .01$), in frequencies of modal types of the D line ($P < .01$) and in frequencies of the sydney lines ($P < .05$). We cannot say at this time whether these three differences are due to random variation, to regional differences or due to differential age composition. In any way, we do not believe that the three significant differences among females are sufficient to provide dermatoglyphic discrimination between the Salamis and the random samples. Therefore, in the detailed analysis of the data and the presentation of bilateral results, we pooled the two regions into one Greek sample.

Dermatoglyphic frequencies of the Greeks are presented in tables 2-12. In the last table the results are summarized (left and right hands combined) for comparison with those of other caucasian populations. Our discussion in the text, on the observed dermatoglyphic frequencies, will be limited to those of the average of the two hands (table 12) unless otherwise stated.

Digital Patterns: Digital pattern frequencies and the pattern intensity index (PII) for male and female Greeks are given in Tables 2 and 12. The overall comparisons between males and females in arch, loop, and whorl frequencies (table 2) show no significant differences between sexes. The bilateral frequencies of the four main digital pattern types are presented, for each digit separately, in table 3. In this table, the pattern frequencies for each digit of the left hand are listed along the horizontal axis (rows), and those of the right hand along the vertical axis (columns). The values at each point of intersection between columns and rows give the frequencies of each pattern combination on the corresponding left and right hand digits of the same individual. All values along the diagonal indicate the percent bilateral symmetry. Values parallel to the diagonal give the frequencies of bilateral asymmetry. Values under the heading "left total" (sum of each row) and "right total" (sum of each column) give the total frequencies of each pattern for the left and right hands, respectively, regardless of bilateral symmetry. Tables 4, 5, 6 and 11 are read in the same manner. Among males, digit I shows the highest percentage of bilateral symmetry followed by digit V. Among females the highest percent of bilateral symmetry is seen in the V digit followed by digit IV. The largest differences in bilateral symmetry between males and females occur in digit I. The average percent bilateral symmetry for all digits, 74.1 for males and 73.6 for females, show little sex difference.

Table 4 illustrates the percent distribution of hands with none, one, two, three, four or five whorls bilaterally. The two extremes indicate that on the average 3.2% of the Greeks (2.7% of males and 3.6% of females) have all whorls on their fingers and 21.2% have no whorls at all. Frequencies of individuals with 2, 3,...9 whorls may also be derived by adding the appropriate intersects of the vertical and horizontal axes.

Main Line Terminations: The main line terminations were studied in terms of modal types of the C line (absent, proximal, ulnar, and radial), modal types of the D line (7,

9, and 11), and main line index (MLI). The results are presented in tables 5 and 12. Greek males have higher frequencies of radial modal types than ulnar types of the C line (table 5) with a moderately high radial/ulnar (R/U) ratio of 1.31. The R/U ratio of the females (0.80) is lower than that of the males (table 12). Bilateral distributions of C line modal types show the usually observed trends (Plato, 1970) in which right hands demonstrate higher frequencies of radial types than left hands, while left hands have higher frequencies of ulnar types than right hands. Eventhough there is no significant difference in the degree of total bilateral asymmetry between males and females, (table 5) there is significant difference ($P < .01$) between sexes in regards to the frequencies of the modal types of the C line (table 12).

The distribution of modal types of the D line (tables 6 and 12) also show the usually observed bilateral differences, with right hands having higher frequencies of type 11 at the expense of both types 7 and 9. Sex differences in D line modal types were statistically significant ($P < .05$) with the males having higher frequencies of type 11 and lower type 7 (table 12).

Palmar Patterns: The percent distribution of patterns in the hypothenar and thenar/I areas are presented in tables 7 and 12. In the hypothenar area, 40.2% of the palms of males and 38.1% of the palms of females have some type of pattern including vestiges. The frequency of hypothenar radial loops is 2 times higher than that of hypothenar ulnar loops. The frequency of all patterns in the thenar/I area is 12.4% in males and 14.1% in females. There are no significant bilateral or sex differences in the distribution of patterns in either the hypothenar or the thenar/I area.

The frequency of patterns in the II, III and IV interdigital areas are shown in tables 8 and 12. Males and females have similar frequencies (5.5% and 5.9%, respectively) of patterns in the II interdigital area (table 12) most of which are found in the right palms (table 8). The III interdigital area shows high frequencies of patterns most of which are radial loops (table 8). There are significant bilateral differences ($P < .01$) with the right III interdigital areas having higher frequencies of loops than the left. There is also significant difference between males and females with the former having more patterns in this area of the palm (table 12). A high frequency of patterns (59.5% among males and 66.8% among females), composed mainly of loops, is found in the IV interdigital area. The average frequency of ulnar and radial loops (both hands combined) are significantly different ($P < .05$) in males, who have more ulnar than radial loops but are not different in females (table 8). Table 9 presents the bilateral frequencies of patterns in the five palmar configurational areas. The highest frequency of bilateral patterns is found in the IV interdigital area of the females (25.7%) and the III interdigital area of the males (23.4%).

<u>Accessory Triradii</u>: The frequency of accessory triradii observed in the hypothenar (axial) and in the II, III, and IV interdigital areas are given in tables 10 and 12. Accessory triradii in the second and third interdigital areas are very rare and when present are unilateral. Accessory triradii are found most commonly in the hypothenar and IV interdigital areas with similar frequencies in males and females and left and right hands (table 10).

<u>Palmar Creases</u>: Bilateral frequencies for complete and aberrant simian and sydney creases are given in table 11. A complete simian crease is a single transverse crease, while a complete sydney crease is an extension of the proximal palmar crease to the ulnar margin of the palm. Aberrant types include all atypical forms of simian and sydney creases (Wertelecki, 1979). Sydney creases, complete as well as aberrant, are more prevalent in Greeks than simian creases and neither show significant bilateral or sex differences.

DISCUSSION

The average dermatoglyphic frequencies of the present Greek sample (males and females combined) were compared to those of other caucasian populations reported in the literature (table 13). Table 13 gives the digital pattern frequencies of the present sample "Greek", the range of frequencies (that is the lowest and highest) reported among South European and Mediterranean whites (Plato, unpublished data), which includes previously studied Greek samples, Italians, Turks, Spaniards and Jews. The arithmetic average of all samples studied is given in parenthesis. The same is done for all caucasians. These data were extracted from table 12 of the 1975 report on the dermatoglyphics of American Caucasians (Plato et al. 1975). All values in this table represent male and female frequencies combined. The digital frequencies of the present sample are 35.8% for whorls, 53.7% ulnar loops, 4.1% radial loops, 6.5% arches and pattern intensity index is 12.3%. These values are well within the range of the Mediterranean and Caucasian populations and very close to the average.

The frequencies of the modal types of the C line of the present Greek sample fall within the range of other white groups but the present sample has higher frequencies of proximal and ulnar types and lower frequencies of radial type than other South European samples. The distributions of the modal types of the D line also show differences between our sample and the other groups but the differences are not as large as those of the C line. The Greek sample has higher frequency of type 11 than other caucasian groups, whereas the main line index which is considered a very good indicator of palmar ridge transversality is very similar.

Comparisons of the frequencies of patterns in the hypothenar, thenar/I, the II, III and IV interdigital configurational areas show that the Greek sample has higher frequencies of patterns in the III and IV interdigital area but they too fall within the range of the more general Caucasian distributions. The next entry of table 13 shows the frequencies of palmar accessory triradii. The present sample has a very high frequency of accessory axial triradii in the hypothenar area. This was not a result of one sample or sex. Males and females of both samples as well as that of the two Cypriot samples reported earlier (Plato 1970) have very high frequency of accessory axial triradii. It is possible that this may be a diagnostic trait among Greeks. Our sample also has high frequencies of accessory triradii in the IV interdigital area, but not as pronounced as in the hypothenar. The last entry of table 13 presents the frequencies of palmar creases. The frequency of complete simian creases was 2.7%, which is relatively low, and for complete sydney creases 6.2%, which is higher than those of Greek Cypriots and other caucasians.

SUMMARY

The present study presents the dermatoglyphic frequencies of two samples from Greece. The first was obtained from adult male and female inhabitants of the island of Salamis. The second is a sample of school children from various parts of Greece. Comparisons of the dermatoglyphic frequencies of the two samples showed no significant differences among males. Female comparisons resulted in significant differences in digital pattern frequencies, modal types of the D line and Sydney creases. These three significant differences among females only, were not considered sufficient to provide dermatoglyphic discrimination between the two samples and therefore were pooled into one Greek sample.

In general the dermatoglyphic frequencies of the present Greek sample fell within the range of, and very close to the mean of, other Caucasian populations. Notable differences were observed, however, in the frequencies of accessory axial triradii and complete Sydney creases in both of which the Greeks had higher frequencies.

REFERENCES

Cummins H and Midlo C (1943). "Finger Prints, Palms and Soles." Philadelphia: Blackiston Co.

Heet H (1982). Dermatoglyphics of the Greeks. (Manuscript in preparation).

Plato CC (1970a). Dermatoglyphics and flexion creases of the Cypriots. Am J Phys Anthrop 33:421-428.

Plato CC (1970b). Polymorphism of the C line: with a new classification of the C line terminations. Am J Phys Anthrop 33:413-420.

Plato CC, Cereghino JJ and Steinberg FS (1975). The dermatoglyphics of American caucasians. Am J Phys Anthrop 42:195-210.

Plato CC and Wertelecki W (1972). A method for subclassifying the interdigital patterns: a comparative study of the palmar configurations. Am J Phys Anthrop 37:97-110.

Roberts DF (1965). Finger prints in a Greek sample. Man 65:21-22.

Steinberg FS, Cereghino JJ and Plato CC (1975). The dermatoglyphics of American Negroes. Am J Phys Anthrop 42:183-194.

Weninger M and Rothenbuchner G (1974). Fingerund Handabdrucke von Griechenb (Finger and palmar dermatoglyphics of Greeks). "Berolkerungsbiologie" S. 255-264.

Wertelecki W (1979). The simian and Sydney crease. In Wertelecki W and Plato CC (eds): "Dermatoglyphics -- Fifty Years Later," New York, Allan R. Liss, Inc., pp 455-471.

Table 1

Digital and Palmar Dermatoglyphic Pattern Frequency Comparisons between Greeks (RAN-random sample, SAL-salamis sample)

Average of Both Hands

	MALE		FEMALE	
	PERCENT		PERCENT	
	RAN	SAL	RAN	SAL
Finger Print Patterns				
Whorls	37.7	37.3	29.7	38.4
Ulnar Loops	52.2	52.6	57.6	51.4
Radial Loops	4.0	3.7	3.9	4.7
Arches	6.1	6.4	8.8	5.5
%Bilateral Symmetry				
I.P. Index	13.2	13.1	12.1	13.0
Modal Types of the C Line				
Absent	6.9	2.8	3.1	10.0
Proximal	17.2	8.5	6.1	10.0
Ulnar	33.2	37.7	51.2	43.3
Radial	42.7	50.9	39.6	36.7
Radial/Ulnar Ratio	1.29	1.35	0.77	0.85
Modal Types of the D Line				
7	13.5	13.9	24.7	17.2
9	35.2	25.9	38.6	28.1
11	51.3	60.2	36.7	54.7
11/7 Ratio	3.81	4.33	1.49	3.18
Main Line Index	8.86	9.28	8.24	9.42
Palmar Patterns				
Hypothenar	40.1	40.2	39.2	37.0
Thenar /I	13.8	10.4	11.0	17.3
II Interdigital	4.7	6.9	5.4	6.5
III Interdigital	62.1	60.4	45.7	48.3
IV Interdigital	60.8	56.6	70.1	62.5
Accessory Triradii				
Hypothenar (acial)	21.1	15.8	17.5	17.4
II Interdigital	3.0	5.6	3.0	1.2
III Interdigital	1.3	0	1.8	0.8
IV Interdigital	14.5	11.9	15.1	12.3
Palmar Creases				
Simian Complete	1.3	3.1	1.2	5.3
Simian Aberrant	1.3	3.1	1.2	5.3
Sydney Complete	7.6	5.9	6.0	7.5
Sydney Aberrant	4.2	5.9	6.6	5.0

Table 2. Percent Distribution of Digital Patterns and Pattern Intensity Index of Greeks

Pattern Types	Male (N = 205)			Female (N = 190)		
	Left Hand	Right Hand	Both Hands	Left Hand	Right Hand	Left Hands
All Arches	6.3	5.8	6.0	8.4	5.3	6.9
Plain	4.2	2.9	3.6	6.3	4.1	5.2
Tented	2.1	2.9	2.5	2.1	1.2	1.7
All Loops	59.4	53.6	56.5	58.7	59.4	59.1
Radial	2.9	4.0	3.5	5.2	3.3	4.2
Radial Transitional	0.2	0.5	0.4	0.2	0	0.1
Ulnar	53.7	46.0	49.8	50.7	53.3	52.0
Ulnar Transitional	2.6	3.1	2.8	2.6	2.8	2.7
All Whorls	34.4	40.5	37.5	32.9	35.2	34.1
Composite	5.4	5.9	5.7	4.0	5.8	4.9
Double Loop	3.8	2.4	3.1	3.6	1.7	2.7
Whorl	25.1	32.2	28.7	25.3	27.7	26.5
Pattern Intensity Index	6.06	6.47	12.53	5.91	6.27	12.18
S.E.	0.14	0.14	0.14	0.16	0.15	0.16

Table 3. Bilateral Percent Distribution of Digital Patterns of Greeks

		MALE (N = 205)					FEMALE (N = 190)				
		RIGHT HAND				Total	RIGHT HAND				Total
Digit	Hand and Pattern	Arch	Rad. Loop	Uln. Loop	Whorl	Left Hand	Arch	Rad. Loop	Uln. Loop	Whorl	Left Hand
I	Left Arch	3.1	0	2.5	0	5.6	1.2	0	1.8	0	3.0
	Left Radial Loop	0	0	0	0.6	0.6	0	0	0	0.6	0.6
	Left Ulnar Loop	0	0	36.8	13.5	50.3	0.6	0	38.4	14.0	53.0
	Left Whorl	0	0	1.8	41.7	43.5	0	0	11.6	31.7	43.3
	Total Right Hand	3.1	0	41.1	55.8	81.6*	1.8	0	51.8	46.3	71.3*
II	Left Arch	5.9	2.5	2.5	0	10.9	6.4	1.1	5.4	0.5	13.4
	Left Radial Loop	3.0	5.5	3.5	1.0	12.9	2.2	6.4	8.1	4.3	21.0
	Left Ulnar Loop	2.0	8.9	15.4	10.0	36.3	0	4.8	15.1	6.5	26.3
	Left Whorl	1.0	4.5	5.0	29.3	39.8	0.5	2.7	4.3	31.7	39.2
	Total Right Hand	11.9	21.4	26.4	40.3	56.1*	9.1	15.0	32.9	43.0	59.6*
III	Left Arch	3.9	0	4.4	0	8.3	5.5	0	7.6	0	13.1
	Left Radial Loop	0.5	0	1.0	0	1.5	0	0.5	2.2	0	2.7
	Left Ulnar Loop	3.0	0	54.2	8.4	65.6	1.6	0	54.1	6.6	62.3
	Left Whorl	0	0	7.4	17.2	24.6	0	0	7.7	14.2	21.9
	Total Right Hand	7.4	0	67.0	25.6	75.3*	7.1	0.5	71.6	20.8	74.3*
IV	Left Arch	3.0	0	0	0	3.0	3.3	0	4.5	0	7.8
	Left Radial Loop	0	0	0	0	0	0	0	0.6	0.6	1.2
	Left Ulnar Loop	0.5	0.5	33.5	14.0	48.5	0.6	0	36.3	9.5	46.4
	Left Whorl	0	0	6.5	42.0	48.5	0	0	6.7	38.0	44.7
	Total Right Hand	3.5	0.5	40.0	56.0	78.5*	3.9	0	48.1	48.1	77.6*
V	Left Arch	2.2	0	1.1	0	3.3	3.1	0	0.6	0	3.7
	Left Radial Loop	0	0	0	0	0	0	0	0	0	0
	Left Ulnar Loop	1.6	0	64.3	13.0	78.9	1.2	0	70.2	5.0	76.4
	Left Whorl	0	0	5.4	12.4	17.8	0	0	8.1	11.8	19.9
	Total Right Hand	3.8	0	70.8	25.4	78.9*	4.3	0	78.9	16.8	85.1*

* Sum of the diagonal Values (% Bilateral Symmetry)

Table 4. Bilateral Percent Distribution of the Number of Whorls per Hand Among the Greeks

Hand	Number of Whorls	Male (N = 205)							Female (N = 190)						
		Right Hand						Left Hand Total	Right Hand						Left Hand Total
		0	1	2	3	4	5		0	1	2	3	4	5	
Left Hand	0	19.6	6.8	3.4	0.7	0	0	30.5	22.9	4.3	2.9	0.7	0	0	30.8
	1	3.4	12.2	6.1	1.4	2.0	0	25.1	7.1	5.0	6.4	0.7	0	0.7	19.9
	2	0.7	3.4	3.4	4.0	2.7	0	14.2	1.4	2.1	4.3	5.7	2.1	0	15.6
	3	0	0.7	1.4	4.0	5.4	2.0	13.5	0.7	2.9	5.0	2.9	2.1	1.4	15.0
	4	0	0.7	2.0	2.0	4.0	4.0	12.7	0	0	0.7	2.9	4.3	1.4	9.3
	5	0	0	0	1.4	0	2.7	4.1	0	0	0	3.6	2.1	3.6	9.3
Right Hand	Total	23.7	23.8	16.3	13.5	14.1	8.7	45.9*	32.1	14.3	19.3	16.4	10.7	7.1	43.0*

* Sum of the diagonal values (% Bilateral Symmetry)

Table 5. Bilateral Percent Distribution of the Modal Types of the C Line of Greeks

Hand Modal Type	Male (N = 205)					Female (N = 190)				
	Right Hand				Left	Right Hand				Left
	Absent	Proximal	Ulnar	Radial	Hand Total	Absent	Proximal	Ulnar	Radial	Hand Total
Left Absent	4.1	0	0	0.6	4.7	2.1	0	1.4	2.8	6.3
Left Proximal	0	3.6	0.6	15.4	19.6	0	0	4.9	8.5	13.4
Left Ulnar	1.2	5.3	20.1	18.3	44.9	3.5	1.4	31.7	16.9	53.5
Left Radial	1.2	0.6	3.6	25.4	30.8	0	0.7	4.2	21.8	26.8
Right Total Hand	6.5	9.5	24.3	59.7	53.2*	5.6	2.1	42.2	50.0	55.6*

* Sum of the diagonal Values (% Bilateral Symmetry)

Table 6. Bilateral Percent Distribution of the Modal Type of the D Line of Greeks

Hand	Modal Type	Male (N = 205) Right Hand 7	Male Right Hand 9	Male Right Hand 11	Male Left Hand Total	Female (N = 190) Right Hand 7	Female Right Hand 9	Female Right Hand 11	Female Left Hand Total
Left	7	5.3	6.5	5.9	17.7	8.2	11.	7.5	27.2
Left	9	1.8	10.6	32.0	44.4	6.1	10.2	25.2	41.5
Left	11	2.4	3.0	32.5	37.9	1.3	4.8	25.2	31.3
Right Total		9.5	20.1	70.4	48.4*	15.6	26.5	57.9	43.6*

* Sum of the diagonal Values (% Bilateral Symmetry)

Table 7. Percent Distribution of Patterns in the Hypothenar and Thenar/I Areas of the Palms of Greeks

A

H Y P O T H E N A R						
	Male (N = 198)			Female (N = 164)		
Type of Pattern	Left	Right	Both	Left	Right	Both
Open/Arch	60.1	59.6	59.8	65.9	57.9	61.9
Vestige	0.5	1.5	1.0	0.6	3.1	1.8
Single Loop	37.4	34.9	36.7	31.7	29.9	30.8
Ulnar	12.1	9.6	10.9	10.4	6.1	8.2
Radial	21.2	18.7	20.0	17.1	19.5	18.3
Distal	3.0	5.6	4.3	3.0	2.5	2.8
Proximar	1.0	1.0	1.0	1.2	1.8	1.5
Double Loop	1.5	2.5	2.0	1.8	6.7	4.3
Whorl	0.5	1.5	1.0	0	2.4	1.2

B

T H E N A R / I				
	Male (N = 205)		Female (N = 190)	
Type of Pattern	Left	Right	Left	Right
Open/Arch	82.8	92.5	84.0	87.8
Vestige	7.1	2.0	2.5	1.8
Loop	5.1	2.5	4.9	1.8
Loop/Vestige	2.5	2.5	2.5	3.7
Loop/Loop	1.5	0	4.3	4.3
Whorl	1.0	0.5	1.8	0.6

Table 8. Percent Distribution of Patterns in Interdigital Areas II, III, and IV of Greeks

Type of Pattern	Male (N = 205)						Female (N = 190)					
	II Interdigital		III Iterdigital		IV Interdigital		II Interdigital		III Interdigital		IV Interdigital	
	Left	Right	Left	Right	Left	Right	Left	Right	Left	Right	Left	Right
Open/Arch	97.4	91.7	48.5	28.4	25.4	55.6	97.5	90.6	57.0	49.3	25.4	40.9
Vestige	0.6	2.2	20.7	10.7	20.7	8.9	1.3	3.8	14.8	3.5	14.1	3.5
Loops	2.2	5.9	30.8	61.0	53.9	35.5	1.2	5.6	28.2	47.2	60.5	55.6
Ulnar	0	1.6	0.6	1.2	24.9	14.8	0	0.6	0	2.8	22.5	26.1
Radial	0	0	29.6	58.0	14.2	10.6	0.6	1.2	26.1	43.0	22.5	15.5
Adjacent	0	0	0	0.6	3.0	0.6	0	0	0	0.7	4.2	1.4
Ulnar/Radial	0	0	0	0	1.2	0	0	0	0	0	0	0
Accessory/Triradius	0.6	1.6	0.6	1.2	4.1	7.1	0	0	0.7	0	1.4	6.3
Triradius/Ulnar	1.6	2.7	0	0	0	0	0.6	3.8	0.7	0	0.7	0
Triradius/Radial	0	0	0	0	6.5	2.4	0	0	0.7	0	7.8	5.6
Whorl	0	0	0	0	0	0	0	0	0	0.7	1.4	0.7

Table 9. Bilateral Percent Distribution of Palmar Patterns in the Hypothenar, and Thenar/I, and the II, III, and IV Interdigital Areas of the Palms of Greeks

Presence of Patterns	Male (N = 205)					Female (N = 190)				
	Hypothenar	Thenar/I	II	III	IV	Hypothenar	Thenar/I	II	III	IV
BOTH PALMS										
Absent	22.2	40.7	45.6	11.8	10.4	24.7	41.4	45.3	19.0	8.8
Present	12.3	3.1	1.1	23.4	19.9	12.8	5.5	1.2	15.9	25.7
Same Pattern	9.3	1.8	0.3	13.6	9.8	6.4	1.2	0.3	9.2	8.8
Different Pattern	3.0	1.3	0.8	9.8	10.1	6.4	4.3	0.9	6.7	16.9
ONE PALM ONLY										
Left	19.7	5.1	1.4	25.7	37.3	16.8	6.7	1.3	21.5	37.3
Right	19.4	2.8	4.1	35.9	22.2	19.5	5.2	4.7	25.4	29.6

Table 10. Percent Distribution of Accessory Triradii in the Hypothenar and the Interdigital Areas of the Palms of Greeks

Palmar Area	Male (N = 205)			Female (N = 190)		
	Left Hand Only	Right Hand Only	Both Hands Average	Left Hand Only	Right Hand Only	Both Hands Average
Hypothenar (axial)	18.7	18.7	18.7	16.0	18.4	17.2
II Interdigital	2.1	5.8	4.0	0.6	3.7	2.2
III Interdigital	0.6	1.1	0.8	2.0	0.7	1.4
IV Interdigital	15.9	11.4	13.6	12.8	14.9	13.8

Table 11. Bilateral Percent Distribution of the Simian and Sydney Palmar Creases in Greeks

SIMIAN CREASE

Male (N = 205)					Female (N = 190)				
Hand-Type	Right Normal	Right Aberrant	Right Complete	Left Total	Hand-type	Right Normal	Right Aberrant	Right Complete	Left Total
Left Normal	94.8	0	0	94.8	Left Normal	93.0	1.0	1.0	95.0
Left Aberrant	2.2	0	0.8	3.0	Left Aberrant	2.0	0	0	2.0
Left Complete	2.2	0	0	2.2	Left Complete	2.0	1.0	0	3.0
Right Total	99.2	0	0.8	94.8*	Right Total	97.1	2.0	1.0	93.0*

SYDNEY CREASE

Male (N = 205)					Female (N = 190)				
Hand-type	Right Normal	Right Aberrant	Right Complete	Left Total	Hand-type	Right Normal	Right Aberrant	Right Complete	Left Total
Left Normal	82.4	2.2	3.7	88.3	Left Normal	78.6	6.8	6.8	92.2
Left Aberrant	2.2	0.7	0.7	3.6	Left Aberrant	1.0	1.0	1.0	3.0
Left Complete	3.7	2.2	2.2	8.1	Left Complete	2.9	1.9	0	4.8
Right Total	88.3	5.1	6.6	82.4*	Right Total	82.5	9.7	7.8	79.6*

* Sum of the diagonal values (% Bilateral Symmetry)

Table 12. Frequency of Digital and Palmar Dermatoglyphic Patterns in Greeks

Dermatoglyphic Feature	Percentages Male	Percentages Female
Finger Print Patterns		
Whorls	37.5	34.1
Ulnar Loops	52.7	54.7
Radial Loops	3.8	4.3
Arches	6.0	6.9
%Bilateral Symmetry		
P.I. Index	12.5	12.2
Modal Types of the C Line		
Absent 0	5.6	6.0
Proximal 1	14.5	7.8
Ulnar 2	34.6	47.9
Radial 3	45.3	38.4
Radial/Ulnar Ratio	1.31	0.80
Modal Types of the D Line		
7	13.6	21.4
9	32.3	34.0
11	54.1	44.6
11/7 Ratio	3.98	2.08
Main Line Index	9.03	8.85
Palmar Patterns		
Hypothenar	40.2	38.1
Thenar /I	12.4	14.1
II Interdigital	5.5	5.9
III Interdigital	61.5	46.8
IV Interdigital	59.5	66.9
Accessory Triradii		
Hypothenar (axial)	18.7	17.2
II Interdigital	4.0	2.1
III Interdigital	0.9	1.4
IV Interdigital	13.6	13.9
Palmar Creases		
Simian		
Complete	1.5	2.0
Aberrant	1.5	2.0
Sydney		
Complete	7.4	6.3
Aberrant	4.4	6.3

TABLE 13. DIGITAL AND PALMAR DERMATOGLYPHIC PATTERN FREQUENCIES COMPARISONS BETWEEN GREEKS & OTHER CAUCASIAN POPULATIONS.*

DERMATOGLYPHIC FEATURE	GREEK	S.EUROPE & MEDITERRANEAN[1]		ALL CAUCASIANS[2]	
	MEAN	RANGE	MEAN	RANGE	MEAN
FINGER PRINT PATTERNS					
WHORLS	35.8	27-42	(34.5)	26-49	(37.5)
ULNAR LOOPS	53.7	51-64	(57.9)	50-66	(58.0)
RADIAL LOOPS	4.1	4-6	(5.3)	4-7	(5.3)
ARCHES	6.5	2-8	(5.1)	2-9	(5.5)
P.I. INDEX	12.3	12-14	(13.0)	11-14	(12.7)
MODAL TYPES OF THE C-LINE					
ABSENT	5.8	3-7	(5.0)	3-12	(7.5)
PROXIMAL	11.2	1-14	(7.5)	1-16	(8.5)
ULNAR	41.3	24-37	(30.3)	24-58	(41.0)
RADIAL	41.9	43-62	(52.7)	31-62	(46.5)
MODAL TYPES OF THE D-LINE					
7	17.5	12-26	(19.0)	11-26	(18.5)
9	33.1	32-48	(40.0)	28-48	(38.0)
11	49.4	30-51	(40.5)	30-59	(44.5)
MAIN LINE INDEX	8.9	8-10	(9.0)	7-10	(8.5)
PALMAR PATTERNS					
HYPOTHENAR	39.2	34-52	(43.0)	21-52	(36.5)
THENAR/I	13.3	6-15	(10.5)	6-20	(13.0)
II INTERDIGITAL	5.7	3-11	(7.0)	0-11	(5.5)
III INTERDIGITAL	54.2	40-58	(49.0)	25-58	(41.5)
IV INTERDIGITAL	63.2	51-64	(57.5)	37-68	(52.5)
ACCESSORY TRIRADII					
HYPOTHENAR (AXIAL)	18.0	5-7	(6.0)	5-12	(8.5)
II INTERDIGITAL	3.1	0-7	(3.5)	0-7	(3.5)
III INTERDIGITAL	1.2	1-4	(2.5)	1-4	(2.5)
IV INTERDIGITAL	13.8	7-16	(11.5)	7-16	(11.5)

*See text for explanation

[1]From Plato unpublished data

[2]From Plato et al 1975

Progress in Dermatoglyphic Research, pages 269-284

GENETICAL VARIATION IN PALMAR FEATURES

NASR F. ABDULLAH

Dept. of Biology, College of Education,
Baghdad University,
Baghdad - IRAQ.

INTRODUCTION

The existence of genetic variation in the population of Iraq was suggested in the digital features (Roberts & Abdullah 1979). But the quantitative palmar features do not show such apparent variation between regions. Yet there is no information about the palmar qualitative features in Iraq. It is of interest therefore to put on record the results of the qualitative palmar features in this country. Several comparisons have been made in order to know whether these dermatoglyphic features can provide any relevant information. For instance, comparisons between unrelated normal samples in the main geographical regions in the country; comparisons between unrelated and related normal samples in Baghdad; as well as between overall unrelated series in Iraq and the similar recorded data for the population in Lebanon (Naffah, 1974). Moreover comparison has been made between overall unrelated series in Iraq and a widely different population in Northumbria which is situated in the North East of England.

On the other hand, the study of palmar features has clinical and diagnostic importance in certain diseases. In this case a group of patients with a particular abnormality can be compared with their normal relatives and with the random controls in the same local geographical region. The purpose of such comparisons is to find some clues to etiology or early diagnosis. For instance Walker (1958)was able to diagnose Mongolism by means of dermatoglyphics only. Roberts et al (1978) found a reduction of palmar patterns in the dermatitis herpetiformis patients as compared with the controls. This indicates a retardation in the development of dermal ridges in the patients. It seems that the present analysis of palmar features could serve as a control for the comparison with the dermatoglyphics of the diseases in this country.

MATERIALS AND METHODS

Palmar prints were obtained from unrelated and related individuals in Iraq. Records on age and birth place of each individual and his parents were taken. The ages in the unrelated series ranged from 6-47 years; whilst the age range in the related series is more wide. From the information in these records each subject of the 107 unrelated individuals was assigned to appropriate geographical area. There were four regional samples. Two represent the southern part of the country, one collected from the shatt Al Arab area (13 males and 12 females) on the east bank of the river, the other from Basrah (23 males and 14 females) on west bank of the shatt Al Arab river, the third sample (20 males and 10 females) originated from Baghdad and the surrounding areas, and the fourth sample derived mainly from Mosul in the northern part of Iraq consisted of 15 males only. The related series consisted of 94 members (52 males and 42 females) of the Al - Mulali sect of the Alanga tribe in Baghdad. All of whom were apparently healthy at the time of the survey.

Palmar prints were obtained from both hands by the Kleenprint method. Then, each palm was analysed using the methods described by Cummins & Midlo (1943), and Penrose & Loesch (1970).

The palmar traits which have been analysed in the present study are the patterns in the four interdigital areas including thenar and hypothenar areas. Additionally, the palmar main line terminations and the palmar axial triradii had been also analysed.

RESULTS

1. Palmar patterns.

Frequencies of palmar patterns in the thenar/1st interdigital areas (Th/I_1), second interdigital area (I_2), third interdigital area (I_3), and fourth interdigital area (I_4) of the random and tribal series are set out in (Table 1). Bimanual differences in the incidence of palmar patterning in these areas were found in both sexes. Left hands showed higher incidence of patterns in Th/I_1 and I_4; whilst the right hands showed higher incidence of patterning in I_2 and I_3.

a. Comparisons among the unrelated samples in Iraq. There is no significant regional difference in the occurrence of these palmar interdigital patterns in both hands combined among the unrelated samples, neither in males nor in females sampled.

b. Comparisons between unrelated and tribal samples. In Th/I_1 areas, patterns (including vestiges) in both hands combined of the females in the tribal series are significantly higher than in the unrelated series (13 out of 84 and 4 out of 72 respectively; $X^2=3.94$, $P<0.05$). In I_2 and I_3 there is no significant difference in any comparison, but in I_4, patterns (excluding vestiges) in both hands combined of the males in the tribal series are significantly higher than in the unrelated series (68 out of 104 and 74 out of 142 respectively; $X^2=4.33$, $P<0.05$). This amount of differences indicate the existence of heterogeneity between the random and tribal series in Iraq.

c. Comparisons between Iraqi and Lebanese populations. Th/1 and I_3 areas in Iraqi males showed significantly higher incidence of patterns as compared with the Lebanese males. But there is no significant difference between females in both populations. In Th/1 areas, patterns in both hands combined in the Iraqi males are significantly higher than in the Lebanese males (21 out of 142 and 30 out of 480 respectively; $X^2=10.63$, $P<0.01$). In I_3 patterns in right and left hands combined in the Iraqi males are significantly higher than in the Lebanese males (84 out of 142 and 200 out of 480 respectively; $X^2=13.51$, $P<0.001$).

d. Continental Variations. The overall unrelated series in Iraq was compared with a widely different population in Northumbria which is situated in the North East of England.

Table 1

Distribution of palmar interdigital patterns in Iraq

	RANDOM SERIES														ALANGA TRIBE			
	S.Al-Arab				Basrah				Baghdad				Mosul		Baghdad			
	M=13		F=12		M=23		F=14		M=20		F=10		M=15		M=52		F=42	
Th/1	R	L	R	L	R	L	R	L	R	L	R	L	R	L	R	L	R	L
V	1	-	1	-	1	1	-	-	-	1	-	-	-	-	1	2	4	1
L	-	-	-	-	-	-	-	-	1	1	-	-	-	-	2	-	-	-
W	-	-	-	-	-	-	-	-	1	-	-	-	-	-	-	1	-	1
O/L	-	-	-	-	-	-	-	-	-	-	-	-	-	1	-	1	-	-
L/V	-	-	-	-	-	1	-	-	-	1	-	-	1	-	2	2	-	-
L/L	-	-	-	1	1	2	-	-	-	-	-	-	-	-	-	-	-	-
L^c/L	-	-	-	1	-	-	-	-	-	2	-	-	-	1	-	1	1	2
L^c	-	-	-	-	-	-	-	-	-	1	-	-	2	-	1	-	-	1
L^c/V	-	-	-	-	-	-	-	1	1	-	-	-	-	-	1	-	2	-
w/v	-	-	-	-	-	-	-	-	-	-	-	-	-	-	-	1	-	-
w/L	-	-	-	-	-	-	-	-	-	-	-	-	-	-	-	1	-	1
												-		-				
All	1	-	1	2	2	4	-	1	3	6	-	-	3	2	7	9	7	6
0	12	13	11	10	21	19	14	13	17	14	10	10	12	13	45	43	35	36

I2																		
D	1	-	1	-	3	2	-	-	4	3	-	-	1	1	4	1	4	2
0	12	13	11	12	20	21	14	14	16	17	10	10	14	14	48	51	38	40
I3																		
T	1	5	-	2	4	6	1	4	2	5	1	2	2	-	7	9	4	5
l	-	-	-	1	1	-	-	1	1	1	-	-	2	-	-	2	1	-
L	5	3	6	1	12	6	6	2	13	3	5	1	7	4	21	8	21	8
D	-	-	-	-	-	-	-	-	1	-	-	-	-	-	1	-	2	1
W	-	-	-	1	-	-	-	-	-	-	-	-	-	-	-	1	-	1
All	6	8	6	5	17	12	7	7	17	9	6	3	11	4	29	20	26	15
0	7	5	6	7	6	11	7	7	3	11	4	7	4	11	23	32	14	27
I4																		
L	7	3	5	5	6	5	5	6	4	6	3	4	4	7	15	26	11	17
D	-	2	2	3	5	3	2	1	5	6	-	-	2	2	8	12	11	12
L/D	-	1	-	-	-	1	-	-	-	1	-	1	-	1	3	2	-	1
IV^u	-	-	-	-	-	1	-	-	-	-	-	-	-	-	-	-	-	-
l	-	-	-	-	-	-	-	-	-	-	-	-	-	1	-	-	-	-
d	-	-	-	-	-	-	-	-	-	-	-	-	-	-	1	-	-	-
l/D	-	-	-	1	-	-	-	-	-	-	-	-	-	1	-	-	-	-
l/d	-	-	-	-	-	-	-	-	-	-	-	-	-	-	1	-	-	-
All	7	6	7	9	11	10	7	7	9	13	3	5	6	12	28	40	22	30
0*	6	7	5	3	12	13	7	7	11	7	7	5	9	3	24	12	20	12

* including vestiges

M = males; F = females; R = right; L = left

Th = thenar; I = interdigital; 0 = unpatterned

The Iraq sample showed higher incidence of patterns in Th/1, I_2 and I_4 as compared with the English population particularly in males. In Th/1 area, patterns in the Iraqi males are significantly higher than in the Northumbrian males, but not in females (21 out of 142 and 10 out of 216 respectively; X^2=11.16, P<0.001). In I_2 area, patterns in the Iraqi population are significantly higher than in the Northumbrian population. For both sexes (16 out of 214 and 14 out of 440 respectively; X^2=6.06, P<0.02). In I_3 there is no significant difference between both populations, though it contains rather lower frequency of patterns in Iraqis. In I_4 area there is significant difference in males only. They showed higher incidence of patterns as compared with the Northumbrian males (74 out of 142 and 85 out of 216 respectively; X^2=5.64, P<0.02).

2. Hypothenar patterns.

Number of hypothenar patterns by hand and sex in the four unrelated samples as well as in the tribal sample are set out in Table 2. Patterns in this area had been classified according to Penrose method, in addition to the known rules of palmar classification (Cummins and Midlo, 1943). Unlike other palmar areas, there is no remarkable difference between right and left hands in the occurrence of patterns. There is no significant regional variation among unrelated samples and also between these overall unrelated samples and tribal sample. Similarly, there is non significant variation between Iraq and Lebanese populations from one side and Iraq and Northumbriam population on the other.

3. Palmar main lines.

Terminations of main lines A and D by hand and sex in the four unrelated series and tribal series are set out in Table 3. Those concerned lines B and C are set out in Table 4.

a. Regional variation. Line C in right and left hands combined of the males in Mosul showed significantly lower incidence in X, x and o terminations and relatively higher incidence in other terminations as compared with the other pooled unrelated samples (3 out of 30 and 34 out of 112 respectively; X^2=5.1, P<0.05).

b. Variation between unrelated and tribal series. Comparisons have been made between particular exits of main line (sum both hands) in the overall unrelated series and tribal series. The males in the latter showed significantly higher incidence in (1-5) exits of line B as compared with the males in the unrelated series (68 out of 104 and 67 out of 142 respectively; $X^2=8.03$, $P<0.01$). The males in the tribal series also showed significantly higher incidence of Line D exits in position 9 by comparison with the unrelated series (47 out of 104 and 45 out of 142 respectively; $X^2=4.68$, $P<0.05$). But there is no significant variation between female samples in these main line exits. Lines A and C did not show such pronounced variation between these samples neither in males nor in females.

c. Continental variation. The Iraqi unrelated females showed significantly higher incidence in (1-5) exits of line B as compared with the Northumbrian females (37 out of 72 and 83 out of 222 respectively; $X^2=4.41$, $P<0.05$). But there is neither significant difference between females in the exits of the remaining main lines, nor between males in the exits of all main lines (A, B, C and D).

4. Palmar axial triradii.

Positions of the axial triradii t, t' and t" and their combinations by hand and sex in the unrelated and tribal series are set out in Table 5. Position t' is situated above the normal position of t, but below the more distally replaced triradius t". Combinations of t t', t t" and t t' t" triradial expression have been found in the present analysed samples, whilst the triradial suppression has been found on the right palm of a male in the tribal series. The single expression of triradius t has been compared with the expression of other types of triradii in the unrelated samples, no significant difference was found. Similarly there was no significant difference between overall unrelated and tribal series in this comparison.

DISCUSSION

Results of the present qualitative analysis provide dermatoglyphic information from Iraq. There are as yet

Table 2

Distribution of palmar hypothenar features in Iraq

		S. Al-Arab				Basrah				Baghdad				Mosul		Alanga Triba			
		M =13		F =12		M =23		F =14		M =20		F =10		M =15		M =22		F =42	
Marker	P	R	L	R	L	R	L	R	L	R	L	R	L	R	L	R	L	R	L
L^u	H-	-	1	-	-	1	1	-	-	1	1	-	-	-	-	-	-	1	1
A^u/L^u	H-	1	2	-	1	1	1	-	-	3	1	-	-	1	1	3	2	2	3
V/L^u	H-	-	-	-	-	-	1	-	-	-	-	-	-	-	-	-	-	-	-
A^c/L^u	H-	-	-	-	-	-	-	-	1	-	-	-	-	-	-	2	2	-	-
T^r/L^u	H-	-	-	-	-	-	-	-	-	1	-	-	-	-	-	-	-	-	-
L^u/L^u	H^2	-	-	-	-	-	1	-	-	-	-	-	-	-	-	-	-	-	-
L^r/L^u	HH	-	-	1	-	-	1	-	1	-	1	-	-	-	-	1	1	1	-
W	HH	-	-	-	-	-	-	-	-	-	-	1	-	2	-	-	-	1	-
W^s	HH	-	-	-	-	-	-	-	1	-	-	-	-	-	-	-	-	-	-
W^d	HH	-	-	-	-	-	-	-	-	-	-	1	-	-	-	1	-	1	2
A^u/W^s	HH	-	-	-	-	1	-	-	-	-	-	-	-	-	-	-	-	-	-
W/L^u	H^2H	-	-	-	-	-	-	-	-	-	-	-	1	-	-	-	-	-	-
Total	H-	1	3	1	1	3	6	-	3	5	3	2	1	3	1	7	5	6	6

L^r	-H	3	2	2	2	2	4	2	2	1	3	3	3	2	4	6	10	8	9
L^r/A^c	-H	1	-	1	1	-	-	1	1	1	2	1	-	-	1	1	1	1	2
L^c	H^r-	-	1	1	-	-	-	1	-	1	-	-	-	-	-	-	-	1	-
A^u	H^r-	-	-	-	-	-	-	-	-	-	-	-	-	-	-	1	-	-	-
Total	H^r+H	4	3	5	3	3	5	4	5	3	6	6	4	4	5	9	13	13	13
A^u		7	7	6	4	12	11	7	6	7	8	2	3	7	7	27	23	17	17
A^c	o	-	-	-	-	1	-	1	1	-	-	1	-	-	-	1	-	1	-
A^r	t	-	-	-	-	-	-	-	-	-	-	-	-	-	-	1	-	-	-
A^u A^c	h	-	-	1	2	5	3	2	1	4	4	1	2	3	1	7	10	6	6
T^r	e	1	-	-	-	-	-	-	-	-	-	-	-	-	-	-	-	-	-
V	r	-	-	-	-	-	-	-	-	1	-	-	1	-	1	2	2	1	2
V/A^c	s	-	-	-	1	-	-	-	-	-	-	-	-	-	-	-	-	1	-
O		-	-	-	1	-	-	-	-	-	-	-	-	-	-	-	-	-	-
		8	7	7	8	18	14	10	8	12	12	4	6	10	9	38	35	26	25

P = Penrose classification; M = males; F = females; L = left

Table 3

Terminations of the palmar main lines A & D in the population of Iraq

	Unkelated Series																		Alanga Tribe			
	S. Al-Arab				Basrah				Baghdad				Mosul		Overall				Baghdad			
Main	M=13		F=12		M=23		F=14		M=20		F=10		M=15		M=71		F=36		M=52		F=42	
line exits	R	L	R	L	R	L	R	L	R	L	R	L	R	L	R	L	R	L	R	L	R	L
Line A																						
1	-	1	-	1	-	4	-	-	-	4	-	1	-	-	-	9	-	2	-	1	-	1
2	-	-	-	-	-	-	-	-	-	-	-	-	-	1	-	1	-	-	-	-	-	-
3	2	4	4	3	3	6	-	6	4	8	-	4	5	5	14	23	4	13	9	26	2	11
4	1	3	-	3	2	5	-	1	-	-	1	1	-	2	3	10	1	5	4	1	3	4
5′	9	4	6	5	14	7	13	7	14	7	8	4	10	7	47	25	27	16	36	23	35	25
5″	1	1	2	-	4	1	1	-	2	1	1	-	-	-	7	3	4	-	3	1	2	1
6	-	-	-	-	-	-	-	-	-	-	-	-	-	-	-	-	-	-	-	-	-	-
7	-	-	-	-	-	-	-	-	-	-	-	-	-	-	-	-	-	-	-	-	-	-

Line D																						
0	-	-	-	-	-	-	-	-	-	-	-	-	-	-	-	-	-	-	-	-	-	1
7	1	1	2	4	1	3	1	4	-	4	-	1	2	3	4	11	3	9	4	14	2	10
8	-	-	-	-	2	1	1	-	-	-	-	-	1	-	3	1	1	-	2	1	4	3
9	1	7	3	3	4	10	4	3	5	8	5	5	-	10	10	35	12	11	21	26	15	20
10	-	-	-	1	-	1	-	2	2	2	-	1	1	-	3	3	-	4	-	1	2	1
11	11	5	7	4	16	8	8	5	13	6	5	3	11	2	51	21	20	12	24	10	19	7
13	-	-	-	-	-	-	-	-	-	-	-	-	-	-	-	-	-	-	-	-	-	-
X	-	-	-	-	-	-	-	-	-	-	-	-	-	-	-	-	-	-	-	-	-	-

M = Males; F = females; R = right; L = left

Table 4

Terminations of the palmar main lines B & C in the population of Iraq

	Unrelated Series																		Alanga Tribe			
Region	S.Al-Arab				Basrah				Baghdad				Mosul		Overall				Baghdad			
Main	M=13		F=12		M=23		F=14		M=20		F=10		M=15		M=71		F=36		M=52		F=42	
line exits	R	L	R	L	R	L	R	L	R	L	R	L	R	L	R	L	R	L	R	L	R	L
Line B																						
1	-	-	-	-	-	-	-	-	-	-	-	-	-	-	-	-	-	-	-	-	-	-
2	-	-	-	-	-	-	-	-	-	-	-	-	-	-	-	-	-	-	-	-	-	-
3	-	-	-	-	-	-	-	-	-	-	-	-	-	1	-	1	-	-	-	-	1	-
4	-	-	-	-	-	1	-	-	-	-	-	-	-	-	-	1	-	-	-	-	-	-
5′	-	1	-	3	1	6	-	2	-	1	-	-	2	1	3	9	-	5	1	10	1	4
5"	3	7	5	5	7	8	6	5	5	11	5	6	1	11	16	37	16	26	26	31	18	31
6	-	-	-	1	-	1	-	2	2	2	-	1	1	-	3	3	-	4	-	1	1	-
7	9	5	7	3	15	7	6	5	13	6	5	2	10	12	47	20	18	10	24	10	17	7

8	1	-	-	-	-	-	2	-	-	-	-	-	-	-	1	-	2	-	1	-	3	-
9	-	-	-	-	-	-	-	-	-	-	-	1	1	-	1	-	-	1	-	-	1	-
10	-	-	-	-	-	-	-	-	-	-	-	-	-	-	-	-	-	-	-	-	-	-
11	-	-	-	-	-	-	-	-	-	-	-	-	-	-	-	-	-	-	-	-	-	-
0	-	-	-	-	-	-	-	-	-	-	-	-	-	-	-	-	-	-	-	-	-	-
Line C																						
x	-	1	-	-	-	1	-	1	-	1	-	1	1	-	1	3	-	2	-	1	-	-
X̸	1	4	-	2	4	5	-	3	2	4	1	-	1	-	8	13	1	5	6	8	4	5
5′	-	-	-	-	1	-	-	-	-	-	-	-	-	1	1	1	-	-	-	-	-	-
5"	1	1	2	4	1	3	1	4	-	4	-	1	2	3	4	11	3	9	5	14	1	11
6	-	-	-	-	2	1	1	-	-	-	-	-	1	-	3	1	1	-	2	1	4	3
7	6	3	2	2	3	2	3	2	4	3	3	5	1	7	14	15	8	9	14	12	5	5
8	-	-	-	1	-	-	-	-	-	-	-	-	-	-	-	-	-	1	-	-	-	-
9	4	3	7	2	12	6	5	3	14	4	4	1	8	3	38	16	16	6	20	11	19	8
10	1	-	-	-	-	-	2	-	-	-	-	-	-	-	1	-	2	-	1	-	3	-
11	-	-	-	-	-	-	-	-	-	-	1	-	1	-	1	-	1	-	-	-	-	-
0	-	1	1	1	-	5	2	1	-	4	1	2	-	1	-	11	4	4	4	5	6	10

M = males; F = females; R = right; L =left

Table 5

The incidence of palmar axial triradii expression in Iraq.

	Unrelated Series																				Alanga Tribe			
Region	S. Al-Arab				Basrah				Baghdad				Mosul		Overall				Baghdad			
Sex	M=13		F=12		M=23		F=14		M=20		F=10		M=15		M=71		F=36		M=52		F=42	
Triradius	R	L	R	L	R	L	R	L	R	L	R	L	R	L	R	L	R	L	R	L	R	L
t	10	9	8	7	14	16	9	8	9	11	5	7	9	12	42	48	22	22	36	37	28	29
t'	2	-	2	4	5	3	3	2	6	6	2	2	3	2	16	11	7	8	8	9	7	7
t"	-	1	1	-	1	-	2	1	-	-	1	-	-	-	1	1	4	1	1	-	1	-
tt'	1	2	1	1	2	3	-	-	4	2	-	-	1	1	8	8	1	1	4	5	3	4
tt"	-	1	-	-	1	1	-	3	1	1	2	-	2	-	4	3	2	3	2	1	3	2
tt't"	-	-	-	-	-	-	-	-	-	-	-	1	-	-	-	-	-	1	-	-	-	-
0	-	-	-	-	-	-	-	-	-	-	-	-	-	-	-	-	-	-	1	-	-	-

M=males; F=females; R=right; L=left; O=suppressed triradius

unavailable data in this respect. But they are of interest also for other purposes. It appears that some of these palmar features can be used to detect variations at different levels as the genetic structure of the studied regional, tribal and continental groups tend to differ. First, there is the difference in the main line C exits between the unrelated northern male sample in Mosul and the pooled unrelated males sampled in the central and southern regions in the country. The former showed significantly lower incidence of (X,x and o forms) as compared with the latter. Concerning the suppression of line C (o form), Abdullah (1978) found that the suppression of this line and its related triradius is monogenic, dominant, but with some reduced penetrance. It was found that the suppression form of this line is more frequent in the unrelated Iraqi series than in the British series particularly in the Iraqi tribal one, reaching to about 24% . Secondly, comparisons have been made between the unrelated and tribal series in Iraq. The females in the tribe exhibited significantly higher incidence of palmar patterning in the thenar/first interdigital as compared with the unrelated females. The males in the tribe exhibited significantly higher incidence of patterns in the fourth interdigital area and significantly higher incidence of terminations in numbers 1-5 positions of line B and number 9 position of line D by comparison with the unrelated males. The high percentage of inbreeding in this tribe probably mainly responsible for the observed differences from the unrelated series. Thirdly, the unrelated Iraqi males showed significantly higher incidence of patterns in the thenar/first and third interdigital areas as compared with the similar reported patterns for the Lebanese males (Naffah,1974). Fourthly, when comparisons have been made between widely different populations structure such as the Iraq and English populations, more variations have been revealed. The Iraqis showed significantly higher incidence of patterns in thenar/first and fourth interdigitals in males only, and in the second interdigital area in males and females as compared with the Northumbrians. On the other hand, the Iraqi females showed higher incidence of line B exits in positions 1-5 as compared with the Northumbrian females. There is obvious need to analyse further dermatoglyphic material from the various ethnic groups in Iraq in order to see whether there is any existence of heterogeneity between them as previously reported by Abdullah (1976) in ABO blood groups.

REFERENCES

Abdullah, N.F. (1976) Human blood groups in Basrah. Man (N.S.) 11: 239-242.

Abdullah, N.F. (1978) Inheritance of palmar triradii suppression. In : Dermatoglyphics - 50 years later (Ed. by W. Wertelecki, C.C. Plato and D. Bergsma). Alan R. Liss, New York.

Cummins, H. and Midlo, C. (1943) Finger prints, Palms and Soles. Blakiston, Philadelphia.

Naffah, J. (1974) Dermatoglyphics and flexion creases in the Lebanese population. Am. J. Phys. Anthrop., 41 : 391-410.

Penrose, L.S. and Loesch, D. (1970) Topological classification of palmar dermatoglyphics. J. Ment. Defic. Res. 14: 111-128.

Roberts, D.F., Abdullah, N.F., Marks, J. and Shuster, S. (1978) Dermatoglyphics in dermatitis herpetiformis. British J. of Dermatology, 99 : 627-634.

Roberts, D.F. and Abdullah, N.F. (1979) Dermatoglyphic variation in Iraq. Man (N.S.) 14 : 349-353.

Walker, N.F. (1958) The use of dermal configurations in the diagnosis of mongolism. Pediat. Clin. N. Amer. 5 : 531-543.

Progress in Dermatoglyphic Research, pages 285-293

A POPULATION STUDY OF FINGER DERMAL PATTERNS AND RIDGE COUNTS

M.P. Mi , A.M. Budy & M.N. Rashad

Department of Genetics and Cancer
Center of Hawaii, University of Hawaii
Honolulu, Hawaii 96822

Dermal ridge configurations on fingers, palms and soles are important characteristics in the study of human populations. (Holt, 1961). These dermal formations are fully developed by the fourth month of fetal life and remain unchanged during the postnatal period. Dermatoglyphic investigations of different human populations in the world have shown great variations. Summaries have been made on published results by Cummins and Midlo (1961), Biswas (1963), Holt (1968), and Pollitzer and Plato (1979). Since these investigations varied in sampling procedure and sample size, a rigid statistical testing of differences in dermatoglyphic traits among populations has not been attempted. This study is a statistical analysis of dermatoglyphic characteristics on fingers among various racial groups represented in Hawaii.

MATERIALS AND METHODS

A population-based fingerprint file was available, which was established by the Office of Civil Defense for the Population Registration of all residents in the Territory of Hawaii during World War II. A random sample was selected from the file representing one percent of the total population of approximately 300,000 on the island of Oahu. The sampling was based on the sequential registration number grouped by household. The first of each hundred households was used from which a single individual was randomly selected.

Depending upon the number of triradii on each finger (Penrose, 1968), the dermal pattern was classified into six types, namely: true whorl, double loop, ulnar loop, radial loop, tented arch, and simple arch. Finger ridge count was also recorded, which was the number of dermal ridges intersecting a straight line drawn from the central point of a triradius to the core of an adjacent pattern. For true whorl and double loop there were two ridge counts, one for each triradius. For loop patterns only one ridge count was made. In the absence of a core, arches always had zero ridge count. The total ridge count of an individual was the sum of ridge counts on all ten fingers, using the larger count only from each finger. The absolute ridge count was the sum of ridge counts for all the separate triradii on the ten fingers.

The racial composition of the Hawaii population was described by Lind (1967) and Nordyke (1977). For the present study, six racial groups were chosen. These were: Caucasian, Hawaiian, Chinese, Filipino, Japanese and Part-Hawaiian. The last group represented outcrosses involving Hawaiian, Caucasian and Oriental, mainly Chinese (Morton et al., 1967).

The dermatoglyphic traits used for analysis included counts of the six dermal pattern types, and total and absolute ridge counts on individuals. Because the number of observations for each race-sex subclass was disproportionate, the least-squares method (Harvey, 1960) was employed. The statistical model underlying the analysis allowed for the partition of the total variation of a trait into four sources. These were variations due to differences: (1) between two sexes; (2) among racial groups; (3) interactions between sex and race; and (4) among individuals of the same sex and race. The last source of variation was used as a term of residual errors for the testing of statistical significance. If the sex differences remained approximately the same from one race to another, the interaction between the two main effects, namely sex and race, would be deleted from the model. One or both main effects could be deleted if the null hypothesis of no difference was accepted. All hypotheses were tested at the 1% significance level ($p<0.01$). Least-squares estimates of means and standard errors were obtained from the best fitted model. The dermatoglyphic patterns were also analyzed by hand and by digit.

RESULTS AND DISCUSSION

The total number of individuals included in the final analysis was 2,983 (Table 1). There were: 31.6 percent Caucasian, 6.0 percent Hawaiian, 8.1 percent Chinese, 8.4 percent Filipino, 42.0 percent Japanese and 3.9 percent Part-Hawaiian. The sex ratio of the total sample was 1.15 but it varied greatly from race to race, ranging from 0.69 in the Hawaiian group to 2.18 in the Filipino group.

There was no evidence that the interaction between sex and race was an important source of variation in all dermal pattern types and ridge counts. It implied that sex differences were of the same magnitude in the six racial groups studied. The interacting terms were then deleted from the model in subsequent analyses.

TABLE 1. NUMBER OF INDIVIDUALS BY SEX & RACE

Race	Males	Females	Total
Caucasian	541	403	944
Hawaiian	73	106	179
Chinese	121	120	241
Filipino	172	79	251
Japanese	638	615	1253
Part-Hawaiian	48	67	115
Total	1593	1390	2983

In Table 2, the mean number of various dermal pattern types on individuals are given with their standard errors. The overall mean was an unbiased estimate for the population mean by holding sex and racial effects constant. Ulnar loops were the most common pattern type and tented arches were the least common. Since each individual contributed ten readings, one for each finger, the mean number of a dermal pattern on individuals could be divided by ten and read as relative frequency in the population. Thus, ulnar loops represented 47.2 percent of all finger prints in Hawaii while the combined true whorls and double loops contributed 47.8 percent. For the remaining five percent there were radial loops, simple arches and tented arches.

Table 2. Least-squares means of number of various dermal patterns on individuals

		True Whorl	Double Loop	Ulnar Loop	Radial Loop	Tented Arch	Simple Arch
Overall mean		3.15±.07	1.63±.05	4.72±.07	0.24±.02	0.06±.01	0.17±.02
Sex:	Male	---	1.77±.06	4.57±.09	0.27±.02	0.05±.01	0.11±.03
	Female	---	1.49±.06	4.88±.09	0.21±.02	0.08±.01	0.23±.03
Race:	Caucasian	1.97±.10	1.00±.07	6.01±.13	0.45±.03	0.15±.02	0.42±.04
	Hawaiian	4.48±.17	2.08±.12	3.27±.20	0.07±.04	0.00±.03	0.05±.06
	Chinese	---	1.92±.10	---	---	---	---
	Filipino	---	---	---	---	---	---
	Japanese	2.89±.09	1.44±.06	5.09±.12	---	---	---
	Part-Hawaiian	---	---	---	---	---	---

--- Least-squares estimates not significantly different from the overall mean

Sex difference was statistically significant in all pattern types except true whorls. Males had a slightly higher frequency of double loops and radial loops. There was also a difference in ulnar loops, simple arches and tented arches between two sexes, all in favor of females.

Racial variations were found to be significant in all pattern types. The Caucasian group was the lowest in the frequency of true whorls and double loops, and the highest in all loop and arch types. The Hawaiians showed a completely different distribution of dermal patterns. They had high frequencies in true whorls and double loops but were low in all other pattern types. The Chinese and Filipino groups did not differ significantly from the overall mean in all patterns with one exception; both were significantly higher in double loops than the overall mean. The frequency distribution of various dermal patterns in Japanese was remarkably different from other Asian groups. They were lower in the frequency of true whorls and double loops but higher in all other patterns than the overall mean. The Part-Hawaiian group did not deviate significantly from the overall mean in all patterns.

When right and left hands were analyzed separately, it was found that sex difference was statistically significant in the frequency of true whorl. On the right hand, male subjects had more whorls. On the left hand, the females were higher in frequency. This would explain the lack of sex difference in the frequency of true whorl on individuals when two hands were combined. There were three other pattern types in which sex difference was not consistent between right and left hands. Males were significantly lower in the frequency of ulnar loop on the right hand. Radial loops occurred more frequently on the right hand of males than that of females. For these two loop patterns, there was no difference between males and females on the left hand. While there was no sex difference in the frequency of tented arch on the right hand, males were found to have a significantly lower frequency than females on the left hand.

The distribution of various dermal pattern types among fingers was also analyzed. Table 3 gives the frequencies of various patterns for each finger by holding sex and race effects constant. Due to extremely low frequencies, tented arch and simple arch were combined. True whorl was common on finger IV, being 0.57 on the right hand and 0.45 on the left. Double loop was moderately low varying from 0.10 to 0.16 in all fingers except the thumb on which the frequency reached 0.28 and 0.32 percent on two hands. Fingers III and V had the highest frequency of ulnar loop, while most radial loops were found on finger II. Arches appeared more frequently on fingers II and III.

Sex difference was less consistent on a finger basis particularly on the left hand. When present, all differences remained in the same direction in favor of one sex except for true whorl. On fingers I, III and V of the right hand, true whorls appeared more frequently in males than in females. On fingers IV and V of the left hand, females had more whorls. There was no sex difference on other fingers. Statistically significant racial variation was observed on most fingers in dermal pattern distribution. For most pattern types, four clusters could be readily identified. The Caucasian and Hawaiian groups occupied the two opposite extremes. In the middle there were Chinese, Filipino and Part-Hawaiians. The Japanese group was intermediate between the Caucasians and the middle cluster of three racial groups.

TABLE 3. FREQUENCIES OF DERMAL PATTERNS ON FINGERS*

Finger		True Whorl	Double Loop	Ulnar Loop	Radial Loop	Arch**
Right	I	0.313	0.279	0.390	0.002	0.015
	II	0.338	0.164	0.344	0.100	0.052
	III	0.262	0.116	0.587	0.011	0.022
	IV	0.571	0.103	0.311	0.006	0.005
	V	0.263	0.086	0.644	0.001	0.006
Left	I	0.202	0.322	0.451	0.002	0.024
	II	0.332	0.160	0.364	0.105	0.052
	III	0.251	0.138	0.563	0.009	0.038
	IV	0.450	0.149	0.385	0.002	0.012
	V	0.170	0.117	0.701	0.002	0.008

* Least-squares estimates holding sex and race effects constant

** Tented and simple arches combined

The estimates of ridge counts are shown in Table 4. Both sex and race effects were found highly signficant statistically. Male subjects had higher ridge counts than females. The difference was 11.1 for the total ridge count and 17.6 for the absolute ridge count. The Hawaiian group ranked the highest in total ridge count and the Caucasian group was the lowest, both deviating signficantly from the population mean. The difference between these two groups was 42 in total ridge count and 92 in absolute ridge count. The Hawaiians were approximately 33 and 57 percent higher in the two ridge counts than the Caucasian group. The other three groups, Chinese, Filipino and Part-Hawaiian were not significantly different from the mean. The Japanese group was found to have a much lower ridge count than the population mean, but significantly higher than the Caucasian group.

TABLE 4. LEAST-SQUARES MEANS OF RIDGE COUNTS

		Total	Absolute
Overall Mean		144.7±1.2	201.6±2.2
Sex:	Males	150.3±1.4	210.4±2.7
	Females	139.2±2.0	192.8±2.7
Race:	Caucasian	126.6±2.0	159.5±3.8
	Hawaiian	168.7±3.2	251.0±6.0
	Chinese	---	---
	Filipino	---	---
	Japanese	134.0±1.9	184.6±3.6
	Part-Hawaiian	---	---

The importance of sampling in dermatoglyphic investigations has been emphasized by Holt (1968). The use of a total population registration for sampling in the present study not only assures a high degree of randomness but also minimizes the likelihood of including individuals related by descent in the sample. In random sampling the probability of selecting an individual of certain characteristics is proportional to the frequency of individuals of these characteristics in the population. It is expected that the sample size for each race-sex group varies under random sampling reflecting the population structure. Data with unequal subclass numbers are statistically non-orthogonal and present difficulties in data analysis. It is necesssary to resort to simultaneous consideration of all fixed effects. The procedure of least-squares analysis is the method of choice. The estimates of mean and standard error derived form the best fitted model in the present study may be used to construct confidence intervals for further comparison.

SUMMARY

Sex and racial variations in dermatoglyphic traits were analyzed using fingerprint records selected from a population file in Hawaii. Both sources of variation were found to be statistically significant. Least-squares means were presented for all finger dermal patterns and ridge counts.

ACKNOWLEDGEMENT

This work was supported in part initially by U.S. PHS Grant HD-04275 and currently by HL-23386.

REFERENCES

Biswas PC (1963). Ethno-geographic variations in dermatoglyphics. Proc. II Intern. Congr. Human Genet. 3:1430-1449.

Cummins H, Midlo A (1961). "Fingerprints, Palms and Soles." New York: Dover Publications, Inc., 319p.

Harvey WR (1960). "Least-squares Analysis of Data with Unequal Subclass Numbers." US: USDA Agricultural Research Service, 157p.

Holt SB (1961). Dermatoglyphic patterns. In Harrison GA (ed): "Genetical Variation in Human Populations," New York: Pergamon Press, p 79.

Holt SB (1968). "The Genetics of Dermal Ridges." Springfield: Charles C Thomas, 195p.

Lind AW (1967). "Hawaii's People." Honolulu: The University Press of Hawaii, 121p.

Morton NE, Chung CS, Mi MP (1967). "Genetics of Interracial Crosses in Hawaii." Basel: S. Karger, 158p.

Nordyke EC (1977). "The Peopling of Hawaii." Honolulu: The University Press of Hawaii, 221p.

Penrose LS (1968). Memorandum on dermatoglyphic nomenclature. Birth Defects Original Article Series 4:3.

Pollitzer WS, Plato CC (1979). Anthropology and dermatoglyphics. In Wertelecki W, Plato CC (eds): "Dermatoglyphics-Fifty Years Later," Birth Defects Original Article Series 15:211. New York: Alan R. Liss, Inc., p 211.

Progress in Dermatoglyphic Research, pages 295-301

RIDGE COUNT OF FINGER DERMAL PATTERNS

M.P. Mi , A.M. Budy & M.N. Rashad

Department of Genetics and Cancer
Center of Hawaii, University of Hawaii
Honolulu, Hawaii 96822

It is well established that the total ridge count of an individual is a highly heritable quantitative trait (Holt, 1952). This measurement is the sum of ten counts, one from each finger. When two counts are possible on a finger as for true whorl and double loop patterns, the larger count is used. Arches always have zero ridge counts. Statistically the differences in total ridge count among individuals is determined by two sources of variation. One is the total number of non-zero-count dermal patterns such as true whorl, double loop, ulnar loop and radial loop present on each individual and the other is the number of counts of each pattern. Mi et al. (1981) reported statistically significant differences in ridge counts and in the frequency of various dermal pattern types between males and females and among several racial groups represented in Hawaii. Holt (1961) analyzed the relationship between ridge count and pattern type from data on 100 males and 100 females sampled in Great Britain. The average total ridge count for whorls was 19.6 in males and 18.3 in females. The corresponding values for loops were 12.9 and 12.1, respectively. The frequency distributions on ridge count of whorls and loops overlapped to a great extent indicating an incomplete agreement between pattern size and pattern type. The present study was designed to elucidate sources of variation in ridge count of each dermal pattern using data derived from a multi-racial population in Hawaii.

MATERIALS & METHODS

The data used for the present study are described in another report (Mi et al., 1981). Four patterns, i.e., true whorls, double loops, ulnar loops and radial loops were chosen. For true whorl and double loop patterns, two measurements of ridge count were used for analysis. The first measurement, designated as single count, represented the larger of the two counts of a pattern on the finger. The second measurement, designated as combined count, was the sum of the counts for all the separate triradii of a pattern. The latter was the basis for the absolute ridge count of an individual when the sum of ten fingers were used (Penrose, 1968). Because the number of observations for each race-sex-hand subclass was disproportionate, the method of least-squares analysis of data with unequal subclass numbers (Harvey, 1960) was employed. Analysis was made of each pattern by finger. The two measurements of ridge count were analyzed separately. The linear statistical model underlying the analysis defined four sources of variation: (1) difference between male and female subjects, (2) difference between right and left hand, (3) variations among six racial groups, and (4) a residual variation among individual observations. Interactions between the main effects, namely: sex, hand, and race were assumed negligible. All hypotheses were tested at the 1% significance level ($p<0.01$). Least-squares estimates of means and standard errors were obtained from the best fitted model.

RESULTS & DISCUSSION

The number of fingers sampled for the analysis of each dermal ridge pattern is shown in Table 1, reflecting the variations in the frequency among fingers. The smallest sample consisted of 559 double loops on finger V while the 4,254 ulnar loops on the same finger constituted the largest sample.

TABLE 1. NUMBER OF FINGERS FOR ANALYSIS BY DERMAL PATTERNS

Pattern	Finger I	Finger II	Finger III	Finger IV	Finger V
True whorl	1,476	1,703	1,199	2,736	1,080
Double loop	1,498	863	669	663	559
Ulnar loop	2,829	2,160	3,728	2,447	4,254
Radial loop	---	792	---	---	---

Table 2 shows the analysis of true whorl pattern type by each finger. Least-squares estimates not significantly different from the overall mean are not shown. The true whorl on finger I was the largest with a mean total ridge count of 20.1 and the smallest was on finger V with a count of 15.0 ridges. With respect to pattern intensity and pattern size as measured by the sum of the two counts, the highest was found on finger I, followed in decreasing order by IV, III, II and V. The combined count of a true whorl represented an increase of 62 to 75 percent over the single count on different fingers. It indicated that the two triradii of a true whorl were located unequally from the core point.

Sex differences were found in both single and combined counts on fingers I, IV and V. Males had a larger pattern than females. The difference varied from 0.52 counts on finger IV to 1.92 counts on finger I. A bilateral difference was only found on finger I, being higher on the right hand. The difference was 1.16 for the single count and 2.15 for the combined ridge count. Racial variation was found to be statistically significant in all fingers except finger V. Hawaiians had the highest counts, while the Caucasian or Japanese were the lowest. The Chinese, Filipino and Part-Hawaiian groups did not differ much from the overall mean in most comparisons.

For the double loop pattern, there was no difference between males and females, between right and left hand, and among six racial groups in all fingers except finger I. The mean single count was 19.07, 18.42, 16.67, 15.80 and 15.61 for fingers I, IV, III, V and II, respectively. The combined count for the fingers was 30.09, 28.87, 27.35,

TABLE 2. RIDGE COUNT OF TRUE WHORL PATTERN

FINGER		I	II	III	IV	V
		Single Count (larger of the two counts)				
Overall Mean		20.11±.16	16.55±.14	17.56±.16	17.89±.11	15.01±.15
Sex:	Male	21.07±.20	---	---	18.15±.14	15.45±.19
	Female	19.15±.20	---	---	17.62±.14	14.57±.19
Hand:	Right	20.69±.20	---	---	---	---
	Left	19.53±.20	---	---	---	---
Race:	Caucasian	---	---	16.61±.33	---	---
	Hawaiian	21.07±.43	17.66±.34	19.27±.37	19.17±.29	---
	Chinese	---	---	---	17.26±.29	---
	Filipino	---	16.15±.35	---	---	---
	Japanese	19.14±.26	15.80±.24	17.08±.28	17.56±.19	---
	Part-Hawaiian	---	---	---	---	---
		Combined Count (sum of the two counts)				
Overall Mean		35.11±.30	28.18±.24	30.77±.31	30.95±.21	24.27±.26
Sex:	Male	36.85±.37	---	---	31.47±.27	25.06±.33
	Female	33.37±.37	---	---	30.43±.27	23.48±.33
Hand:	Right	36.16±.37	---	---	---	---
	Left	34.01±.37	---	---	---	---
Race:	Caucasian	34.15±.56	27.28±.46	28.47±.65	29.21±.41	---
	Hawaiian	37.03±.80	30.33±.61	33.92±.72	33.34±.54	---
	Chinese	---	---	---	---	---
	Filipino	---	---	---	---	---
	Japanese	33.70±.49	26.92±.42	---	---	---
	Part-Hawaiian	---	---	---	---	---

--- Least-squares estimates not significantly different from the overall mean

23.18 and 25.18. Finger V had a slightly higher single ridge count but a lower combined count than finger II. As shown in Table 3, there was a significant difference of 1.57 and 2.50 in the two counts between males and females on finger I in favor of the males. There was also a significant bilateral difference of 1.75 and 2.60 in the two counts, the right hand being higher. Hawaiians had the largest double loop pattern, while the Japanese ranked the smallest.

TABLE 3. RIDGE COUNT OF DOUBLE LOOP PATTERN ON FINGER I

		Single Count	Combined Count
Overall Mean		19.07±.15	30.09±.25
Sex:	Male	19.86±.19	31.34±.32
	Female	18.29±.19	28.84±.32
Hand:	Right	19.95±.19	31.39±.32
	Left	18.20±.19	28.79±.32
Race:	Caucasian	18.55±.28	---
	Hawaiian	20.90±.38	32.45±.63
	Chinese	18.12±.36	28.60±.61
	Filipino	19.91±.37	31.65±.62
	Japanese	17.96±.27	28.44±.45
	Part Hawaiian	---	---

--- Least-squares estimates not significantly different from the overall mean

Table 4 gives the least-squares estimates of ridge count for the ulnar loop pattern. Finger I had the highest count, followed in decreasing order by finger IV, V, III and II. Sex difference was found to be significant on all fingers varying from 0.58 on finger II to 1.74 on finger I, all in favor of the males. A significant bilateral difference was found on fingers I, III and IV. On finger I the right hand had a higher ridge count, but on the other two fingers the difference was reversed, the left hand being higher. Invariably the Hawaiians had larger ulnar loops; either the Caucasian or Japanese had the smallest pattern. On fingers I, III, and IV, the Part-Hawaiian group was signficantly different from the overall mean approaching the Hawaiian means. On the same fingers, the Chinese had smaller ulnar loops which were comparable to

TABLE 4. RIDGE COUNT OF ULNAR LOOP PATTERN

FINGER		I	II	III	IV	V
Overall Mean		15.04±.16	10.37±.15	11.66±.11	13.33±.19	12.06±.11
Sex:	Male	15.86±.19	10.66±.18	12.06±.14	13.80±.22	12.40±.13
	Female	14.12±.19	10.07±.18	11.26±.14	12.86±.22	11.72±.13
Hand:	Right	15.86±.19	---	11.42±.14	12.94±.22	---
	Left	14.21±.19	---	11.90±.14	13.72±.22	---
Race:	Caucasian	---	9.24±.26	10.47±.19	12.29±.30	---
	Hawaiian	16.79±.47	12.51±.44	13.60±.35	15.66±.62	12.88±.33
	Chinese	13.69±.41	---	10.92±.28	12.53±.44	---
	Filipino	---	---	---	---	---
	Japanese	13.84±.26	9.52±.25	10.74±.19	11.90±.30	11.15±.18
	Part-Hawaiian	16.23±.43	---	12.94±.31	14.64±.58	---

--- Least-squares estimates not significantly different from the overall mean

the Japanese or Caucasians. It should be pointed out that the ulnar loop for the Chinese group was the smallest on finger I.

For the radial loop pattern on finger II, there was no race or sex difference. Radial loop on the right hand had 1.7 more counts than that on the left, the difference being statistically significant.

The present study clearly demonstrates a great variation in ridge count among fingers for the same pattern type, as well as among different patterns on the same finger. Sex and racial variations are also noted in pattern size and pattern intensity.

SUMMARY

The variations of ridge count in four dermal patterns were analyzed using multi-racial population data in Hawaii. These patterns were true whorls, double loops, ulnar loops and radial loops. For each pattern, the ridge count varied greatly from finger to finger. Sex and racial differences in pattern size and intensity were found on most fingers.

ACKNOWLEDGEMENT

This work was initially supported in part by U.S. PHS Grant HD-04275 and currently by HL-23386.

REFERENCES

Harvey WR (1960). "Least-squares Analysis of Data with Unequal Subclass Numbers." US: USDA Agricultural Research Service, 157p.

Holt SB (1961). Dermatoglyphic patterns. In Harrison GA (ed): "Genetical Variation in Human Populations," New York: Pergamon Press, p 79.

Holt SB (1952). Genetics of dermal ridges: Inheritance of total ridge count. Ann. Eugen. (Lond.) 17:140-161.

Mi MP, Budy AM, Rashad MN (1981). A population study of finger dermal patterns and ridge counts.

Penrose LS (1968). Memorandum on dermatoglyphic nomenclature. Birth Defects Original Article Series 4:3, 13p.

Progress in Dermatoglyphic Research, pages 303-315

DIGITAL RIDGE-COUNT VARIATIONS IN SOME CASTES OF INDIA

R.D. Singh

Department of Sociology and Anthropology
University of Windsor
Windsor, Ontario, Canada N9B 3P4

Some geographic trends in the (nature of) distribution of dermatoglyphic configurations have been suggested in many human populations (Cummins & Midlo, 1943; Rife, 1953; Newman, 1960; Singh, 1963, 1968; Roberts and Coope, 1972; Marquer and Jakobi 1976); Sarkar (1976) has noticed some mixed situations as well. Such trends have been supported by anthropometric and serological traits also, more specifically in the populations of India (Mahalanobis, et al., 1949; Majumdar, 1951; Majumdar and Rao, 1958; Karve and Dandekar, 1951; Karve, 1954, 1968). Thus, keeping in mind the factor of environmental influences, four castes were selected from one area to study the nature of distribution of dermatoglyphic configurations. A qualitative analysis of the finger-ball patterns did not reflect the social hierarchical position for any of the groups except that the lower castes had larger bimanual differences than the higher castes. However, the castes were heterogeneous for certain specified traits and the significant differences could be seen in the left hands only (Singh, 1978). Hence, a further study of the same data is attempted to examine the nature of the finger ridge-count variations in the same context, i.e., each caste as a reproductive isolated population living in a homogeneous geographic environment, and the manner in which they differ from one another.

MATERIALS AND METHODS

The four caste groups, the Brahmin (237), the Kurmi (224), the Pasi (213) and the Chamar (172) belong to the district Bara Banki Uttar Pradesh, India. The total sample of 846 individuals reported here was collected from 43 villages. Impressions of both the hands were obtained by traditional ink method; blood relatives were not included in the sample. The three basic patterns (the whorl, the loop, and the arch) were identified after Cummins and Midlo (1943) for the ten fingers of each individual of the four groups. The ridge-counting of these patterns was done on the line connecting the triradius and the core, according to rules described by Holt (1968). The higher count has been used in the case of whorls because this indicates the measure of a single trait, i.e., the size of the pattern (Holt, 1968). No case of extralimital triradii is found in the sample. The total finger ridge-count has been obtained by adding up the single counts on the fingers of an individual in both the hands. Table 1 gives the mean values, standard deviations, and ranges of the ridge-counts on the individual digits in the two hands and all digits in the right and left hands of the four groups.

RESULTS

The higher values of standard deviations indicate large intracaste variability. The highest mean ridge-count is found for the first and the fourth digits of both hands in all the four groups. The lowest counts occur on second and third digits while the highest are encountered on the first right digit. With regard to this latter finding, the Brahmin and the Kurmi are found to have the highest means (18.7), followed by the Chamar (18.6), and the Pasi (17.9). A similar order is maintained in respect to the higher limits of their ranges of distribution. The Kurmis have a range of 0-33, the Brahmins 0-32, the Chamars 0-31, and the Pasis 0-30.

TABLE 1

The mean values and their standard errors, standard deviations, and ranges of the ridge-counts on the individual digits of the four groups

BRAHMIN = 237

Rt. Digit	Mean	S.D.	Range	Lt. Digit	Mean	S.D.	Range
I	18.7±0.39	6.1	0-32	I	16.5±0.39	6.0	0-31
II	12.2±0.43	6.7	0-27	II	12.0±0.42	6.5	0-27
III	12.9±0.36	5.6	0-28	III	13.5±0.37	5.8	0-25
IV	17.3±0.36	5.6	0-28	IV	16.8±0.36	5.7	0-28
V	14.4±0.30	4.6	0-25	V	14.5±0.30	4.6	0-28
All	75.6±1.46	22.5	9-126	All	73.2±1.48	22.8	8-124

KURMI = 224

Rt. Digit	Mean	S.D.	Range	Lt. Digit	Mean	S.D.	Range
I	18.7±0.41	6.2	0-33	I	17.5±0.39	6.0	0-29
II	11.3±0.43	6.6	0-23	II	11.4±0.46	6.9	0-24
III	13.5±0.34	5.1	0-24	III	13.9±0.38	5.9	0-27
IV	16.8±0.35	5.3	0-29	IV	17.1±0.34	5.1	0-28
V	14.0±0.32	4.8	0-24	V	14.4±0.31	4.8	4-31
All	74.3±1.46	21.9	20-115	All	74.4±1.49	22.4	20-123

(continued)

Rt. Digit	Mean	S.D.	Range	Lt. Digit	Mean	S.D.	Range
PASI = 213							
I	17.9 ± 0.43	6.3	0-28	I	16.0 ± 0.43	6.4	0-30
II	10.8 ± 0.44	6.5	0-24	II	10.3 ± 0.45	6.6	0-25
III	12.9 ± 0.39	5.7	0-25	III	13.2 ± 0.38	5.6	0-24
IV	16.2 ± 0.29	4.3	2-27	IV	15.6 ± 0.33	4.9	0-25
V	14.3 ± 0.28	4.2	1-25	V	14.2 ± 0.29	4.2	5-25
All	72.2 ± 1.45	21.3	9-113	All	69.2 ± 1.42	20.8	23-114
CHAMAR = 172							
I	18.6 ± 0.47	6.2	0-31	I	16.9 ± 0.51	6.8	0-29
II	12.4 ± 0.42	5.6	0-26	II	11.5 ± 0.46	6.1	0-23
III	12.8 ± 0.46	6.1	0-32	III	13.0 ± 0.45	5.9	0-27
IV	15.6 ± 0.39	5.2	0-30	IV	15.8 ± 0.42	5.6	0-30
V	14.1 ± 0.35	4.6	0-23	V	13.7 ± 0.35	4.6	0-24
All	73.2 ± 1.77	23.2	0-136	All	70.9 ± 1.78	23.4	0-119

1. There is no missing data for any of the fingers for ridge counts.

2. Means and standard deviations for individual digits and all the five digits in each hand were calculated from individual distributions.

The lowest mean value, 10.3, occurs on the Pasi second left digit; and the second digit in all the groups, for both the hands, maintains the lowest count.

These observations are in general agreement with those of Singh (1961), Mukherjee (1962), Mavalwala (1963), Srivastava (1965), Sarkar (1969), and others.

The bimanual comparisons in ridge-count show higher values for the right hand over the left, in general. The Brahmin, the Pasi, and the Chamar follow the general tendency (Holt, 1954), but the Kurmi have a larger count in their left hand.

The critical value of <u>t</u> calculated after Sokal and Rohlf (1969) for the corresponding digits in the two hands of the four groups to examine the bimanual differences are presented in Table 2. These values indicate that there is a significant difference between the right and left hand counts of each group in the first digit only which, however, is obscured in the total ridge-count.

DISCUSSION

As noted elsewhere (Singh, 1978) the different pattern types occur in different digits in varying frequencies, and that each digit has a characteristic frequency for these types. This characteristic is to a large extent reflected in the finger ridge-count distribution also. Since whorls on the average are the patterns which are larger in size (ridge-count) than loops, the digits which have higher frequencies for whorls are expected to have larger counts as well. The corresponding digits in the right and left hand are also expected to follow the general trend. With these two general trends, the mean ridge-count is also expected to vary accordingly. The frequency distributions of the main patterns suggest that the whorls are lowest in the fifth digit and, therefore, the lowest count should logically occur there. Instead, the mean count on fifth digit is higher than those

TABLE 2

Values of *t* for the significance of difference between means of total ridge-count in the right and left hands of the four groups

	Brahmin	Kurmi	Pasi	Chamar
Digit I	4.000	2.104	5.843	2.330
II	0.334	0.191	0.750	1.434
III	1.171	0.581	0.402	0.252
IV	0.995	0.174	0.976	0.431
V	0.082	0.925	0.324	0.781
All Digits	1.121	0.015	1.162	0.923

t = 1.96; significant with $P \leq .05$ for large samples

on the second and the third digits. This increase can be explained by the fact that the arches which have zero value have their highest concentration on second and third digits and least on fifth digits (Singh, 1978). Also, the loops on the fifth digits are relatively smaller in size. These results confirm Holt's (1968) observations that the agreement between pattern-type and pattern-size is far from complete and, therefore, the ridge-count is likely to vary.

The means and range of distribution of ridge-counts in the right hand digit one, as mentioned earlier, suggest that there is a kind of ordering of the castes in this respect. But the mean ridge-counts in other digits, however, do not show the same order, because sometimes a digit in the right hand shows higher count than the corresponding digit in the left hand; at other times, a left hand digit has a higher count than the corresponding digit in the right hand. Thus, in a digit-to-digit comparison, there is no one order among the castes. The total count for each hand shows that the Chamar right hand has the largest count (136) whereas the minimum (113) occurs in the Pasi right hand. The Brahmin and the Kurmi fall in between.

In their total ridge-count for both hands considered together, the Chamar is characterized by the highest range, from 0-255. For the upper limit the descending order is: the Chamar (255), the Brahmin (250), the Kurmi (238), and the Pasi (227). On the ascending scale the positions of the Kurmi and the Pasi are changed in the following order: Chamar (0), Brahmin (17), Pasi (32), and Kurmi (40). Thus, in their wider range, the Chamar and the Brahmin fall on one side, and the Pasi and the Kurmi on the other.

Although the pattern-size follows the general tendency of being larger in the right hand, a comparison of the corresponding digits in the two hands shows exceptions for the second digit in the case of the Brahmin, the Chamar, and the Pasi. The former two groups have also exceptions in their fifth and fourth digits respectively; the Kurmi has only one exception for the first digit.

The ridge-counts on the ten fingers are intercorrelated (Holt, 1951, 1959; Mavalwala, 1962). The highest correlations occur between homologous fingers, while the adjacent fingers, with some exceptions in the case of first digits, are more highly correlated than those further apart. In general, as the distance between the fingers increases, the correlation between them decreases (Holt, 1968).

The correlation coefficients were calculated for all possible combinations for each group separately. The correlations in each group are high, ranging from 0.407 between right fourth and left second digits to 0.818 for the homologous digit one in the Pasi; the other groups fall within this range. Invariably the highest correlation occurs between the homologous digits and the data supports the findings by Holt. The range of high correlation between the digits for the four groups is as follows:

Brahmin Right V and left I 0.425; homologous IV 0.786
Kurmi Right I and III 0.418; homologous III 0.793
Pasi Right IV and left II 0.407; homologous I 0.818
Chamar Right I and left II 0.408; homologous IV 0.803.
The pattern of correlation for adjacent fingers is also confirmed, in general. The high correlation values for homologous digits two fall along the hierarchical pattern among the castes (Brahmin 0.718; Kurmi 0.753; Pasi 0.691; Chamar 0.680).

Since the range of high correlation coefficients is large, it was considered necessary to explore further whether or not some significant differences also exist among various pairs. This was done using the correlation coefficients and confidence intervales at the .05 level as suggested by Walker and Lev (1953). Although significant differences do exist in many pairs, no systematic pattern seems to emerge except for the homologous digits four and five among the four groups. These are invariably significantly different than most other correlation coefficients. Among the remaining pairs more than half of them are significantly different from others.

The test of significance (t) of the differences between means among the four groups based upon the total ridge-count (Table 3) does indicate that there are significant differences between the Brahmin and the Pasi, the Brahmin and the Chamar, the Kurmi and the Pasi, and the Kurmi and the Chamar. No significant difference is noticed, however, between the Brahmin and the Kurmi, or between the Pasi and the Chamar. Socially, the Brahmin and the Kurmi are closer to one another in the upper echelons of Hindu society, whereas the Chamar and the Pasi occupy a position lower down in the social pyramid.

A comparison of these castes with other similar groups is not without interest. For instance, the $Brahmin_1$ and $Brahmin_3$ of West Bengal studied by Sarkar (1969) and Banerjee (1970) respectively are part of the same major caste, but live in different geographic areas. The $Brahmin_2$ of Uttar Pradesh (Singh, 1961) belong to several districts, and, in a way, may be considered representing the Brahmin population of the province. Similar is the case with the Rajput, the Ahir, and the Muslims representing their respective groups (Singh, 1961). The Rajput are second in status under the Brahmin in social hierarchy, and the Ahir are considered to have an equal status to the Kurmi, but below the Rajput. The Muslim have a separate status. The Mahars of Maharashtra (Mukherjee, 1962) are an equivalent caste group of the Chamars of North India. The Parsis of Bombay (Mavalwala, 1963) form an endogamous group within themselves and have maintained their identity as a population.

The Mech of West Bengal are of tribal origin, maintain endogamy, and are located in one geographic area (Sarkar and Biswas, 1972). Banerjee, Sarkar and Biswas found significant differences in the total ridge-counts of their male and female samples, hence only the male sample has been compared. Since there is no significant difference in the Parsi male and female ridge-counts, the two samples have been

TABLE 3

Values of *t* for the significance of the difference between means of total ridge-count in various groups from India

	Brahmin	$Brahmin_1$	$Brahmin_3$	Chamar	Kurmi	Mahar	Mech	Parsi	Pasi
Ahir	-	-	-	1.89	-	-	2.73	2.82	3.14
Brahmin	-	-	-	-	-	-	3.93	-	3.57
$Brahmin_1$	-	-	-	-	-	-	3.75	-	-
$Brahmin_2$	-	-	-	-	-	-	3.69	1.85	-
$Brahmin_3$	-	-	-	-	-	-	2.96	1.90	1.92
Chamar	2.01	-	-	-	1.97	-	4.99	-	-
Kurmi	-	-	-	-	-	-	3.94	-	3.52
Mahar	-	-	-	-	-	-	2.26	-	2.13
Muslim	4.55	4.34	3.43	5.84	4.61	2.43	-	5.92	7.54
Rajput	-	-	-	-	-	-	3.28	1.81	-
Parsi	3.49	-	1.90	-	3.44	2.14	5.66	-	-
Pasi	3.57	-	1.92	-	3.52	2.13	6.51	-	-

1. $t=1.96$; significant with $P \leq .05$ for large samples
2. Out of total pairs of 72, only 30 have significant values
3. Brahmin (present study) and $Brahmin_2$, both of Uttar Pradesh (Singh, '61); $Brahmin_1$ of Nadia (Sarkar, '69); $Brahmin_3$ of Bengal (Banerjee, '70)

pooled together.

The values of *t* for these groups as well as of the four groups of the present study show that the Parsi differ significantly from the Brahmin, the Kurmi, the Mech, the Muslim, the Ahir, and the Mahar but the $Brahmin_2$, $Brahmin_3$ and the Rajput are quite close to the significant level of variation. The Mahar on the other hand differ significantly from the Pasi, Mech, Ahir and the Muslim. The tribal background of the Mech separates them significantly from all the groups compared here except the Muslim. And the Muslim in their own turn differs significantly from eight other groups which include the higher as well as lower caste groups. The Kurmi differ from the Pasi, the Chamar, the Muslim and the Parsi, whereas the Pasi differ from the Muslim, the Ahir, and the Mahar. A separate identity of the Uttar Pradesh Muslims need to be further examined in the context of the history of the expansion of Islam through conversions from the middle caste groups of the region. In this process the Muslims,by and large, avoided large scale acceptance from the lower ranks of the society. The nature of sub-sections of the Muslim population included here in the sample belong mostly to weaver, barber, butcher, herdsmen (*Gujar*), oil-pressers (*teli*) and other similar groups. Wherever there has been mass conversion from the lower ranks of the society, e.g., the sweepers (*Bhangi*), invariably such groups have maintained their social identity, that is, they have remained in the form of a caste under Islam. However, it should be noted that the Muslim caste structure is not as rigid as that of the Hindus. Therefore, a study of Muslim populations designed along different caste groups would be more revealing from the point of view of population variations.

Since the Brahmin groups from different geographic locations do not seem to differ with one another, but they do differ with some other local groups in their respective regions, it appears that this dermatoglyphic trait is the result of a biogenetic expression rather than that of physical environment. However, the limitations of the data in terms of sample size need not be overlooked.

REFERENCES

Bannerjee DK (1970). Finger dermatoglyphics of some Bengali castes. Man in India 50:161-176.

Cummins H, Midlo C (1943). "Finger Prints, Palms and Soles." Philadelphia: The Blakistan Company.

Holt SB (1951). The correlation between ridge counts on different fingers. Ann Eugen 16:287-297.

_______ (1954). Genetics of dermal ridges: bilateral asymmetry in finger ridge counts. Ann Eugen 18:211-231.

_______ (1959). The correlations between ridge-counts on different fingers estimated from a population sample. Ann Hum Genet 23:459-460.

_______ (1968). "The Genetics of Dermal Ridges." Springfield Illinois: C.C. Thomas.

Karve I (1954). Anthropometric measurements in Karnatak and Orissa and a comparison of these two regions with Maharashtra. J Anthrop Soc Bombay: No 8.

Karve I, Dandeker VM (1951). "Anthropometric Measurements of Maharashtra." Poona: Deccan College Monograph Series 8.

Karve I, Malhotra KC (1968). A biological comparison of eight endogamous groups of the same rank. Current Anthropology 9:109-124.

Mahalanobis PC, Majumdar DN, Rao CR (1949). "Anthropometric Survey of the United Provinces." Calcutta: Sankhya 9(2 and 3).

Majumdar DN (1951). "Race Realities in Cultural Gujarat." Bombay: Gujarat Research Soc.

Majumdar DN, Rao CR (1958). "Race Elements in Bengal." Bombay: Asia Publishing.

Marquer P, Jakobi L (1976). Dermatoglyphics and endogamy in Bearn, France. Man 11:367-383.

Mavalwala JD (1962). Correlation between ridge-counts on all digits of the Parsis of India. Ann Hum Genet 20:137-138.

_______ (1963). The dermatoglyphics of the Parsis of India. Zeitschrift fur Morphologie und Anthropologie 54:173-189.

Mukherjee DP (1962). The Mahar hand prints—a preliminary report. Current Science 31:66-67.

Newman MT (1960). Populational analysis of finger and palm prints in Highland and Lowland Maya Indians. Am J Phys Anthrop 18:45-58.

Rife DC (1953). Finger prints as criteria of ethnic relationship. Am J Hum Genet 5:389-399.

Roberts DF, Coope E (1972). Dermatoglyphic variation in South Midlands. Heredity 29:293-305.

Sarkar D (1969). Dermatoglyphic study among three Bengal castes. Man in India 49:80-92.

_______ (1976). A dermatoglyphic study of four Hindu Castes of Midnapur. Man in India 56:158-164.

Sarkar D, Biswas JN (1972). A dermatoglyphic study among the Mech of Jalpaiguri, West Bengal. Man in India 52:268-275.

Singh RD (1961). Digital pattern frequency and size variations in some castes of Uttar Pradesh. The Eastern Anthropologist 14:169-181.

_______ (1963). A note on arch/whorl index as a tool for classifying human populations. The Eastern Anthropologist 21:28-46.

_______ (1968). Finger dermatoglyphics of the Pasis (India). In "Proceedings volume of international symposium on dermatoglyphics 1966," University of Delhi: 241-247.

_______ (1978). Dermatoglyphic variations in four castes of Uttar Pradesh, India. Human Biology 50:251-260.

Sokal RR, Rohlf FJ (1969). "Biometry: the principles and practice of statistics in biological research." San Francisco: W H Freeman and Co.

Srivastava RP (1965). A quantitative analysis of the finger prints of the Tharus of Uttar Pradesh. Am J Phys Anthrop 23:99-106.

Walker HM and Lev J (1953). "Statistical Inference." New York: Henry Holt, p255.

Progress in Dermatoglyphic Research, pages 317–323

FINGER RIDGE COUNTS AND TFRC AMONG THE FIVE TURKMAN GROUPS IN IRAN

M.Sharif Kamali

Centre for Iranian Anthropology
Markaz Mardom Shenasi Iran
Ministry of Culture and Higher Education
Baharestan Tehran Iran

The quantitative dermatoglyphic features have got more attention in the recent years.Of the various quantitative dermatoglyphic features the total finger ridge count(TFRC)has,however,received major attention.A number of studied carried out on TFRC;mostly from European and Indian data; reveal marked vaiation among the various populations studied(Note among them;Holt,55;Book,54; Matsunaga et al.,76;Malhotra et al.,78;Singh,67; Weninger et al.,76;Kamali,79;Kamali and Bhanu,80).

On Iranian populations so far only few studies are available for their quantitative finger dermatoglyphics(Kamali,79;Kamali and Bhanu,80).

The purpose of this paper,therefore,is to report the finger ridge counts and TFRC among the five Tukman groups in Iran.An attempt has also been made to report their intragroup differences.

MATERIALS AND METHODS

Bilateral finger prints of 240 males belonging to the five Turkman groups viz. Garkaz,Jargalan, Hootan,Aqtaqeh and Korand Turkmans have been collected and analized.The sample size were 84,40, 4o,36 and 40 from the above groups,repectively.

Turkmans are supposed to be a Mongol tribe which migrated to Turkmanistan(USSR)and Turkman

Sahra(Iran) 700 years ago.Their physical characteristics support this and their language is composed of Mongol and Turkish dialects.They have been a nomad group before 1917.Their nomadic ways were Turkman Sahra and Turkmanistan.After 1917,s Revolution of USSR,because of the political situation,they could not continue their nomadic life,therefore,they settled both in Turkman Sahra and Turkmanistan.

Turkmans constitute a big exogamous tribe which contains many small endogamous groups.Each group lives in a village,and usually do not get married with the other Turkmans or non-Turkmans. They are patrilocal and patrilieal with more or less extended families.They usually have small land for cultivation and their ladies are carpet weavers.

The present data have been collected in 1978 and analized for the finger ridge counts and TFRC.The ridge counting method used was that of Holt(68).The t values have been used for the intragroup differences.

RESULTS AND DISCUSSION

The distribution of the TFRC among the groups studied;pooled data;are given in table-1.Total ridge counts of 200 and over occurred only in 8 out of 240 individuals studied and 117individuals are reported with a total ridge count of less than 100.Thus the results are not in agreement with Holt,s and Mavalwala,s findings.In those results, the number of individuals with TFRC of 200 and over occurred more and the number of individuals with less than 100 TFRC occurred much less compared with the present data.

The mean ridge counts on the individual fingers and TFRC among the groups studied are given in table-2.It is evident that TFRC values vary among the groups studied.The Aqtaqeh showed the highest(160.08) and the Garkaz Turkmans showed the lowest TFRC(127.95).

Table-1
Distribution of TFRC among the Turkman groups studied

Class	No	%
0-9	3	1.25
10-19	4	1.67
20-29	2	0.83
30-39	2	0.83
40-49	6	2.50
50-59	14	5.83
60-69	17	7.08
70-79	26	10.83
80-89	29	12.08
90-99	14	5.83
100-109	11	4.58
110-119	9	3.75
120-129	17	7.08
130-139	16	6.67
140-149	15	6.25
150-159	15	6.25
160-169	13	5.42
170-179	7	2.92
180-189	10	4.17
190-199	6	2.50
200-209	3	1.25
210-219	5	2.08
TFRC	137.65±2.79	

The highest mean finger ridge count is that for the right finger I among the four groups studied,while the mean ridge count of left fingerI among the Aqtaqeh Turkmans,is the highest.Holt (58) reported the mean ridge cout in the decreasing order of magnitude among the Britishers are those for finger I,IV,V,III,II.In the present series,however,only left hand of the Garkaz Turkmans conform to this pattern,while in the remaining nine hands,the sequence is variable. The sequences are I,IV,II,III,V among the right hands of the Jargalan,Hootan and Aqtaqeh Turkmans;I,IV, III,V,II among the right and left hands of Garkaz and Hootan Turkmans,respectively; I,IV,III,II,V

Table-2
Mean ridge couts of the individual fingers and TFRC among the groups studied

Side	Digit	Garkaz	Jargalan	Hootan	Aqtaqeh	Korand
	I	15.58±0.69	17.15±0.83	17.60±0.71	18.28±0.60	18.55±0.54
	II	11.45±0.78	13.43±0 77	12.25±0.77	16.39±0.99	12.95±0.92
R	III	11.64±0.78	12.93±0.77	11.53±0.82	15.14±0.92	11.05±0.79
	IV	14.40±0.57	15.73±0.81	13.97±0.79	16.72±0.89	13.25±0.96
	V	11.48±0.53	12.40±0.67	11.48±0.66	12.97±0.66	13.30±0.44
	I	14.24±0.72	16.55±0.79	16.00±0.84	18.47±0.81	17.50±0.67
	II	11.57±0.68	12.85±1.06	11.30±0.83	15.47±0.92	13.10±0.89
L	III	11.83±0.64	13.00±0.93	11.70±0.80	15.64±0.79	11.75±0.72
	IV	14.05±0.59	15.28±0.91	14.35±0.36	16.22±0.96	13.88±0.63
	V	12.01±0.50	12.75±0.62	11.43±0.59	14.31±0.79	12.20±0.45
TFRC		127.95±5.53	141.2±6.62	132.1±5.58	160.08±6.98	138.23±5.08

Table-3
Bimanual differences of the mean ridge counts on the individual fingers

Digit	Garkaz	Jargalan	Hootan	Aqtaqeh	Korand
I	+1.13	+0.60	+1.60	-0.19	+1.05
II	-0.12	+0.58	+0.95	+0.92	-0.15
III	-0.19	-0.07	-0.17	-0.50	-0.70
IV	+0.35	+0.45	-0.38	+0.50	-0.63
V	-0.53	-0.35	+0.05	-1.34	+1.10

among the left hands of Jargalan and Aqtaqeh Turkmans;I,V,IV,II,III among the right hands of Korand Turkmans,and finally I,IV,II,V,III among the left hands of Korand Turkmans.

Table-3 gives the differences in mean ridge counts between the fingers of the right and left hands.In the British samples(Holt,58)the mean ridge counts are higher on right hands than left, with the single exception of R III,and in the Parsi samples(Mavalwala,63) the values on right hands are greater only on digits I and II.However, the present data shows more ridge counts on right digits I and IV among the Garkaz;I,II and IV among the Jargalan;I,II and V among the Hootan; II and IV among the Aqtaqeh,and finally I and V among the Korand Turkmans.

Table-4 gives percent frequencies of persons in the sample with higher counts on the right hand,on the left hand,and with equal counts on both hands.Persons with higher ridge counts are almost as frequent as those with higher counts on right hand and even in two groups;Jargalan and Aqtaqeh Turkmans;are more than on the right hands. There are comparatively few with equal counts on both hands among the three out of the five groups studied.Equal counts on both hands are nil among the Garkaz and Hootan Turkmans.

Table-5 gives the intragroup differences for TFRC among the five Turkman groups studied.It is evident that the three out of the ten paired groups studied(30.00%)showed significant differences.The results,thus,showed homogeneity among the Turkmans of Iran in respect of TFRC.

REFERENCES

Holt SB(1968)."The Genetics of Dermal Ridges." USA: Charles C.Thomas.

Kamali M Sharif(1979)."Bio-Anthropological Profiles of the People of South Iran."University of Poona:Ph.D.Thesis.

Kamali M Sharif,Bhanu BV(1980).Summed finger

Table-4
Percent distributions of right/left differences of the finger ridge counts among the groups studied

R/L fference	Jarkaz	Gargalan	Hootan	Aqtaqeh	Korand
R L	55.42	45.00	57.50	44.45	65.80
R L	44.58	52.50	42.50	47.22	27.50
R L	00.00	2.50	00.00	8.33	7.50

Table-5
Intragroup differences of TFRC among the groups studied

Groups	Garkaz	Jargalan	Hootan	Aqtaqeh	Korand
Garkaz					
Jargalan	1.57				
Hootan	0.54	1.05			
Aqtaqeh	3.68*	1.96	3.11*		
Korand	1.41	0.36	0.81	2.53+	

*P<0.001 +P<0.05

ridge counts and ATFRC among the five Turkman groups groups in Iran.Unpublished.

Malhotra KC,Chakraborty R,Bhanu BV,Rao JM(1978). Distribution and inter-population differences of TFRC,ATFRC and PII among the 9 endogamous groups of Maharashtra,India.Tech.Rep.No.Anthrop /4/78 ISI.

Mavalwala J(1963).Quantitative analysis of finger ridge counts of the Parsi Community in India. Ann.Hum.Genet. 26:305

Singh S(1967).Quantitative analysis of finger ridge counts in Australians of European Ancestry Hum.Biol. 39:368

Progress in Dermatoglyphic Research, pages 325-334

DERMATOGLYPHICS IN SEIZURE DISORDERS

B. Schaumann, S.B. Johnson, and R.L. Jantz

Veterans Administration Medical Center, Minneapolis, Minnesota and University of Tennessee, Knoxville, Tennessee USA

Nearly all (Féré 1905, Abel 1936, Portius 1937, Brown and Paskind 1940, Katzenstein-Sutro 1945, Lübbe 1966, Rosner 1967, Pelkhofer 1969, Figueroa 1974, Razavi 1975, Sivanandan and Sambasivan 1975, Inada 1977a, Inada 1977b, Lopez and Lopez 1977, Tay 1979) of the 17 previous studies reviewed have indicated significant associations between dermatoglyphics and seizure disorders. In comparing the results of these studies, several problems arise, such as the comparability of diagnostic terminology, sample size, the level of significance of results, and the type and number of controls used. Some of these problems may explain seemingly contradictory results, such as the reported increase in ulnar loops on the left second digit in females with idiopathic seizures (Rosner 1967) and the decrease of the same in "genuine" seizures (Figueroa 1974) or both the increase (Portius 1937) and the decrease (Inada 1977b) in the total finger ridge count in unclassified seizures.

MATERIALS AND METHODS

The present study was undertaken to determine characteristic deviations of dermatoglyphic traits in seizure disorders using a cohort of 197 white, male epileptics compared with 200 white, male controls. The epileptics in the study were all patients with a confirmed diagnosis of one or more seizures and under treatment at the Epilepsy Treatment Center of the Minneapolis Veterans Administration Medical Center. Diagnosis was determined by patient history, neurological examination and electroencephalogram results. None of the patients suffered a significant congenital anomaly. The controls were healthy, North American Caucasian males from a geographically similar area (Minnesota) as the patients.

The patients were divided by etiology of seizures into the following eight groups:
(1) post-traumatic (trauma)--patients suffered a head injury serious enough to result in a loss of consciousness with a first seizure occurring within ten years after the injury;
(2) alcohol related--the convulsive disorder was related to alcohol either as a toxic-metabolic agent or due to alcohol withdrawal;
(3) familial--patient had a first or second degree relative(s) who had experienced a convulsion or seizure of any etiology;
combinations of the above factors in an individual patient, i.e.,
(4) trauma + alcohol,
(5) trauma + family,
(6) alcohol + family,
(7) trauma + alcohol + family; and
(8) other--seizures were of idiopathic or other etiologies, such as a cerebrovascular accident.

Because of the large number of variables, the dermatoglyphic data were grouped into smaller and more managable categories for multivariate analysis as follows:
Finger ridge counts (20 variables),
Finger pattern types, (10 variables),
Palmar quantitative traits (a-b ridge-count, atd angle and main line index; 6 variables), and
Palmar patterns (hypothenar, thenar/first interdigital, second, third and fourth interdigital areas; 10 variables).

All analyses were carried out using the Statistical Analysis System (SAS Institute 1979). Summary statistics were calculated for all variables. Then each of the above mentioned categories was subjected to one-way multivariate analysis of variance (MANOVA) using the general linear models procedure (GLM). Treatment classes were the eight etiological categories plus controls, a total of nine groups. The GLM procedure carries out a univariate analysis of variance for each variable followed by several multivariate tests for intergroup heterogeneity. Wilks' criterion and the associated F approximation were used to judge overall significance. For those analyses where the overall group effect was significant, we further evaluated residual variation after removing successive eigenvalues, using Bartlett's procedure (Seal 1964). Group scores were then obtained on canonical variates associated with significant eigenvalues to provide a picture of intergroup relationships in reduced dimensions.

RESULTS AND DISCUSSION

Mean frequencies of fingertip patterns are given in Table 1. Although some of these patterns appear to occur in different frequencies when compared by etiology to the controls (such as the radial and ulnar loops and the whorls of the alcohol + family or the arches in the trauma + alcohol categories), none of these differences were found to be statistically significant. Fingertip patterns showed one digit (left fourth) to be significant in the univariate analysis but the multivariate test was not significant. Since this is likely to have been a chance occurrence, or at best an exceedingly weak relationship, we have not considered it further.

The mean frequencies of the palmar patterns are found in Table 2. Again, the differences seen, such as the decreased frequencies of patterns in the third interdigital and hypothenar areas in the patients with a family history of seizures or the increased frequency of patterns in the fourth interdigital area in patients with an etiology of trauma + alcohol, were not significant.

Table 3 shows the mean total finger ridge counts, a-b ridge counts, the main line index, and the atd angle. When considered by etiology, none of the values was significant. However, when each variable was considered by hand in the epileptic cohort as a whole, univariate F ratios were significant for both the right and the left a-b ridge counts ($p<.001$) and the right main line index ($p<.01$). Using Wilke's criterion, the overall test for the six variables (left and right main line index, left and right atd angles, and left and right a-b ridge counts) was highly significant. Tests of the individual eigen values showed only one as being significant. This eigenvalue accounted for 71.8% of the intergroup variation. Canonical coefficients associated with this eigenvalue were used to obtain canonical variate scores for each individual and these were used to examine intergroup relationships. The contribution of the original variables to the canonical variate was ascertained by correlating the canonical variate scores obtained for each individual with the original variables (Table 4). The highest correlation of the canonical variate score was found in the left a-b ridge count. This variable was responsible for more of

TABLE 1

FREQUENCY BY PERCENT OF FINGERTIP PATTERN TYPES
IN PATIENTS WITH EPILEPSY AND CONTROLS

Epilepsy Type	Number of Digits	Pattern Type			
		Arch	Radial Loop	Ulnar Loop	Whorl
Post-traumatic	480	4.6	7.5	64.6	23.3
Alcohol-related	257	3.1	6.2	62.6	28.0
Idiopathic	486	4.5	6.4	58.2	30.9
Familial	230	1.7	6.1	69.1	23.0
Trauma + alcohol	90	1.1	6.7	56.7	35.6
Trauma + family	210	1.4	4.3	61.9	32.4
Alcohol + family	110	2.7	3.6	45.5	48.2
Trauma + alcohol + family	100	4.0	6.0	66.0	24.0
TOTAL	1963	3.4	6.2	61.6	28.7
CONTROLS	2000	6.7	5.0	59.9	28.4

TABLE 2
FREQUENCY BY PERCENT OF PALMAR PATTERNS
OF PATIENTS WITH EPILEPSY AND CONTROLS

Epilepsy Type	Number of Palms	Palmar Area				
		Thenar/ I_1	I_2	I_3	I_4	Hypothenar
Post-traumatic	96	2.1	7.3	37.5	49.0	34.4
Alcohol-related	52	3.8	7.7	30.8	55.8	36.5
Idiopathic	98	10.2	2.0	38.8	40.8	28.6
Familial	46	6.5	6.5	23.9	47.8	17.4
Trauma + alcohol	18	0.0	0.0	33.3	61.1	50.0
Trauma + family	42	2.4	2.4	33.3	50.0	26.2
Alcohol + family	22	9.1	0.0	40.9	40.9	22.7
Trauma + alcohol + family	20	0.0	5.0	40.0	35.0	45.0
TOTAL	394	3.8	4.6	35.0	47.2	31.2
CONTROLS	400	7.5	3.0	40.5	47.5	36.2

TABLE 3

MEAN VALUES OF TOTAL FINGER RIDGE COUNT, a-b RIDGE COUNT, MAIN LINE INDEX AND atd ANGLE IN PATIENTS WITH EPILEPSY AND CONTROLS

EPILEPSY TYPE	n	TFRC	a-b	MLI	atd
Post-traumatic	48	124.6	75.3	8.8	43.2
Alcohol-related	26	123.4	76.7	8.3	41.1
Idiopathic	49	137.4	78.5	8.6	43.5
Familial	23	134.7	79.0	8.3	41.9
Trauma + alcohol	9	151.8	82.9	7.6	47.1
Trauma + family	21	140.3	79.6	8.1	45.3
Alcohol + family	11	152.4	80.3	7.6	43.9
Trauma + alcohol + family	10	127.0	77.2	9.0	43.0
TOTAL	197	133.4	77.9	8.4	43.3
CONTROLS	200	142.9	84.0	8.3	42.8

TABLE 4
CORRELATION OF PALMAR PATTERNS
WITH THE CANONICAL VARIATE

Variable	Epilepsy (mean)	Controls (mean)	Univariate F	Correlation with CV1
L MLI	7.505	7.960	1.72	0.464
R MLI	9.366	8.680	2.61*	-0.222
L ATD	43.005	43.250	1.15	-0.017
R ATD	43.561	42.310	0.81	0.174
L AB	39.531	42.520	4.72**	-0.656
R AB	38.531	40.760	2.87**	-0.438

Wilks Criterion = 0.735, F=2.52, p<0.001

* p<0.01
**p<0.001

TABLE 5
MEANS AND STANDARD DEVIATIONS BY
ETIOLOGY ON THE CANONICAL VARIATE

Etiology	N	CV Mean	SD
Alcohol + Trauma	9	0.360	2.455
Alcohol	26	0.443	1.487
Alcohol + Family	11	0.565	1.938
Family	23	0.623	1.608
Other	47	0.625	1.313
Trauma + Family	21	0.878	1.725
Trauma + Alcohol + Family	9	1.045	1.330
Trauma	48	1.141	1.496
Control	200	-0.735	1.610

the intergroup variation than any other single variable. Both right and left a-b ridge counts had negative correlations with the canonical variate, i.e., epileptic patients were characterized by lower a-b ridge counts than controls.

The main line index correlations were of opposite signs, left being positive and right being negative. This may be taken to signify asymmetry of main line indices as the primary source of their intergroup heterogeneity. In general, it appears that epilepsy patients are characterized by higher right and lower left main line indices than controls.

Group means and standard deviations on the canonical variate are shown in Table 5. All epileptic patients, regardless of etiological category, were characterized by positive scores on the canonical variate, while controls had a negative score. This implies that epileptics of all etiological categories are more similar to each other than to controls. In an attempt to differentiate among different etiological categories of epileptics, a one-way analysis of variance was performed, using their scores on the canonical variate and omitting controls. The test showed no heterogeneity. Therefore, if there is heterogeneity among different etiological categories, it is not detectable with present sample sizes. It may be important, however, that those categories characterized by trauma and not alcohol have consistently higher canonical variate means than those groups characterized by alcohol and not trauma. This matter can only be resolved by larger samples of epileptics.

The above results support the hypothesis of an increased susceptibility to seizures occurring in some patients and/or families. An insult to the brain precipitating a seizure in these individuals would not cause a seizure in a less susceptible individual. Larger, more detailed studies and further analyses, however, are needed to answer such questions as the relationship of dermatoglyphics to this susceptibility and to other parameters such as seizure type; the possible diagnostic value of significant dermatoglyphic parameters both within and outside individual families; and factors which influence the development of epidermal ridge patterns.

SUMMARY

A dermatoglyphic study of 197 adult Caucasian males with a confirmed diagnosis of epilepsy was carried out in an attempt to ascertain possible associations between aberrant dermatoglyphics and seizures and to estimate their diagnostic usefulness. Qualitative and quantitative fingertip and palmar dermatoglyphic traits were evaluated. The data were analyzed by etiology of seizures.

Previous studies and our own earlier data (Schaumann 1979) analyzed by univariate statistical methods indicated the presence of some dermatoglyphic deviations in patients with epilepsy, suggesting the existence of a genetic predisposition to seizures of various etiologies. In the present study, a multivariate analysis was employed on an enlarged patient sample. Three variables were found to be significant: an increased main line index on the right palm ($p<.01$) and decreased a-b ridge counts on both left and right palms ($p<.001$). Tests of the eigenvalues showed only one value to be significant and accounting for 71.8% of the intergroup variation.

REFERENCES

Abel W. Über Störungen der Papillarmuster I. Gestörte Papillarmuster in Verbindung mit einigen körperlichen und geistigen Anomalien. Z Morphol Anthropol 36:1-37, 1936.

Brown M, Paskind HA. Constitutional differences between deteriorated and non-deteriorated patients with epilepsy. III. Dactylographic studies. J Nerv Ment Dis 92:579-604, 1940.

Féré C. Les empreintes digitales dans plusiers groupes des psychopathes. J Anat Physiol (Paris) 41:394-410, 1905.

Figueroa HH, Campos FJ, Lozano MT. Los dermatoglifos en la epilepsia. Estudio de 60 pacientes del Instituto Nacional de Neurologia. Rev Inst Nacl Neurol (Mex) 8:9-16, 1974.

Inada N. Studies on dermatoglyphs in children with disorders of the central nervous system. I. Palmar pattern (Jap.). J Tokyo Wom Med Coll 47:74-105, 1977a.

Inada N. Studies of dermatoglyphs in children with disorders of the central nervous system. II. Digital pattern (Jap.). J Tokyo Wom Med Coll 47:644-654, 1977b.

Katzenstein-Sutro E. Die Papillarmuster von Epileptikern ostschweizerischer Herkunft im Vergleich mit denjenigen der gesunden Population, dargestellt im Bimanuar und Daktylogramm. Arch Jul Klaus-Stift 20:27-50, 1945.

Lopez AR, Lopez TAV. Análisis de las líneas dermopapilares en epilépticos esenciales. Arch Neurobiol (Madr.) 40:347-362, 1977.

Lübbe H. Das Papillarleistensystem bei 100 genuinen Epileptikern. Dissertation, Münster, 1966.

Pelkhofer M. Kerngeschlecht und Papillarmuster bei 100 weiblichen Epileptikern. Dissertation, Erlangen, 1969.

Portius W. Über Anomalien der Beugefurchen an den Händen von Geisteskranken. Erbarzt 4:80-83, 1937.

Razavi L. Cytogenetic and dermatoglyphic studies in sexual offenders, violent criminals, and aggressively behaved temporal lobe epileptics. Proc Am Psychopathol Assoc 63:75-94, 1975.

Rosner F., Steinberg FS, Spriggs HA: Dermatoglyphic patterns in patients with selected neurological disorders. Am J Med Sci 254:695-708, 1967.

SAS Institute, Inc. SAS User's Guide. Raleigh: SAS Institute Inc., 1979.

Schaumann B, Mayersdorf A. Dermatoglyphics in epilepsy. Birth Defects XV(6):627-633, 1979.

Seal H. Multivariate Statistical Analysis for Biologists. London:Methuen and Co. Ltd., 1964.

Sivanandan G, Sambasivan M. Dermatoglyphics in epilepsy. Phronesis 19:37-43, 1975.

Tay JS. Dermatoglyphics in children with febrile convulsions. Br Med J 1:660, 1979.

Progress in Dermatoglyphic Research, pages 335-352

DERMATOGLYPHICS OF JEWISH DOWN PATIENTS

M. Bat-Miriam Katznelson, Ph.D.

Department of Human Genetics, Tel-Aviv University Medical School
Institute of Human Genetics, The Sheba Medical Center, Tel-Hashomer, Israel

INTRODUCTION

Since the discovery of Down Syndrome many investigations into the etiology of Down Syndrome were concerned with the genetical aspects of the subject.

The recognition of non-European populations was an important step in the study of this syndrome and its etiology.

Barbour (1902), Blyer (1925) and Dunlap (1933) recorded Negro patients and Blyer (1932, 1934) noted that it occurred among American and Mexican Indiano. An affected Chinese boy was reported in 1922, many Chinese and Japanese boys were reported in 1934 by Sweet. Cases were mentioned from India and Malaya. In 1955 it was found amongst Bantus of S. Africa and Uganda.

The cytogenetic studies from Japan and other countries proved the Down Syndrome to be all standard trisomies.

Cummins in 1936 was the first to define the characterisitc dermatoglyphic features of Down Syndrome as compared to normal populations. His findings were confirmed by various investigators for different racial and ethnic groups. Walker (1957) for Canadians and Italians (1964). Holt (1951, 1964) and Smith (1964) for the British (1966), Shiono et al. for the Japanese (1969), Bryant for the Chinese (1970), Saksena for Indians (1966)Plato for North Americans (1973). All studied the Down Syndrome patients and compared their results with their corresponding control populations.

The questions raised are whether the typical dermatoglyphic characteristics are superimposed onto the existing basic ethnic differences, and are the dermatoglyphic findings for the Jewish Down Syndrome oriented in the same direction as other Down patients, inspite of the initial ethnic differences between the control populations.

MATERIAL AND METHODS

We established in 1973 the main dermatoglyphic differences between the Ashkenazi Jews and the British populations (Katznelson & Ashbel, 1973).

Two hundred and ninety individuals of both sexes with Down syndrome are being reported. Their ages ranged from 1 day to 50 years. The diagnosis of all of them was confirmed by chromosomal analysis.

The group of the Down patients consists of two main sub-groups: Ashkenazi Jews and Sephardic Jews.This division has a long history to account for, but one can say in very general terms that the Ashkenazi Jews originate in Europe and North America - while the Sephardic Jews come from Spain, North Africa and the Eastern Mediterranean region.

The non-Jewish control populations we used were the British used by Penrose and Smith in their various papers.

Fingers, palms and plantar prints were available for analysis. The methods used for obtaining prints were the Hollister Dry-plate Footprinter and the Faurot Inkless method. A hand lens was used as an aiding tool. For counting ridges and measuring atd angles, a low binocular dissecting microscope was employed.

The general rules for counting ridges were those outlined by Holt (1968). The atd angle, the a-b ridge count and the ridge breadth were calculated according to the Memorandum of Dermatoglyphic Nomenclature by Penrose (1968) and by Penrose and Loesch (1967). The plantar and palmar topology are reported in the manner suggested by Penrose and Loesch (1969, 1970a).

The dermatoglyphic parameters studied were as follows: digital patterns, total ridge count, the a-b ridge count, the ridge width, the maximal atd angle, the main line index. The topological classification of the palmar and plantar patterns.

RESULTS AND DISCUSSION

I. Fingers

a. Pattern frequencies. One of the prominent dermatoglyphic features of Down Syndrome, as described by Cummins (1939), is the excess of ulnar loops. The elevated frequency of ulnar loops is associated with a decrease of whorls, radial loops and arches. Table 1, Figure 1, 2). This finding is common to both the Jewish and British Down patients. The absolute frequencies, however, of the digital patterns in the two control populations differ significantly (Katznelson and Ashbel, 1973). The trend described for Down Syndrome is present uniformly in the two different ethnic Down Syndrome patients groups.

Figure 1

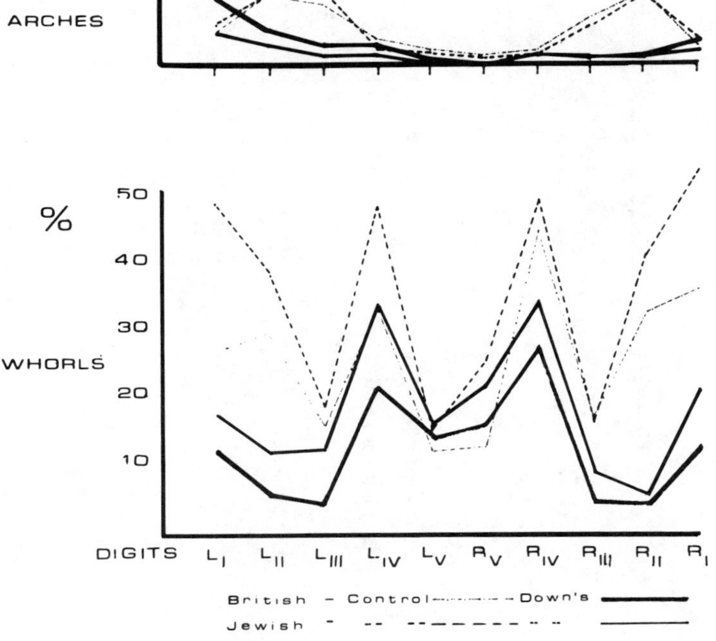

Table 1. PATTERN FREQUENCIES IN D.S. AND CONTROLS

	WHORL		ULNAR LOOP		RADIAL LOOP		ARCH	
	D	C	D	C	D	C	D	C
JEWS								
Ashkenazi	19.50	35.75	82.90	54.05	3.00	5.05	1.70	5.15
Sephardi	18.50		78.90		1.60		1.50	
British	12.68	26.10	82.81	63.50	1.70	5.40	2.74	5.00
Italian	12.60	33.10	81.00	57.20	5.20	3.50	1.10	6.20

D = Down Syndrome

C = Control

Figure 2

LOOP FREQUENCY.

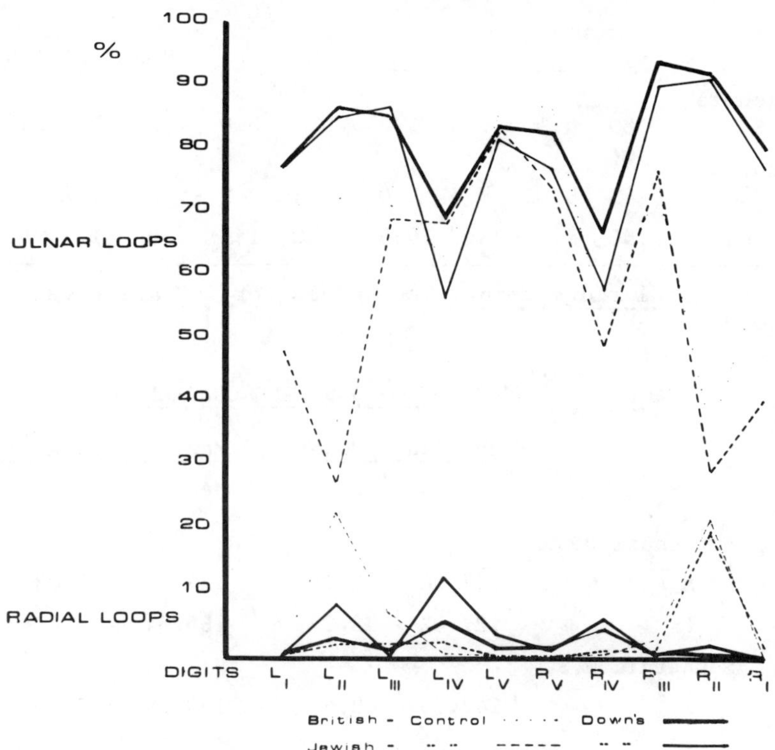

The radial loops tend to increase on digits IV and V and not on digits II and III as is found normally (Table 2). The average frequency of radial loops on digits IV, for both Jewish Down Syndrome patients is 13.8% as compared to 2% found in the control .

The average frequency of radial loops on digits V of Down Syndrome patients is 2% as compared to 0% found in the control population. This observation has been described by other investigators in patients with Down Syndrome of different racial and ethnic origins (Walker, 1957; Holt, 1964; Smith, 1966; Shiono et al, 1969; Bryant et al, 1970).

Table 2.

PERCENT OF RADIAL LOOPS ON DIGITS OF JEWISH D.S. AND CONTROLS

Digits	I		II		III		IV		V	
	R	L	R	L	R	L	R	L	R	L
Ashkenazi D.S.	0.80	0.9	1.8	1.8	0.9	0.9	4.7	12.5	1.8	1.8
Sephardi D.S.	0.45	0.0	8.5	2.0	0.5	0.5	5.7	15.7	1.9	1.5
Control	0.50	1.5	23.0	19.5	2.0	1.5	2.0	1.5	0.0	0.0

b. Total ridge count. The values for TRC are given in Table 3.

Table 3: COMPARISON OF D.S. AND CONTROLS

	Total Ridge Count Mean	S.D.	Maximal atd Angle Mean	S.D.
Ashkenazi D.S.				
M	127.06	± 42.18	154.74	± 32.83
F	127.02	± 38.29	166.54	± 37.40
Sephardic D.S.				
M	142.36	± 38.60	153.99	± 32.88
F	137.86	± 28.85	157.91	± 36.11
British D.S.				
M	130.29	± 41.32	137.30	± 27.50
F	124.44	± 33.28	137.70	± 28.60
Jewish Control				
M	152.17	± 39.93	89.50	± 18.00
F	138.21	± 40.09	88.20	± 14.80
British Control				
M	145.18	± 50.49	85.00	± 15.30
F	126.97	± 52.33	85.90	± 15.70

The TRC is lower in both Jewish groups with D.S. as compared to their control group. The same was found for the British D.S. and its control. The means for the two sexes differ significantly in both Jewish and British control groups (Katznelson and Ashbel, 1973).

The mean total ridge count for the two Jewish groups of males with Down syndrome is 127.06 and 142.36 as compared to 152.17 of the control population. The differences are significant. The mean total ridge count for the two female groups with Down Syndrome are closer to the mean total ridge count of the control. The mean TRC for Sephardic females is 137.86 as compared to 138.21 of the control, the Ashkenazi D.S. females have a mean of 127.20.

There exists a definite tendency toward a uniformity in the values of TRC for both sexes with Down Syndrome of the two different ethnic populations, (Holt, 1951).

II. Palms

a-b ridge count. The mean sum of the a-b count in Down Syndrome is significantly lower in both sexes (Table 4),

Table 4: COMPARISON OF D.S. AND CONTROLS

	a-b Count			Ridge Width		
	Mean		S.D.	Mean		S.D.
Ashkenazi D.S.						
M	74.20	±	15.76	365.34	±	124.19
F	72.90	±	12.09	353.85	±	97.49
Sephardic D.S.						
M	76.65	±	13.92	330.16	±	174.66
F	74.30	±	11.44	324.96	±	86.92
British D.S.						
M	76.88	±	11.42	499.00	±	42.00
F	79.18	±	8.62	472.00	±	34.00
Jewish Control						
M	82.90	±	12.23	558.00	±	44.60
F	81.43	±	11.15	507.00	±	74.30
British Control						
M	83.01	±	9.7	565.00	±	41.00
F	80.04	±	10.3	514.00	±	39.00

than in controls. The variance in the mongol males, both Jewish and British, is higher than in females. The mean a-b value for Ashkenazi males with D.S. is 74.20 with standard deviation of 15.76, and 76.65 for Sephardic males with D.S., the standard deviation being 13.92. The corresponding value for control sample is 82.90 with standard deviation of 12.23.

The mean value for female Ashkenazi D.S. is 72.90 with standard deviation of 12.09 and the value obtained for the Sephardic female with D.S. is 74.30 with standard deviation of 11.44. The value for normal Jewish female is 81.43 $\pm$ 11.35. The mean sum of the a-b counts of both D.S. groups is significantly lower than the controls.

Fang (1949) found that the mean sum of the a-b ridge count of patients with D.S. differ significantly from that of the control population. Holt (1968) did not confirm Fang's finding in her series. Both Jewish mongol groups show the same trend as described by Fang (1949), that the a-b ridge count of the patients with D.S. is lower than the controls of both sexes. Shiono and Kadowaki (1974) found the a-b ridge count for Japanese patients slightly lower than the normals, but not significantly.

Cummins (1936, 1939) found a high axial triradius (t") in 72% of his patients, which was 8 times more than in normal individuals. Penrose (1954) introduced the quantitative measurement of the atd angle and found it to be significantly higher in mongols than in controls. He found this quantitative parameter to be age and sex dependent, thus he divided his results to three age groups: 0-4 years, 5-14 years and from 15 years on. Penrose's mean of maximal atd for adult British mongols is 137.3^{o}. The mean obtained for Jewish mongols is 154.70^{o} for males and 166.50^{o} for females, but the samples are of all ages from 1 day to 50 years of age. However, there is no doubt that the value of the maximal atd angle for mongols is higher than the control group.

According to Penrose and Loesch (1970a) topological classification the frequency of triradius t" (Table 7) is 69% in Ashkenazi D.S. and 82.5 in Sephardic mongols, and both differ significantly from the value of 7.8% obtained for the Jewish control group. The values for Canadian mongols and British as reported by Walker (1957) and Penrose (1954) are 90% of t" for Canadians and 72.5% for British. The values reported by other investigators for Japanese and Chinese D.S. (Shiono et al, 1969; Bryant et al, 1970) are lower, 44.5% and 58.5% respectively.

Ridge width (Table 4). Both the Jewish D.S. and the British have significantly narrower ridges than their respective controls. The significant differences between the means of the sexes as were observed for both control groups, (Katznelson and Ashbel, 1973) are diminished in all three D.S. patients groups. The narrow ridges in the cases of Down Syndrome can be considered according to Penrose (Penrose and Loesch, 1967) "to be a reflection of their relatively short statures". When Penrose compared his results of the ridge width with those obatined in control children of comparable stature he found the values to be very similar.

Simian line (Table 5). A single transverse flexion crease occurs at 40% of individuals with Down syndrome. In both Jewish Down syndrome patients the frequency is lower than found for the British Down Syndrome patients. There is no significant difference between the two control groups.

Table 5: COMPARISON OF D.S. AND CONTROLS

<table>
<tr><th></th><th colspan="2">%
III Interdigital</th><th colspan="2">%
Simian Line</th></tr>
<tr><th></th><th>L</th><th>R</th><th>L</th><th>R</th></tr>
<tr><td>Ashkenazi D.S.
M + F</td><td>63.71</td><td>82.86</td><td>27.61</td><td>31.42</td></tr>
<tr><td>Sephardic D.S.
M + F</td><td>59.73</td><td>81.88</td><td>31.54</td><td>30.87</td></tr>
<tr><td>British D.S.
M + F</td><td>52.20</td><td>83.90</td><td>65.60</td><td>71.00</td></tr>
<tr><td>Jewish Control
M + F</td><td>44.50</td><td>57.50</td><td colspan="2">6</td></tr>
<tr><td>British Control
M + F</td><td>27.50</td><td>48.20</td><td>13.0</td><td>8.00</td></tr>
</table>

Main line index. A high main line index is one of the typical dermatoglyphic traits described by Cummins (1939). He stated that "the main line index being unprecedentedly high 11.11".

The main line index for both Jewish Down Syndrome is high, where right is higher than left in both groups Table 6). The same manual differences are much more pronounced in the control group, where the values for the right hand are higher than for left hand.

Table 6. COMPARISON OF D.S. AND CONTROLS

	Main Line Index	
	L	R
Ashkenazi D.S.		
M + F	10.59 ± 1.91	10.93 ± 1.52
M	10.67 ± 0.64	10.81 ± 1.56
F	10.47 ± 2.25	10.47 ± 1.51
Sephardic D.S.		
M + F	10.53 ± 2.08	10.85 ± 1.93
M.	10.28 ± 2.36	10.86 ± 2.12
F	10.89 ± 1.49	10.83 ± 1.68
Jewish Control		
M	8.18 ± 2.06	9.29 ± 1.87
F	8.39 ± 2.20	9.28 ± 2.07

Palmar patterns. Results are given in Table 7. One of the most prominent dermatoglyphic feature of Down Syndrome, as drescribed by Cummins (1939) is the increase in the frequency of the II and III interdigital patterns.

In both Jewish D.S. patients and British D.S. patients there is an elevated frequency of the third interdigital pattern, where the right hand exceeds significantly that of the left hand. This was observed by others for various populations (Fang, 1950, Beckman et al, 1962, Shiono et al, 1969; Bryant et al, 1970; Plato et al, 1973). The differences between D.S. patients and their respective control groups are significantly (Table 10).

Table 7. FREQUENCIES OF PALMAR CHARACTERISTICS IN JEWISH D.S. AND CONTROLS

	Ashkenazi D.S. %	Sephardi D.S. %	Control %
Patterns			
I	0.0	0.0	9.30
I^R	0.0	1.50	8.50
II	7.04	10.50	9.50
$\hat{II}$	0.0	0.0	0.00
III	78.67	75.00	51.50
III^T	19.01	16.00	12.50
IV	11.97	13.00	56.00
$\widehat{IV}$	0.0	0.50	3.50
V	61.27	52.00	12.30
$\hat{V}$	11.27	7.50	26.30
V^R	0.0	0.0	2.00
Total	189.43	176.00	191.90
Triradii			
e,f	0.0	1.5	16.8
t	64.08	64.0	72.0
t'	11.97	8.50	30.5
t"	69.01	82.50	7.8
t'"	0.70	0.0	0.0
t^b	10.56	5.5	26.00
t^u	0.0	0.0	1.5
z'	4.23	4.5	1.0
z"	0.70	1.0	3.0
Total	161.25	167.5	158.6

Abortive C or III^T is found considerably higher in both Jewish D.S. patients but is completely absent in the British D.S. group. This finding corresponds with the results obtained for both control groups, namely a complete absence of III^T in the British control population (Katznelson and Ashbel, 1973).

The hypothenar patterns V, $\hat{V}$, V^R are usually associated with a high atd angle, are significantly more frequent among all the Down Syndrome patients than their respective controls.

Absence of C triradius (z') is significantly higher in both groups of Jewish Down Syndrome patients as compared to the Jewish control population (Table 10). The British Down Syndrome patients do not differ from their control.

There is a significant reduction in the frequency of palmar patterns in the thenar / first interdigital area and also in the IV interdigital area (Table 7). This observation was described by Beckman et al (1962) for Swedish D.S., by Berg (1968) for British and by Plato et al (1973) for North American Down Syndrome patients.

Pattern intensity. There is no marked difference in the frequency of the palmar patterns of Jewish Down Syndrome patients, of both groups, as compared to the Jewish Control.

The pattern intensity of Jewish D.S. patients is either equal or smaller than their control value (1.91 for control population, Ashkenazi D.S. - 1.89, and 1.76 for Sephardic D.S.).

British D.S. have a higher pattern intensity than the control population (1.88 vs 1.67 for British control group).

The pattern intensity of Jews is significantly higher than in British population (Katznelson and Ashbel, 1973).

These results suggest that the frequency of the palmar patterns in Jewish Down Syndrome patients does not differ markedly from that of the control group; however, in the British Down patients there is a significant elevation of the palmar pattern.

III. Soles

The predominant pattern in the hallucal area of Down syndrome patients is the arch tibial and if not arch tibial then a small distal loop with a ridge count of 20 or less. The arch tibial is a very very rare pattern in both normal Jewish and British populations (Table 8).

Another typical dermatoglyphic trait for Down Syndrome is the presence of distal loops in the fourth interdigital plantar area: Consequently the triradius p" occurs more frequently (Table 9).

Table 8. FREQUENCIES OF HALLUCAL PATTERNS

	% A^t		% L^d *	
	L	R	L	R
Ashkenazi D.S.	56.04	64.83	40.66	43.95
Sephardic D.S.	55.63	55.63	34.72	36.62
British D.S	53.80	46.95	30.20	35.80
Jewish Control	0.0	0.0	?	?
British Control	0.0	0.3	9.75	12.30

* L^d small = less than 20 ridges

The frequency of the pattern in fourth interdigital area for Ashkenazi D.S. patients is 25.46 and 20.88 for Sephardic as compared to the 11% (Bat-Miriam, 1970) of the control population. The British have an incidence of 48% as compared to 12.5% of the British control (Table 11), (Smith, 1964).

Contrary to the report by Penrose and Loesch (1970b) about the almost complete absence of zygodactylous triradii in their British patients of Down Syndrome, the Jewish D.S. patients show a marked increase of the zygodactylous triradii (Tables 9 and 11).

The pattern intensity for Sephardic D.S. is lower (1.49) than that of the Ashkenazi D.S. (1.70). The pattern intensity of the British D.S. much lower (1.61) than its control (2.62).

The over all plantar pattern intensity is decreased in all Down Syndrome patients because of a reduced frequency of plantar patterns, except in the fourth interdigital area. Not enough data is available as yet of the pattern types of soles of normal Jewish populations.

Table 9. COMPARISON OF FREQUENCIES OF PLANTAR CHARACTERISTICS OF JEWISH D.S. AND BRITISH D.S.

	Ashkenazi D.S. %	Sephardic D.S. %	British D.S. %
<u>Loops</u>			
I	53.25	45.63	51.09
I^R	0.70	1.94	1.46
II	0.70	1.46	0.73
$\widehat{\text{II}}$	2.82	3.40	2.19
III	56.34	49.51	53.65
$\widehat{\text{III}}$	4.23	2.91	0.73
IV	25.35	19.42	46.35
$\widehat{\text{IV}}$	2.11	1.46	2.55
V	0.0	0.97	0.73
$\widehat{\text{V}}$	24.65	22.33	1.09
Total	170.42	149.03	160.93
<u>Triradii</u>			
e	0.70	1.46	1.46
f	50.70	46.60	50.73
g	0.0	0.97	1.09
h	24.65	22.33	1.09
p	45.07	35.44	34.67
p'	22.54	19.40	35.77
p"	18.31	14.56	30.66
z	4.23	8.74	4.01
z'	4.93	3.40	0.36
z"	2.11	2.43	0.73
Total	173.24	155.83	160.57

Table 10. COMPARISON OF FREQUENCIES OF PALMAR CHARACTERISTICS BETWEEN JEWISH D.S., BRITISH D.S. AND THEIR CONTROL

	Ashkenazi D.S.		Sephardic D.S.		British D.S.	
	Higher Frequency in	Significance of Difference $p \leq$	Higher Frequency in	Significance of Difference $p \leq$	Higher Frequency in	Significance of Difference $p \leq$
Loops						
I	C	.001	C	.001	C	.005
I^R	C	.001	C	.001	C	.02
II					D	.01
III	D	.001	D	.001	D	.001
IV	C	.001	C	.001	C	.001
$\acute{IV}$	C	.05	C	.05	N.S.	
V	D	.001	D	.001	D	.001
$\hat{V}$	C	.001	C	.001	C	.001
Triradii						
e,f	C	.001	C	.001	C	.001
t'	C	.001	C	.001	C	.001
t"	D	.001	D	.001	D	.001
t^b	C	.001	C	.001	C	.001
z'	D	.01	D	.01	N.S.	

D = Down Syndrome

C = Control

SUMMARY

Two Jewish groups with Down Syndrome were studied, and were found to be similar. The findings were compared with those obtained by various investigators for British D.S. and British controls (Penrose, 1954; Holt, 1964, 1968; Penrose and Smith, 1966; Smith and Berg, 1976).(Table 10).

Digital, palmar and plantar parameters were studied.

Inspite of the significant ethnic differences existing between the two control populations, the Jews and the Britons, the Jewish patients with Down Syndrome manifest a uniformity of dermatoglyphic characteristics as do the British patients (Table 11). These typical dermatoglyphic characteristics are superimposed on the ethnic differences.

Table 11. COMPARISON OF FREQUENCIES OF PLANTAR CHARACTERISTICS BETWEEN JEWISH D.S. AND BRITISH D.S.

	Ashkenazi D.S.		Sephardic D.S.	
	Higher Frequency in	Significance of Difference p ≦	Higher Frequency in	Significance of Difference p ≦
Loops				
III	J	.01	J	.05
IV	B	.001	B	.001
V	J	.001	J	.001
Triradii				
h	J	.001	J	.001
p'	B	.005	B	.005
p"	B	.001	B	.001
z	N.S.		J	.05
z'	J	.001	J	.005
z"	N.S.		J	.05

J = Jewish D.S.

B = British D.S.

It seems that Down Syndrome has many features in common the world over, but the details of the differences are important for each ethnic group, and should not be neglected.

Acknowledgment

Heartfelt thanks are extended to Mrs. R. Grossman for her painstaking efforts in preparing this manuscript for publication.

REFERENCES

Barbour PF (1902). Quoted by Penrose LS & Smith GF (1966).

Bat-Miriam M Unpublished data.

Beckman L, Gustavson KH, Norring A (1962). Finger and palm dermal ridge patterns in normal and mongoloid individuals (The Down Syndrome). Acta Genet (Basel) 12:20.

Berg JM (1968). Observations on thenar / first interdigital dermatoglyphic pattern in mongolism. J Ment Defic Res 12:307.

Blyer A (1925) Quoted by Penrose LS & Smith GF (1966).

Brahdy MB (1927) Quoted by Penrose LS & Smith GF (1966).

Bryant J, Emanuel I, Huan SW, Kronmal R & Lo, J. (1970) Dermatoglyphics of Chinese children with Down's Syndrome. J Med Genet 7 :338.

Cummins H (1936) Dermatoglyphic stigmata in Mongoloid imbeciles. Anat Rec 64:11.

Cummins H (1939) Dermatoglyphic stigmata in Mongoloid imbeciles. Anat Rec 73:407.

Cummins H, Talley C, Platov RU (1950) Palmar dermatoglyphics in Mongolism. Pediatrics 5:241.

Dunlap JE (1933) Quoted by Penrose LS & Smith GF (1966).

Fang TC (1949) A comparative study of the a-b ridge count on the palms of mental defectives and the general population. J Ment Sci 95:945.

Fang TC (1950) A third interdigital pattern on the palm of the general British population, mongoloid and non-mongoloid mental defectives. J Ment Sci 96 :780.

Holt SB (1951) A comparative quatitative study of the finger prints of mongolian imbeciles and normal individuals. Ann Eugen (London) 15:355.

Holt SB (1964) Finger print pattern in mongolism. Ann Hum Genet 27:279.

Holt SB (1968)"The Genetics of Dermal Ridges". Springfield, Ill, Charles C Thomas.

Katznelson Bat-Miriam M, Ashbel S (1973) Dermatoglyphics of Jews. Z Morph Anthrop 65:14.

Penrose LS (1954) The distal triradius t on the hands of parents and sibs of mongol imbeciles. Ann Hum Genet 19:10.

Penrose LS, Smith GF (1966) "Down's Anomaly" London: J and A Churchill.

Penrose LS, Loesch D (1967) A study of fermal ridge width in the second (palmar) interdigital area with special reference to aneuploid states. J Ment Defic Res 11:36.

Penrose LS (1968) Memorandum on dermatoglyphic nomenclature. Birth Defects Original Article Series 4. New York: The National Foundation.

Penrose LS, Loesch D (1969) Dermatoglyphic sole patterns: a new attempt at classification. Human Biology 41:427.

Penrose LS, Loesch (1970a) Topological classification of palmar dermatoglyphics. J Ment Defic Res 14:111.

Penrose LS, Loesch D (1970b) Comparative study of sole patterns in chromosomal abnormalities. J Ment Defic Res 14:129.

Plato CC, Cereghino JJ, Steinberg FS (1973) Palmar dermatoglyphics of Down Syndrome: Revisited. Pediat. Res. 7:11.

Saksena DW, Bajpai PC, Dube SK (1966). Quoted by Schaumann B and Alter M (1976.

Schaumann B, Alter M (1976)"Dermatoglyphics in Medical Disorders". New York, Springer Verlag.

Shiono H, Kadowaki J, Kasahara S (1969) Dermatoglyphics of Down's syndrome in Japan. Tohoku J Exp Med 99:107.

Shiono H, Kadowaki J (1971). The palmar a-b ridge count in Japanese: normal population, Down's syndrome and Klinefelter's syndrome. Hum Biol 43 :288.

Smith GF (1964) Dermatoglyphic patterns on the fourth interdigital area of the sole in Down's syndrome. J Ment Defic Res 8:125.

Smith GF, Berg JM (1976) "Down's Anomaly". New York, Churchill Livingstone.

Walker FN (1957) The use of dermal configurations in the diagnosis of mongolism. J Paediat 50:19.

Walker FN, Johnson HM (1964) Comparative studies of the dermatoglyphics of Italian patients with Down's syndrome. Int Copenhagen Cong Scient Study Ment Retard.

Progress in Dermatoglyphic Research, pages 353–370

DEVELOPMENT OF PALM AND MAIN-LINE CONFIGURATIONS IN DOWN'S SYNDROME

DHARMDEO N. SINGH AND KAREN DAVIS

Division of Medical Genetics, Dept. of Pediatrics
Meharry Medical College Nashville, Tennessee
37208, U.S.A.

Since Cummins (1,2) first demonstrated the dermatoglyphic abnormalities associated with Down's Syndrome, a vast number of reports have appeared in the literature.

The emphasis of differentiating between Down's Syndrome and normal has been placed on the presence of increased ulnar loop patterns on the finger tips (3-12), low total ridge count (7,13), distally placed axial triradius (7,10,12,14-16), presence of hypothenar pattern (4,10,17,18), third interdigital loop (4,6,7,10,12,16,18-20), simian crease (4,7,10,12,15,17,18,20), sydney line and single flexion crease on fifth finger (7,10,12,15.17, 20,22-24). Few studies have been conducted (26, 30) on main-line termination positions in Down's Syndrome individuals. The present study has focused on the development of the gross configuration and termination point of all five main lines in Down's Syndrome as compared to normal individuals.

The study was carried out on a sample of 483 individuals consisting of 370 normal controls (197 male and 122 female Blacks and 30 male and 21 female Whites) and 113 Down's Syndrome (32 male and 10 female Blacks and 32 male and 38 female Whites).

The normal control population was derived from the staff and medical students of Meharry Medical College who were proven to be both clinically and cytogenetically normal.

The Down's Syndrome patients referred to our Medical Genetics Laboratory for a chromosomal analysis were diagnosed as all having trisomy 21.

Palmar prints were obtained by the inkless method of printing using materials furnished by Faurot Incorporation. The prints were analyzed for comparison between the two groups as to the pattern types formed and the termination position of D,C,B,A, and T main lines. The results were coded and the data placed in the computer and analysed by the method given in Statistical Package for the Social Sciences (31).

Holt (30) based main line configuration types as to the frequency found, the highest being the α -type in which D-line terminates in interdigital area II, and the least frequent, δ -type, in which D-line terminates in interdigital area I.

As the D line influences the direction of the other main line termination points and pattern thereby formed, we are hereby suggesting a change in the name of the main line configuration types as starting with the D line terminating from radial to ulnar side. The following types are described: α-type, if the termination is in interdigital area I, β -type, in area II, γ -type in area III, δ -type in area IV and ε -type if the termination is in the ulnar border of the palm.

α-Type:

The D-line ridge courses across the distal portion of the palm in a radial direction enclosing C,B and A main lines and terminating at the radial border in the interdigital area I in position 13. By enclosing C,B, and A-lines, it has restricted their possible terminations to the distal border of the palm between positions 7 through 13(Fig. 1).

In Down's Syndrome α-type pattern was found in 1.77 and 4.42 percent in the left and right palms respectively, while in the normals it was absent in the left and present in 0.51 percent in the right palm (Table 1).

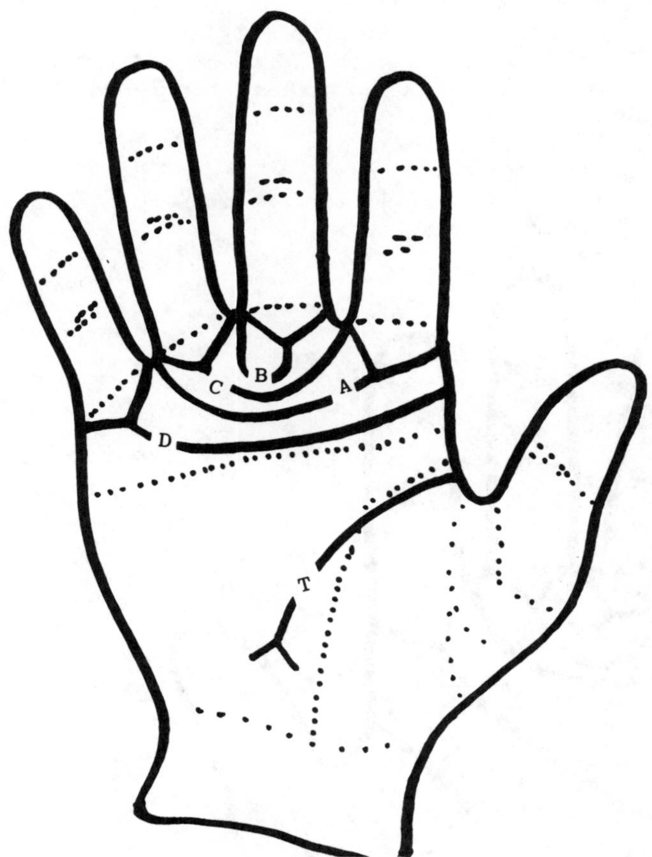

Fig. 1. α-type main line configuration.

β- Type:

The D-line has a radial course, enclosing C and B main lines, and terminating at the distal border of the palm in the interdigital II area in termination position 11. Main lines A has not been enclosed and will have possible termination position of 11, 13 or 1 through 5. Termination positions for C-line are restricted to 7 through 10, X (abortive) or 0 (missing) by either forming an ulnar or radial loop in the interdigital IV or III areas, terminating into b triradius, or having an abortive C-line or absent c triradius. Termination positions for B-line would be from 7 through 11, either by enclosing C-line, or forming a radial loop in interdigital II area or forming an ulnar loop in interdigital III or terminating into c triradius (Fig. 2).

The β-type pattern was found in 61.06 and 61.95 percent in Down's and 17.17 and 37.13 percent in normals in the left and right palm respectively (Table 1).

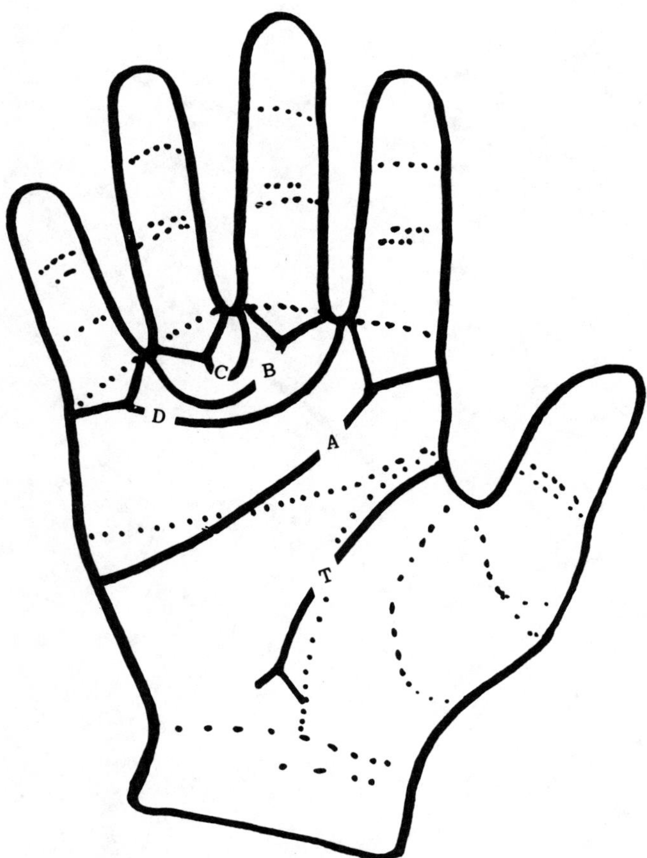

Fig. 2. β-type main line configuration

γ-Type

The D-line has a radial course enclosing C-line only

and terminating at the distal border of the palm in interdigital III area in termination position 9. By this enclosure, D-line has restricted C-line to termination positions of either 7 or 9, forming a ulnar or radial loop in the interdigital IV or III area, or by having an abortive C-line or an absent c triradius. Main lines B and A are not enclosed or restricted by D-line and have termination positions between 1 through 5 or 9 through 13 (Fig. 3).

The ϒ-type pattern was found in 10.35 and 15.93 percent in Down's and 30.56 and 29.80 percent in normals in the left and right palms respectively (Table 1).

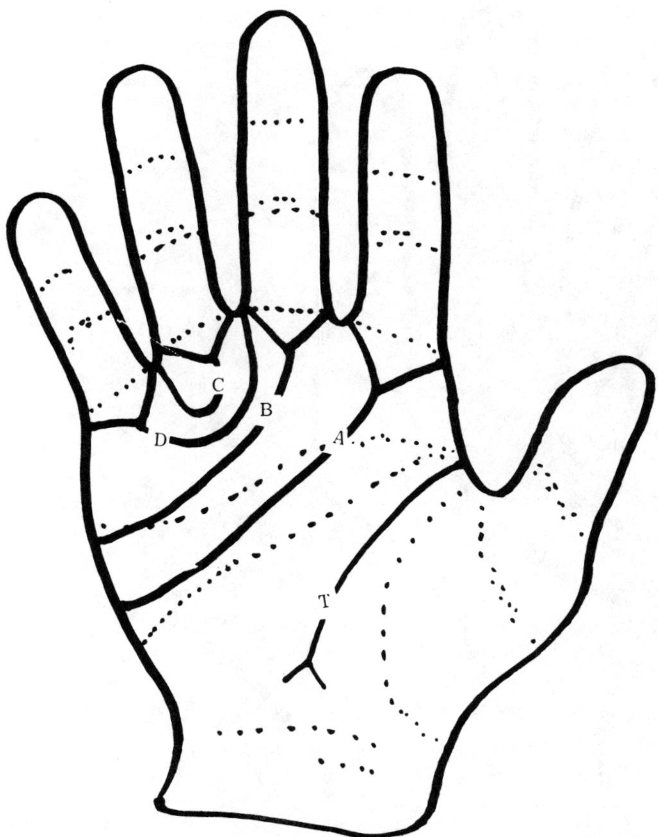

Fig. 3. ϒ -type main line configuration.

δ -Type:

The D-line forms a radial loop in the interdigital IV area and terminate at the distal border of the palm in termination position 7. Main line C, B and A are not enclosed or restricted by D-line and have possible terminations positions between 1 through 5, or 7 through 13 (Fig. 4).

The δ -type pattern was found in 14.14 and 16.81 percent in Down's and 48.74 and 27.53 percent in normals in the left and right palm respectively (Table 1).

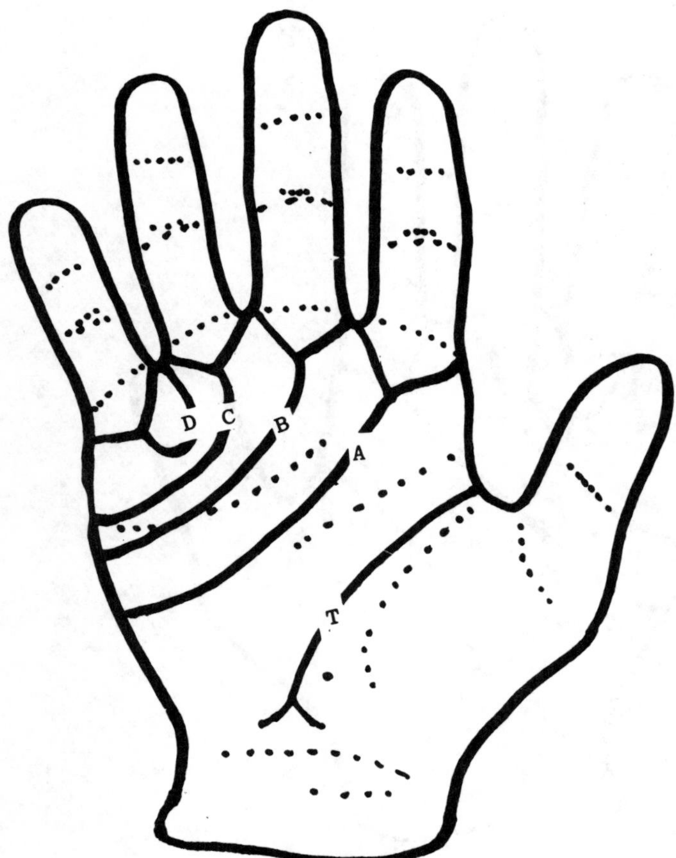

Fig. 4. δ -type main line configuration.

ϵ -Type:

The D-line has formed a loop with an ulnar opening, situated proximially to the d triradius in termination position 5. Main line C, B, and A are not enclosed or restricted by D-line and have possible termination positions between 1 through 5 and 7 through 13 (Fig. 5).

This rare ϵ-type was not found in Down's but was present in 0.51 and 0.76 percent of the normals in the left and right palm respectively (Table 1).

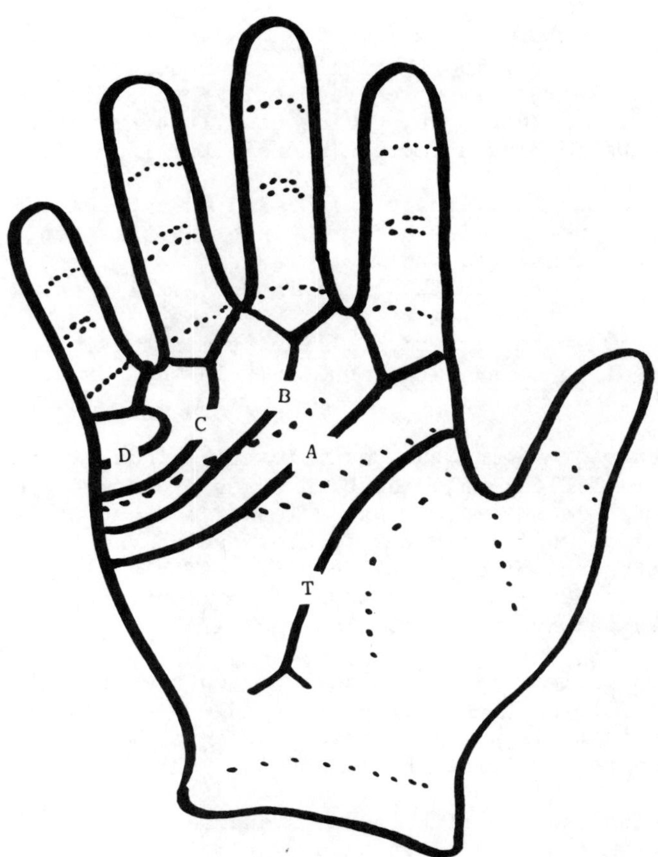

Fig. 5. ϵ -type main-line configuration.

The α-type in which the D line terminates at the radial border of the hand is usually present in male Down's Syndrome in both races, but is extremely rarely present in normal individuals and female Down's Syndrome of both races (Table 5). Similar results were found by Geipel (25), Dallopiceola and Ricci (17) and Holt (26).

The β-type, in which the D line terminates in interdigital area II, is the most frequent pattern found in Down's Syndrome, however in female Down's Syndrome it is significiantly higher (Table 5). In this -type, C line terminates in position 9 forming a third interdigital loop (Table 4).

The γ-type, in which the D line terminates in the interdigital III area, is more frequently found in normals of both races. In this type, C-line usually terminates in position 7 thus forming a fourth interdigital loop (Table 5).

In the normal individuals the γ-and δ-types are more frequently present, forming a fourth interdigital loop, while in Down's Syndrome, the most frequent is a loop, formed by C line only, in the third interdigital area.

The rare ϵ-type, in which D-line terminates into the ulnar border of the hand, was found only in the normal male of both races.

An absence of C-line was significantly higher in both races and normal Black male and both sexes of Down's Syndrome. Normal Black females showed less frequency of abortive C-line, while no Black female Down's Syndrome showed the presence of an abortive C line (Table 4). Similar results were found by others in oriental populations (10,12) and Europeans populations (17).

There is a significantly higher percentage of C and B main lines joining together in Black male Down's Syndrome, while there is no difference between normal male and female White and female Black Down's Syndrome.

In Down's Syndrome of both races and sex, A-line more frequently terminates in position 5 (Table 2), which corresponds with the β-type. In normal individuals, A-line seems to terminate in position 11 due to the formation of either an extra a triradius, or when A line forms a radial loop in the hypothenar area.

In the left palm of Down's Syndrome in both races and sexes, there is a significantly higher percentage of T-line terminating in position 11, while it is absent in the right palm of normal males of both races and both sexes of Black Down's Syndrome(Table 6).

Discussion

The primary dermal ridges and grooves begin to differentiate during the 12th and 13th weeks of gestation, and begin to subdivide into double parallel ridges, or secondary dermal ridges, by the formation of the furrow from about the 18th to 19th week.

Okajima (27) observed dermal ridges on the finger apices of a 13 week fetus that were distinctive enough to be counted. Formation of ridges starts from the apices of the volar pads and gradually extend to cover the whole volar surface with a distinctive pattern. Volar pads regress with age and are considered to be most important for pattern determination.

The dermal ridges are different for every palm of every person and they do not change throughout life and survive superficial injury.

The percise mechanisms involved in pattern type development at this time still remain obscure. There seems, however, to be two major theories. The first theory is dependent upon the underlying peripheral nerve arrangement(28); the second theory is dependant upon the amount of tension and pressure which is set up with skin growth and subsidence of the volar mounds has a determinating effect on the direction of the parallel line system. Parellel lines tend to follow the greatest convexity of the external surface (29).

Because of this early embryonic development of dermal ridges, dermatoglyphic patterns are among the relatively few human characteristics which are not modified by environmental influences after birth. They provide traits which are well suited for genetic and anthropological investigations, particularly when they can be analysed in a quantitative manner. In certain abnormal conditions there are characteristic pattern distortions occuring when an abnormality affects limb growth at an early stage of development. Disturbances can be caused environmentally by diseases such as fetal rubella syndrome or by thalidomide poisoning. Specific peculiarities are sometimes the results of a single abnormal gene which affect the growth of the hands and feet as in the "lobster claw" deformity. Consistent peculiarities of hand shape occur in association with chromosomal aberrations. Down's Syndrome has a very distintive gross appearance of a short, broad, square shaped hand with short fingers and incurved and missing flexion crease on the fifth finger, with a single transverse palmar fexion crease.

In Down's Syndrome α and β types patterns are the most frequently found, whereas in the normal, γ, δ and ε- type patterns are more frequent. So it would seem that there is a definite correlationship of the development of the D,C,B, and A main line exits. Development of the D-line certainly influences the development of A,B and C-lines. When D-line develops first and terminates in the radial border of the palm, as in the α-type it encloses A,B and C-lines to the distal border. In γ-type, A and B-lines develop before the D-line and in δ and ε type, A-B and C-line develop before the D-line.

When A-line develops before D-line, as in type, which is found more frequently in Down's Syndrome, D-line encloses B and C-lines and terminates in position 11. The A-line is pushed distally by the presence of a hypothenar pattern or extra axial triradius, to the distal side of the palm, and to terminates into position 5. Down's Syndrome usually has a hypothenar pattern or a distally placed axial triradius which deters the A-line to terminate in the proximal area of the palm.

A third interdigital loop is formed by C-line terminating in position 9 as seen in β type and most frequently found in Down's Syndrome, whereas in the normal, a fourth interdigital loop is formed by either D and or C-line terminating in position 7, as in γ and δ- types:

This incidence of palmar main line patterns suggest a fundamental difference in origin and development of the palm in-utero between the normal and Down's Syndrome individuals.

1. Cummins H (1936). Dermatoglyphic stigmata in mongolian idiocy. (Abstract). Anat. Rec., 64 (Suppl.3): 11.
2. Cummins H (1939). Dermatoglyphic stigmata in mongoloid imbeciles. Anat. Rec., 73: 407.
3. Walker NF (1957). The use of dermal configurations in the diagnosis of mongolism. J. Pediatr., 50: 19.
4. Beckman L, Gustavson KH, Norring A (1962). Finger and palm dermal ridge patterns in normal and mongoloid individuals (the Down Syndrome). Acta Genet. (Basel), 12:20.
5. Holt SB (1964). Finger-print patterns in mongolism. Ann. Hum. Genet., 27:279.
6. Matsui I, Nakagome Y Higurashi M (1966). Dermatoglyphic study of Down's Syndrome in Japan. Paediatr. Univ. Tokyo, 13:43.
7. Giovannucci ML, Bartolozzi G (1968). La mano nel soggetto con sindrome di Langdon Down. Studio su 135 soggetti ricoverati nella Clinica Pediatrica dell' Universita di Firenze. Minerva Pediatr.,20:729.
8. Gebala A, Jaklinski A, Dobrzanska A, Iwaszkiewicz A, Grzeszyk C (1969). Dermatoglify dloni i palcow w zespole Dwwna z czesciowa trisomia chromosomu 21. Pol. Tyg. Lek., 24:867.
9. Fujita H (1969). A comparative study on finger patterns with Down's Syndrome in Japan. Jap. J. Hum. Genet. 14:193.
10. Shiono H, Kadowaki J, Kasahara S (1969). Dermatoglyphics of Down's Syndrome in Japan. Tohoku J. Exp. Med., 99:107.
11. Zajaczkowska K (1969). Badania dermatoglifow dloni u pacjentow z zespolem Downa i ich rodzicow. Neur. Neurochir. Pol., 3:267.
12. Bryant JI, Emanuel I, Huang SW, Kronmal R, Lo J (1970). Dermatoglyphs of Chinese children with Down's Syndrome. J. Med. Genet., 7:338.
13. Holt SB (1963). Current advances in our knowledge of the inheritance of variations in fingerprints. Proc. Second Intl. Congr. Hum. Genet., 3:1450.
14. Walker NF, Carr DH, Sergovich FR, Barr ML, Soltan HC (1963). Translocation chromosome patterns in related mongol defectives. J. Ment. Defic. Res., 7:150.
15. Soltan HC, Clearwater K (1965). Dermatoglyphics in translocation Down's Syndrome. Am. J. Hum. Genet., 17:476.

16. Walker NF, Johnson HMC (1965). Comparative studies of the dermatoglyphics of Italian patients with Down's Syndrome. Proc. Int. Copenhagen Cong. Scient. Study Ment Retardation, 2:767.
17. Dallapiccola B, Ricci N (1967). I dermatoglifi nella sindrome di Down tipica ed atipica. Acta Genet. Med. Gemellol. (Roma), 16:384.
18. Plato CC, Cereghino JJ, Steinberg FS (1973). Palmar dermatoglyphics of Down's Syndrome: revisited. Pediatr. Red., 7;111.
19. Fang TC (1950). The third interdigital patterns on the palms of the general British population mongoloid and non-mongoloid mental defectives. J. Ment. Sci., 96:780.
20. Saksena PN, Bajpai PC, Dube SK (1966). Evaluation of dermatoglyphics in mongolism. Indian J. Pediatr., 33:293.
21. Purvis-Smith SG (1972). The Sydney line. A significant sign in Down's Syndrome. Aust. Paediatr. J., 8:198.
22. Penrose LS (1931). The creases on the minimal digit in mongolism. Lancet, 2:585.
23. Uchida IA, Soltan HC (1963). Evaluation of dermatoglyphics in medical genetics. Pediatr. Clin. North Am., 10:409.
24. Hall B (1964). Mongolism in newborns. Acta Paediatr. Scand. (Suppl.), 154:1.
25. Geipel G (1961). Das Tastleistensystem der Hande und die Beugefurchen mongoloider Personen. Acta Genet. Med. Gemellol. (Roma), 10:80, 1961.
26. Holt SB (1970). Dermatoglyphics in mongolism. Ann. N.Y. Acad. Sci., 171:602.
27. Okajima M (1975). Development of Dermal Ridges in the Fetus. J. Med. Genet. 12: 243.
28. Bonnevie K (1925). Studies on Papillary Patterns of human fingers. J. Genet. 15:1.
29. Penrose LS and PT Ohara (1973). The Development of the epidermal ridges. J. Med. Genet. 10:201.
30. Holt SB (1968). The Genetics of Dermal Ridges. Charles Thomas Publisher, Springfield, 17.
31. Nie NH, CH Hull, JG Jenkins, K Steinbrenner and DH Bent (1975). Statistical Package for the Social Sciences. McGraw Hill, New York.

Table 1. Total Percentage Frequencies of Terminations of Palmar Main-Lines.

		Left		Right	
		Normal	Down's	Normal	Down's
D-line	7	48.74*	14.16	27.53	16.81
	9	30.56	20.35	29.80	15.93
	11	17.17	61.06 **	37.12	61.95 *
	13	-	1.77 *	0.51	4.42 *
	15	.51	-	0.76	-
C-line	0	8.59	12.39	5.05	7.08
	X	11.36	22.12	8.33	10.62
	5	27.52 *	2.65	17.17*	4.42
	7	20.71	15.04	19.44	8.85
	9	29.04	46.02 *	45.45	64.60 *
B-line	4	17.93 *	2.65	13.38	1.77
	5	59.60 *	27.43	41.41	24.78
	7	21.21	66.37 *	40.40	65.49 *
	8	0.25	1.77	0.51	1.77
A-line	1	3.03	6.19	0.76	-
	2	1.77	3.54	-	-
	3	15.66	11.50	10.61	5.31
	4	69.44	53.98	70.96	57.52
	5	3.03	19.47 **	5.30 *	31.86 **
	9	0.51	-	0.51	-
	11	4.55 *	0.88	8.33 *	0.88
	13	2.02	-	2.78	-
T-line	11	5.05	11.50 *	1.52	3.54 *
	12	0.51	-	-	-
	13	93.18	86.73	98.23	95.58

* $p < 0.01$

** $p < 0.001$

Table 2. Percentage frequencies of terminations of palmar A-main line.

	BLACK				WHITE			
	MALE		FEMALE		MALE		FEMALE	
Position	Normal	Down's	Normal	Down's	Normal	Down's	Normal	Down's
1 L	2.0	6.2	1.6	0	6.6	12.5	4.7	2.6
R			1.6	0				
2 L	2.0	0	0.8	10.0	0	6.2	4.7	2.6
R								
3 L	16.7	9.3	14.7	0	20.0	12.5	19.0	15.7
R	11.6	9.3	10.6	0	10.0	6.2	9.5	2.6
4 L	69.0	50.0	73.7	50.0	56.6	50.0	57.1	60.5
R	74.6	46.8	68.0	30.0	66.6	59.3	52.3	71.0
5 L	1.0	2.8**	4.0	40.0**	6.6	12.5*	9.5	13.1*
R	2.0	34.2**	9.0	70.0**	3.3	28.0**	14.2	23.6*
7 L	0	6.2			0	3.1		
R	1.0	9.3			0	6.2		
9 L					6.6	0		
R					3.3	0	4.7	0
11 L	6.6*	0	4.1*	0	0		0	2.6
R	9.1*	0	7.3*	0	10.0*	0	14.2 *	2.6
13 L	2.5	0	0.8	0	3.3	0	4.7	0
R	1.5	0	3.2	0	6.6	0	4.7	0
X L					0	3.1	0	2.6
R								

* $p < 0.01$
** $p < 0.001$

Table 3. Percentage frequencies of terminations of palmar B-main line.

	BLACK				WHITE			
	MALE		FEMALE		MALE		FEMALE	
Position	Normal	Down's	Normal	Down's	Normal	Down's	Normal	Down's
4 L	19.8	0	14.7	0	16.6	3.1	33.3	5.2
R	14.2	3.1	11.4	0	10.0	3.1	28.5	0
5 L	63.9	34.3	60.5	10.0	49.9	28.0	38.1	26.3
R	42.5	28.1	50.9	10.0	33.3	24.9	9.5	26.2
6 L	0.5	0	0	10.0				
R	2.5	3.1	0.8	0				
7 L	15.2	59.3	22.9	70.0	30.0	68.7	28.5	68.4
R	38.5	56.2	34.4	80.0	46.6	62.5	61.9	71.0
8 L	0	6.2*	0.8	0				
R	0	3.1*	0.8	0	3.3	3.1		
9 L			0.8	10.0	3.3	0		
R	1.5	6.2	0.8	10.0	6.6	6.2	0	2.6
11 L	0.5	0						
R								
X L								
R	0.5	0						

* $p < 0.01$

Table 4. Percentage frequencies of terminations of palmar C-main line.

	BLACK				WHITE			
	MALE		FEMALE		MALE		FEMALE	
Position	Normal	Down's	Normal	Down's	Normal	Down's	Normal	Down's
0 L	10.1	15.6*	9.0	30.0**	3.3	6.2 *	4.7	10.5 *
R	6.6	3.1*	4.9	40.0**	3.3	3.1 *	0	5.2 *
4 L	1.5	0	0.8	0			4.7	0
R	1.0	0					4.7	0
5 L	28.8	3.1	30.2	0	23.3	0	23.8	5.2
R	18.7	6.2	18.8	10.0	10.0	0	14.2	5.2
6 L	0.5	0	3.2	0				
R	1.0	0	1.6	0	3.3	0		
7 L	20.8 *	6.2	18.0 *	20.0	23.3	25.0	23.8**	13.1
R	19.8 *	6.2	21.3 *	20.0	13.3 *	6.2	28.5**	10.5
8 L								
R								
9 L	27.4	43.7*	31.1	50.0 *	20.0	43.7*	23.8	47.3 *
R	44.6	65.6*	43.4	30.0 *	46.6	68.7*	38.1	68.4 *
10 L	0	6.2*						
R	0.5	3.1*	0.8	0	3.3	3.1		
11 L								
R	0.5	6.2	2.4	0	0	3.1		
X L	10.6	25.0*	7.3*	0	30.0	25.0 *	19.0	23.6 *
R	7.1	9.3	6.5*	0	20.0	15.6 *	14.2	10.5 *

* $p < 0.01$

** $p < 0.001$

Table 5. Percentage frequencies of terminations of palmar D-main lines.

Position		BLACK				WHITE			
		MALE		FEMALE		MALE		FEMALE	
		Normal	Down's	Normal	Down's	Normal	Down's	Normal	Down's
0	L			1.6	0				
	R								
3	L								
	R							4.7	0
4	L			0.8	0				
	R			0.8	0			0	2.6
5	L					6.6**	0		
	R	0.5	0			6.6	0		
7	L	54.8 *	25.0	87.5*	0	26.6*	9.3	42.8*	13.1
	R	29.9 *	31.2	31.9*	10.0	13.3*	12.5	23.8*	10.5
8	L	1.0	0	1.6	0				
	R	1.0	0	0.8	0	3.3	0	4.7	0
9	L	29.5*	21.8	25.4*	10.0	43.3*	25.0	42.8 *	18.4
	R	30.4*	15.6	32.7*	10.0	30.0*	18.7	19.0 *	15.7
10	L	0.5	0	0.8	10.0				
	R	3.0	0	0.8	0				
11	L	13.2	46.8*	18.0	80.0*	23.3	59.3*	14.3	68.4*
	R	33.5	43.7*	32.7	80.0*	46.6	62.5*	47.6	71.0*
12	L	0	3.1						
	R								
13	L	0	3.1*			0	3.1*		
	R	0.5	9.3*			0	6.2*		
X	L					0	3.1		
	R	0.5	0						

* $p < 0.01$
** $p < 0.001$

Table 6. Percentage frequencies of terminations of palmar T-main line.

	BLACK				WHITE			
	MALE		FEMALE		MALE		FEMALE	
Position	Normal	Down's	Normal	Down's	Normal	Down's	Normal	Down's
1 L	0.5	0						
R	0.5	0						
3 L	0.5	0	0.8	0				
R								
4 L							0	2.6
R							0	2.6
7 L	0.5	0						
R								
11 L	3.5	6.2*	4.1	10.0*	10.0	18.7*	4.7	10.5*
R			2.4	0	0	6.2*	9.5	5.2*
12 L	1.0	0						
R								
13 L	93.9	93.7	95.0	90.0	90.0	78.1	95.2	86.8
R	99.4	100.0	97.5	100.0	100.0	93.7	90.4	92.1
X L					0	3.1		
R								

*$p < 0.01$

Progress in Dermatoglyphic Research, pages 371-384

DERMATOGLYPHIC STUDIES IN PARENTS OF CHILDREN WITH TRISOMY 21: DETECTION OF HIDDEN MOSAICISM AND ITS ROLE IN GENETIC COUNSELLING +

Alexander Rodewald§,PhD,Monika Bär,Merve Zankl,MD,Heinrich Zankl++,MD,PhD,Sigrid Reicke,MD,and Klaus D Zang,MD
Institute of Human Genetics,University of the Saar,D-6650 Homburg;++Division of Human Biology and Human Genetics,University of Kaiserslautern,Federal Republic of Germany

Although the importance of dermatoglyphics in medical genetics for the identification of many syndromes has been recognized for many years,its usefulness in genetic counselling has been discovered only in the past few years.Quantitative dermal indices such as the Walker,Hopkins,and General indices are promising diagnostic tools,as in the detection of trisomy 21 or of normal/trisomy 21 mosaicism(Bolling et al,1971; Deckers er al 1973;Loesch and Smith,1975;Priest et al,1976; Reed,1981;Rodewald et al,1976;Rodewald et al,1981).

The first dermal index for Down's syndrome,devised by Walker(1957/58),included scores for 16 patterns and discriminated only 80% of persons with Down's syndrome and 66% of controls. The Hopkins methods of analysis by predictive discrimination increased the number of patterns to 30(including left-right symmetry)and gave a high discriminance(over 90%). Our General index(adding the symmetry of the endings of the main lines and their combinations;36 patterns in all)reduces the overlap region between the Down's syndrome and control groups from 6%(in the Hopkins index) to 3.1%.

Some authors(Ayme et al,1979;Penrose,1954,1963;Priest, 1969;Rodewald et al,1981;Turpin and Lejeune,1953;Zajaczkowska, 1969)have found unusual combinations of dermatoglyphic patterns in parents of children with trisomy 21,in comparison with the control populations.These combinations include:increased frequencies of simian creases and Sydney lines,and of large hypothenar patterns(especially of ulnar loops and whorls),high frequencies of t'' triradii,and a transversal direction of

+ This work was supported by the Deutsche Forschungsgemeinschaft Ro 516/1 and Ro 516/2-2.
§Senior and corresponding author

main lines A and D with high main-line values.In this connection,and on the basis of his results,Penrose(1954/1963)postulated that some apparently normal parents of mongoloid children have unrecognized trisomy-21 mosaicism.

To the best of our knowledge, the authors of only one study(Ayme et al,1979)have hitherto investigated the dermatoglyphic patterns of the fingers and palms of 24"informative"parents of Down's syndrome children(that is the father or the mother who had transmitted the supernumerary chromosome 21; called "true parents" by Ayme et al,1979).Those authors found that the "true parents" showed a more distinct dermatoglyphic stigmatization, calculated by an index score based on only three palmar patterns(the simian crease,palmar hypothenar patterns,and the Turpin index)than either the whole group of parents of trisomic children or the controls.They concluded that "some unknown relationship seems to exist between dermatoglyphic patterns and non-disjunction".

It is therefore of medical and clinical interest in relation to genetic counselling to clarify this subject by describing in detail the dermatoglyphic patterns on the fingertips, palms and especially on the soles in a large series of noninformative and "informative" parents of Down's syndrome children.

DERMATOGLYPHIC AND CYTOGENETIC INVESTIGATIONS

The composition and characteristics of each group studied, as well as their sources, are given in Table 1. Complete dermatoglyphic data for fingertips,palms,and soles have been analyzed in 550 controls(280♂;270♀),200 cytogenetically diagnosed Down's syndrome patients with free trisomy 21,286 phenotypically and chromosomally normal parents of these patients(143 fathers and 143 mothers),and in 40 "informative" parents of trisomic children.The dermatoglyphic features studied were:fingertip patterns,patterns in the palmar and plantar areas,axial triradii,atd angles,palmar and plantar creases,and the Turpin index.The patterns were computed separately for males and females. The values for the Walker and General indices were calculated(Rodewald,1974;Rodewald,

TABLE 1.The composition of the groups analyzed(Southern Germany)

Populations		N	Total
Trisomy 21 children	♂	125	200
	♀	75	
	♂	280	550
	♀	270	
Parents of tris.chil.	Mo.	143	286
	Fa.	143	
Informative parents	Mo.	31	40
	Fa.	9	

et al,1976) for all probands.This study,like that of Aime et al.(1979),also included a computation of Turpin's index,i.e. the sum of the values of the proximal radiants of the main lines A,B,C,and D in each individual.Palm and sole prints were made by inking with hydrosoluble ink or by the Faurot photosensitive method(Rodewald and Zankl,1981).The prints were interpreted by two independent observers in accordance with the "Memorandum on Dermatoglyphic Nomenclature"(Penrose,1968).

The information about the informative parents of trisomic children was verified by Q-G banding and silver-staining of the chromosomes in accordance with established cytogenetic criteria(Casperson et al,1970;Kodama et al,1980;Zankl and Bernhardt,1977).In 40 of 90 couples,it could be determined which parent was responsible for the chromosomal non-disjunction (Fig.1).

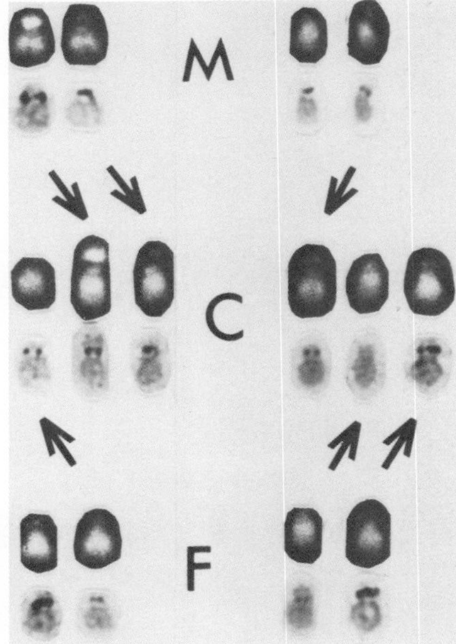

Fig.1.Derivation of the supernumerary chromosome 21 from the mother(M) and the father(F),respectively, in Down's syndrome children(C).(Fluorescence staining above;silver staining below).Nondisjunction in the first meiotic division. (Original)

RESULTS

Dermatoglyphic patterns ocurred with various frequencies in the configurational areas of the palms and soles in the four groups.Comparison of the frequencies of these dermatoglyphic patterns demonstrates a lack of significance for the distributions of ulnar and radial loops on the 2nd finger and of t'' triradii on the palms between the controls and the groups of the parents of trisomic children(fathers/♂ controls;

mothers/♀ controls; $0.10 < p < 0.05$; Tables 2 and 3).

TABLE 2. Frequencies of digital patterns on the 2nd fingers in the four groups($^+$ $p < 0.05$)

Populations			A	U	R	W	TA
Trisomy 21 children		R	2.0	91.0	0.5	6.5	-
		L	2.0	90.0	1.5	6.5	-
Controls	♂	R	7.8	32.3	27.0	33.0	-
		L	10.3	33.3	20.9	35.5	-
	♀	R	15.2	34.4	13.7	36.7	-
		L	14.8	30.7	20.4	34.1	-
Parents of tr.21 childr.	Fa.	R	13.3	32.9	22.4	30.8	0.7
		L	12.6	40.6	18.2	28.7	-
	Mo.	R	11.9	39.2	15.4	33.6	-
		L	13.3	35.0	18.9	32.2	0.7
Informative parents		R	10.0	52.5$^+$	12.5$^+$	25.0	-
		L	10.0	42.5	25.0	22.5	-

TABLE 3. Frequencies of t, t', and t'' triradii in the four groups

Populations			t	t'	t''
Trisomy 21 children		R	12.5	5.5	82.0
		L	14.6	12.1	73.3
Controls	♂	R	71.5	20.1	8.4
		L	73.5	18.6	7.9
	♀	R	63.3	28.0	8.7
		L	65.8	25.9	8.3
Parents of tris. child.	Fa.	R	69.2	17.5	13.3
		L	68.5	22.4	9.1
	Mo.	R	74.1	16.1	9.8
		L	74.8	14.0	11.2
Informative parents		R	57.5	20.0	22.5^{++}
		L	42.5	40.0	17.5$^+$

$^+$ $p < 0.05$; $^{++}$ $p < 0.01$

An increase of ulnar loops on the 2nd finger (left in the fathers and right in the mothers) and of t'' triradii on the palms was found in parents of trisomic children in comparison to the controls. Tables 4-7 show the significant differences in the distribution of palmar and plantar patterns analyzed in the four groups. The parents of trisomic children had significantly more ulnar loops on the palmar hypothenar areas ($p < 0.05$), typical or atypical simian creases ($p < 0.001$; classification of Weninger and Navratil, 1957), Sydney lines ($p < 0.001$), and small distal loops on the hallucal areas of the soles ($p < 0.05$), than did the controls.

The informative parents of the trisomic children had the following dermatoglyphic peculiarities significantly more often than the control population: ulnar loops on the right 2nd finger ($p < 0.01$), t'' triradii ($p < 0.01$), ulnar loops ($P < 0.10$) and carpal arches ($p < 0.01$) on the hypothenars, typical or atypical simian creases and Sydney lines ($p < 0.001$), and small distal loops ($p < 0.001$) on the hallucal areas of the soles (Table 2-7).

TABLE 4. Frequencies of palmar hypothenar patterns in 4 groups

		A^u	A^c	A^r	L^u	L^r	L^c	L^u/L^r	W
Trisomy 21 chil.	R	11.0	18.0	0.5	51.5	3.5	0.5	3.0	12.0
	L	15.0	23.0	0.5	52.5	3.5	1.5	-	4.0
Controls ♂	R	47.5	11.5	2.5	7.5	22.0	1.8	1.1	6.1
	L	45.7	12.7	1.4	5.8	27.6	-	2.5	4.3
Controls ♀	R	31.5	18.1	2.6	8.9	31.1	1.1	1.1	5.5
	L	45.2	17.4	0.4	7.4	23.3	1.1	2.2	3.0
Parents of tris. child. Fa.	R	39.9	12.6	3.5	16.1^+	21.0	2.1	-	4.9
	L	39.9	15.4	-	14.7^+	28.0	0.7	-	1.4
Mo.	R	44.1	15.4	2.1	11.2^+	22.4	2.1	-	2.8
	L	51.0	12.6	1.4	9.8	21.7	0.7	-	2.8
Informa. parents	R	42.5	22.5^+	-	10.0	17.5	2.5	-	-
	L	37.5	32.5^{++}	-	12.5^+	15.0	-	-	2.5

$^+ p < 0.05$; $^{++} p < 0.01$

TABLE 5. Frequencies of simian creases and Sydney lines (S.L.) in the four groups ($^+p < 0.05$; $^{++}p < 0.01$)

		typical		abortive			
		Ia	Ib	IIa	IIb	S.L.	O
Trisomy 21 children	R	14.0	17.0	1.5	27.0	12.5	28.0
	L	13.0	20.5	5.0	23.0	14.0	24.5
Controls ♂	R	0.4	1.9	0.4	5.8	2.4	89.1
	L	-	1.1	0.8	8.3	2.4	87.4
Controls ♀	R	0.4	0.4	0.4	2.6	2.4	93.8
	L	-	1.1	0.4	5.6	3.4	89.5
Parents of tris. children Fa.	R	1.4^+	2.8^+	3.5^+	16.1^{++}	8.4^+	67.8
	L	1.4^+	4.2^+	2.8^+	18.9^{++}	2.1	70.6
Mo.	R	1.4^+	0.7	4.2^+	16.8^{++}	9.1^{++}	67.8
	L	-	4.2^+	3.5^+	16.8^{++}	9.1^{++}	66.4
Informative parents	R	5.0^+	10.0^{++}	10.0^{++}	10.0^+	32.5^{++}	32.5
	L	5.0^+	-	10.0^{++}	10.0^+	20.0^{++}	55.0

Some distinct differences between the noninformative and the informative parents can be noted: the informative parents had more ulnar loops on the right 2nd finger ($p < 0.05$) and less radial loops ($p < 0.05$), more t'' triradii ($p < 0.05$), carpal arches on the hypothenar areas ($p < 0.02$), typical simian creases ($p < 0.05$), and Sydney lines ($p < 0.01$), and more small distal loops ($p < 0.01$) on the hallucal areas on the soles.

In general, the group of mothers and fathers of trisomic children was intermediate between the Down's syndrome children and the control populations with regard to the patterning on the fingertips, and those palmar and plantar patterns known for their reliability in discriminating between normal and Down's syndrome groups. In addition the mean Turpin values were sig-

nificantly higher for the group of parents of trisomic children (t-Tests: $\alpha = 0.01$; Table 7) than for the controls. The mean values for the informative parents were also significantly higher ($\alpha = 0.001$) than those for the noninformative parents.

TABLE 6. Frequencies of hallucal patterns in the four groups

Populations		A^p	A^f	A^t	TA	L^d	l^d	L^f	L^t	W
Trisomy 21 children	R	0.5		38.0	-	12.0	45.0		1.0	3.5
	L	-	0.5	39.0	-	12.5	43.0	-	1.0	4.0
Controls ♂	R	1.4	3.6	-	0.4	42.9	12.8	1.1	8.2	29.8
	L	2.1	1.4	-	0.4	44.7	5.7	0.4	11.0	33.7
Controls ♀	R	1.5	1.9	-	-	54.1	6.7	0.7	8.9	26.3
	L	1.1	2.2	0.4	-	46.3	11.5	0.4	7.8	30.4
Parents of tris. childr. Fa.	R	2.8	2.8	0.7	-	32.2	18.9^+	-	11.2	31.5
	L	2.8	2.1	1.4	-	32.9	10.5^+	0.7	10.5	39.2
Mo.	R	1.4	2.8	-	-	46.9	13.3^+	0.7	8.4	26.6
	L	1.4	4.9	-	.	39.2	13.3	-	13.3	28.0
Informative parents	R	-	-	-	-	37.5	32.5^{++}	-	7.5	22.5
	L	2.5	-	-	-	27.5	27.5^{++}	-	5.0	37.5

$^+ p < 0.05$; $^{++} p < 0.01$

TABLE 7. Mean values of Turpin Index in the 4 groups

		$\bar{x}$	$\pm s$
Trisomy 21 children	R	31.35	2.50
	L	30.20	2.93
Controls ♂	R	28.75	4.14
	L	25.71	4.20
Controls ♀	R	27.82	4.02
	L	25.12	4.11
Parents of tri. child. Fa.	R	29.10^+	3.85
	L	27.11^+	3.61
Mo.	R	28.42^+	3.80
	L	26.46^+	4.09
Informative parents	R	30.37^{++}	3.58
	L	28.62^{++}	3.51

t-Test $^+\alpha < 0.01$; $^{++}\alpha < 0.001$

The combination of digital, palmar, and plantar patterns and the degree of the stigmatisation for Down's syndrome in the four groups was mathematically expressed by the Walker Index (16 patterns) and by the General index (36 patterns: score based on the combination of left and right pattern areas). The Walker index correctly discriminated only 80.7% of the Down's syndrome group and 66.2% of the controls. The General index score was more accurate, correctly discriminating 96% of the Down's syndrome population, and 97% of the controls. The overlap region (range from -2 to +0.5) for the control population was 3%, and for the Down's syndrome group only 4%. The histograms of the Walker and General indices gives a good comparison between the groups analyzed (Figures 2-4). The calculation of the General index scores showed in 14% of the parents (20.3% of the mothers, and in 7,7% of the fathers) of trisomic children values characteristic for Down's syndrome, and in 10.5% of the mothers and in 24.5% of the fathers values in the overlap region.

TABLE 8. Mean values of WALKER and GENERAL indices in the 4 groups

Populations		WALKER $\bar{x}$	WALKER $\pm s$	GENERAL $\bar{x}$	GENERAL $\pm s$
Tris.21 child.		+5.53	2.09	+8.79	2.68
Controls	♂	-3.81	1.96	-7.06	2.83
	♀	-3.68	1.97	-7.14	2.78
	♂+♀	-3.74	1.96	-7.10	2.80
Parents of tri. child.	Fa.+Mo.	-3.02+	2.35	-3.64++	3.80
	Fa.	-3.15+	2.12	-3.79++	3.43
	Mo.	-3.00+	2.56	-3.49++	4.14
Inf. parents		-1.79++	3.11	-0.11++	4.23

' t ' Tests

+ $\alpha < 0.01$

++ $\alpha < 0.001$

The mean Walker and General Index values for the noninformative and informàtive parents, on the one hand, differed significantly from those for the control populations on the other hand (Table 8). t-tests showed significant ($\alpha < 0.01$) and highly significant ($\alpha < 0.001$) differences between the noninformative parents and the control groups for, respectively, Walker and General index. The largest differences, however, were between the controls and the informative parents, where the t-test results for both indices were highly significant ($\alpha < 0.001$).

TABLE 9. Distribution of log values in the parents of Down's syndrome children and in the controls (%).

	Normal area		Overlap. area		Down's area	
	Walker	General	Walker	General	Walker	General
Parents of tris. children N=286	56.4	68.5	41.6	17.5	2.0	14.0
Informative parents N=40	37.5	30.0	52.5	22.5	10.0	47.5
Partner of inf. parents N=40	57.5	72.5	42.5	15.0	-	12.5
Controls N=550	66.2	96.9	33.8	3.1	-	-

The patterning of the palms and soles and the values of the two indices indicate also a higher incidence of a pattern combination typical of or similar to Down's syndrome in the informative parents than in the noninformative parents of trisomic children (Table 9; Figures 2-4). The General index score correctly discriminated 70% of the informative parents and 97% of the control individuals, in contrast to 62.5% and 66%, respectively, by the Walker index (Down's syndrome and overlapping areas together). The data from the General index also indicate that the parents of trisomic children, like the Down's syndrome patients, had greater right/left symmetry of the

Fig.2.Histograms of the Walker index values in fathers(a),and mothers(b)of trisomic children,and in the controls.

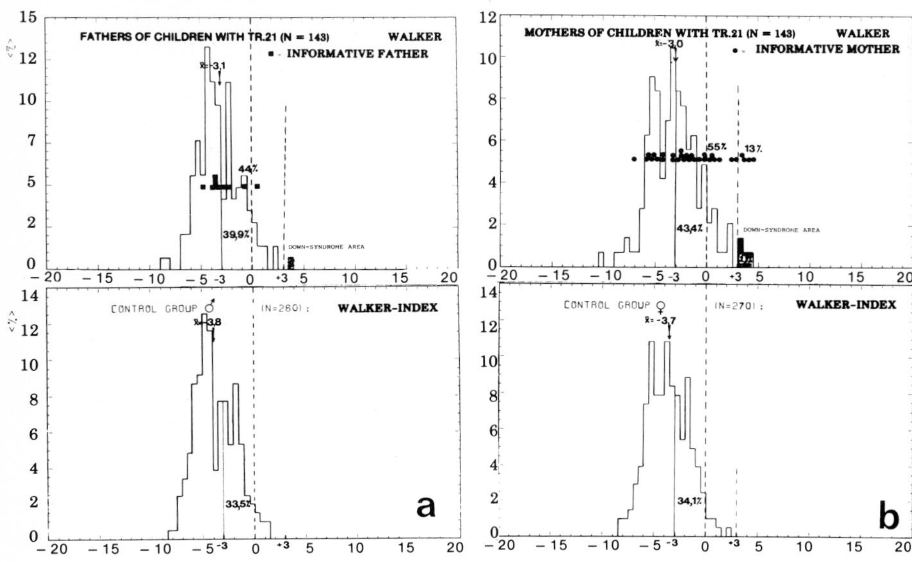

Fig.3.Histograms of the General index values in fathers(a),and mothers(b) of trisomic children, and in the controls.

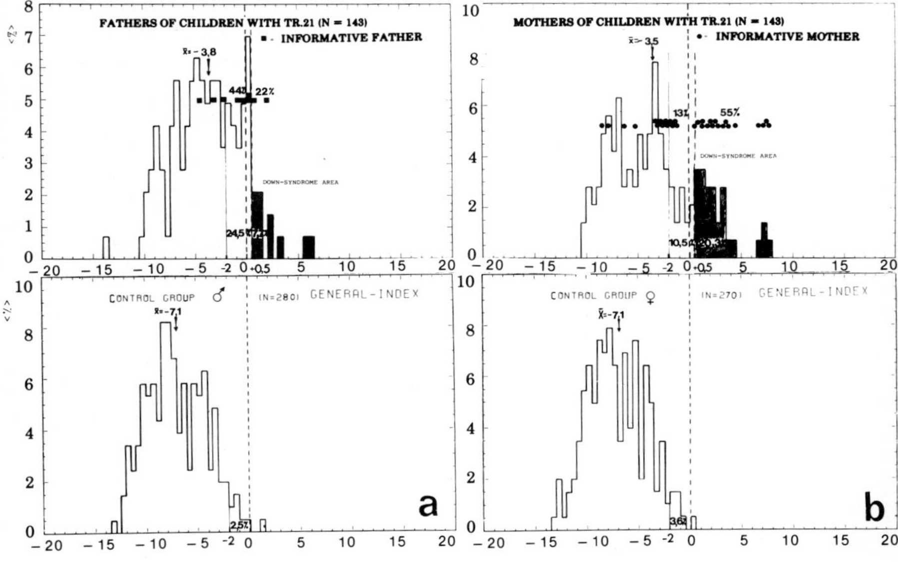

Fig.4.Histograms of the Walker(a),and General(b)index values in parents of trisomic children,and in the controls.

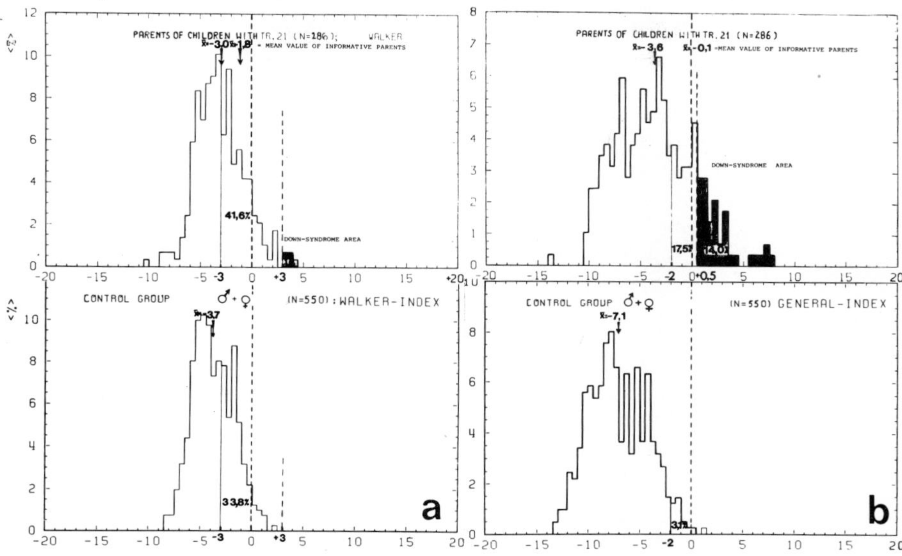

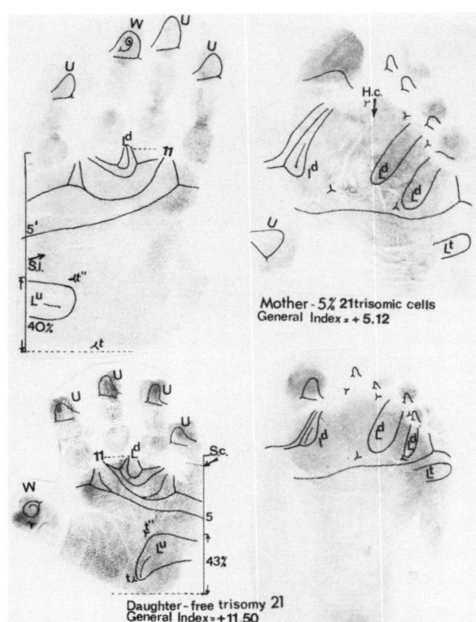

Fig.5.Palmar and plantar prints of a mother with mosaic trisomy 21 and her mongoloid daughter (S.l.=Sydney line; H.c.=Hallucal crease;S.c.=single crease).

patterns on their palms and soles than the control population did(Rodewald,1974;Rodewald et al.1976;Rodewald et al.1981).

DISCUSSION

Our study indicates a significantly higher incidence of certain dermatoglyphic patterns typical for Down's syndrome not only in the "informative" parents, but also in the group of noninformative parents of Down's syndrome children in contrast to the normal populations.On the palms,there were frequent ulnar loops on the 2nd finger,t''axial triradii,ulnar loops on the hypothenar areas,simian creases,and Sydney lines; and on the soles,small loops on the hallucal areas.Significant differences between the parents of trisomic children and the respective control populations were also found in the mean values of the Turpin index.We were able to distinguish a high percentage of parents of trisomic children from the normal populations on the basis of General index values.The high percentage(70%)of correct classifications obtained from our sample of informative parents by the General index method can be attributed to the efficacy of the General index score in the detection and utilization of dermatoglyphic patterns in differentiating normal and abnormal individuals,and it therefore demonstrates its value as a diagnostic aid.

The findings of Aime et al.(1979)concerning the dermatoglyphic stigmatisation of parents of trisomic children were confirmed in the present study,in which even more accurate discrimination between the control and the parent groups was obtained by calculation of the General index scores with the addition of the assessment of the bilateral symmetry of dermatoglyphic patterns on the palms.

A more plausible explanation for the increased occurrence of dermatoglyphic stigmata characteristic of Down's syndrome in some parents of Down's syndrome children,especially in the group of "informative"parents,seems to be the presence of cytogenetically undetected mosaics in the germ lines of these parents,a hypothesis proposed by Penrose(1963).We found by extensive cytological examination of blood cultures(100 mitoses) in three parents of trisomic children with a peculiar dermatoglyphic combination and with General index values characteristic of Down's syndrome(in the range +1 to +8) a sideline with 3-6% 21 trisomic cells(Fig.5).Similar cases were reported by Aime et al.(1979),Loesch(1974),Loesch and Smith(1975),and Taylor(1970). The data presented from these materials agree with Penrose's hypothesis.Moreover,the proportion of 21 trisomic cells in a mosaic patient can change with time,and in some individuals with a high percentage of normal cells,depending on selective forces, the trisomic cell lines in the blood can disappear(Zankl and Rodewald,1977;Rodewald et al.,1981). Frequently these mosaic patients showed a very low proportion of trisomic cells(under 10%),and no physical and/or mental peculiarities, but the palmar and plantar dermatoglyphic stigmata for Down's syndrome were present(Loesch, 1979;Zankl and Rodewald, 1977).

Among other aspects of dermatoglyphics in the informative parents of trisomic children that are relevant to medical genetics and genetic counselling are, in this context, the fact that stigmatisation was more frequent and stronger in the informative mothers(55%) than in the informative fathers(22%)-a quite unusual but not unexpected finding. A more probable explanation for the increased occurrence of dermatoglyphic peculiarities in the mothers of trisomic children described here could be a selection mechanism working more strongly against pathological male than female germ cells.

On the other hand, Aime et al.(1979) postulated that in certain individuals there may be an "unknown" relationship at the genetic level between the ontogenetic development of dermatoglyphics and non-disjunction phenomena or a predisposition to non-disjunction. While their conclusions and ours differ somewhat, they do not necessarily conflict,considering the mechanism of and the reasons for the dermatoglyphic stigmatisation of parents of trisomic children.

The documentation of dermatoglyphics in larger groups of informative parents of trisomic children may lead to a better understanding of genetic factors associated with chromosomal anomalies and the mechanism of their genesis.

We can conclude that dermatoglyphic analyzis could become of great importance in the genetic counselling of such families with trisomic children, particularly in estimating the risk of aneuploidy. According to the Bayesian method,we can calculate a predictive value of "informative" parents General Index score(the probability for Down's syndrome is approximately 1/680 if the age of mothers and fathers is not taken into account; 96.9% of controls have normal negative index score and 70.0% of informative parents of trisomic children have a peculiar index score). Thus,an individual with a negative General index score has a probability of 1/2000(1/2500 in the study of Ayme et al,1979) of giving birth to a child with trisomy 21, whereas the probability is 1/32 (1/160 in the study of Ayme et al,1979) when the General index score is positive (Table 10).

TABLE 10. Predictive value of "informative" parents General index score

a) Negative General index score

$$P = \frac{(0.3000)(0.0015)}{(0.3000)(0.0015)+(0.9690)(0.9985)} = 0.0005 = \frac{1}{2000}$$

b) Positive General index score

$$P = \frac{(0.7000)(0.0015)}{(0.7000)(0.0015)+(0.0310)(0.9985)} = 0.0310 = \frac{1}{32}$$

It may also help by providing an additional indication for prenatal diagnosis if the dermatoglyphic examination suggest the possibility of parental mosaicism in one of the partners.

Last but not least, dermatoglyphic analysis of large groups in normal population is a noninvasive and inexpensive technique, and because it does not suject an individual to any risks or discomfort, it can be used for screening purposes in genetic counselling.

ACKNOWLEDGMENTS

The authors thanks Dr.S.Stengel-Rutkowski,MD and Dipl. Biol.G.Kelterborn(Kinderklinik-University of Munich)for providing us with dermatoglyphic and cytogenetic materials from 18 families with Down's syndrome children. We thank Mr.H. Degitz of the Computation Center,University of Karlsruhe,for assitance in computing the data treated in this paper, and Mr.D Scheck and Mr. N Pohlmann for cytogenetic screening.

REFERENCES

Ayme S,Mattei M-G, Mattei JF, Aurran Y, Giraud F (1979).Dermatoglyphics in parents of children with trisomy 21.Evaluation of their interest in genetic counsellling.Clin Genet 15:78.

Bolling DR, Borgaonkar DS, Herr HM, Davis M(1971).Evaluation of dermal patterns in Down's syndrome by predictive discrimination II-Composite score based on the combination of left and right pattern areas. Clin Genet 2:163.

Casperson T, Zech L, Johanson C, Modest EJ (1970).Identification of human chromosomes by DNA-binding fluorescing agents. Chromosoma(Berl) 30:215.

Deckers JFM, Oorthuys MA, Doesburg WH (1973).Dermatoglyphics in Down's syndrome.I-Evaluation of discriminating ability of pattern areas.Clin Genet 4:311.

Kodama Y, Joshida MC, Sasaki M (1980).An improve silver staining technique for nucleolus organizing regions by using nylon cloth. Jap J Hum Genet 25:229.

Loesch D (1974).Dermatoglyphic characteristics of 21-trisomy mosaicism in relation to the fully developed syndrome and normality.J ment Defic Res 18:209.

Loesch D (1979).Dermatoglyphic distances and position of 21 trisomy mosaics.J ment Defic Res 23:253.

Loesch D, Smith CA (1975).Discriminant functions and 21-trisomy mosaicism. Ann Hum Genet 39:127.

Penrose LS (1954). The distal triradius t on the hands of parents and sibs of mongol imbeciles. Ann Hum Genet 19:10.

Penrose LS (1963). Dermatoglyphics in mosaic mongolism and allied conditions.Proc 11th Internat Cong Genet,The Hague.

Penrose LS (1968). Memorandum on dermatoglyphic nomenclature. Birth Defects:Orig Article Series Vol IV, No 3.

Priest JM (1969).Parental dermatoglyphics in age-independent mongolism.J med Genet 6:304.

Reed T (1981). Review: Dermatoglyphics in medicine-Problems and use in suspected chromosome abnormalities.Am J Med Genet 8:411.

Rodewald-Rudescu A (1974). Das Hautleistensystem beim Down-Syndrom mit einem Beitrag zur Differentialdiagnose.Doctoral Dissertation,University of Munich.

Rodewald A, Zang KD, Ziegelmayer G (1976). Bilateral symmetry of qualitative dermatoglyphic patterns in the Down's syndrome. Z Morph Anthropol 67:333.

Rodewald A, Zang KD, Zankl H, Zankl M (1981).Dermatoglyphic peculiarities in Down's syndrome.Detection of mosaicism and balanced translocation carriers.In Burgio GR, Fraccaro M, Tiepolo L, Wolf U (eds):"Trisomy 21. An international Symposium", Springer-Verlag, Berlin Heidelberg New York,p 41.

Rodewald A, Zankl H (1981). "Hautleistenfibel".Stuttgart: Gustav Fischer Verlag, p 37.

Taylor AI (1970). Futher observations of cell selection in vivo in normal/G-trisomic mosaics. Nature 227:163.

Turpin R, Lejeune J (1953).Etude dermatoglyphique de la paume des mongoliens et de leurs parents et de leurs germains. Sem Hop Paris 29:3955.

Walker NF (1957).The use of dermal configurations in the diagnosis of mongolism. J Pediatr 50:19.

Walker NF (1958).The use of dermal configurations in the diagnosis of mongolism. Pediatr Clin North Am 5:531.

Weninger M, Navratil L (1957). Die Vierfingerfurche in ätiologischer Betrachtung. Mitt Anthropol Ges Wien 87:1.

Zajaczkowska F (1969).Palmar dermatoglyphics in patients with Down's syndrome and their parents. Pol Med 8:1477.

·Zankl H, Bernhardt S (1977). Combined silver staining of the nucleolus organizing regions and Giemsa banding in human chromosomes. Hum Genet 37:79.

Zankl H, Rodewald A (1977). Diagnostische Probleme beim Mosaik-Down-Syndrome. Klin Pädiatr 189:430.

SUMMARY

The combination of dermatoglyphic patterns and the number and intensity of traits characteristic of Down's syndrome can be statistically expressed by the Walker Index and the General Index. In one study more than 96% of a Down's syndrome series and a control series were clearly separated by the General Index. We studied cytogenetic and dermatoglyphic features of 200 patients with trisomy 21, 286 of their parents (143 mothers and 143 fathers), and 550 control persons (280 ♂ and 270 ♀). In 14% of the families with trisomic children, one parent (7.7% of fathers and 20.3% of mothers) had a higher than usual General index value, similar to the value in Down's syndrome. One possible explanation for the dermatoglyphic similarities between these parents and their trisomic children is that the parents may have hidden mosaicism. The detection of 3-6% of 21-trisomic blood cells in three of the "informative" parents with an unusual dermatoglyphic combination agrees with this hypothesis.

In 27 of 40 parents of Down's syndrome children with an informative chromosome 21, the father or the mother who showed the more distinct dermatoglyphic stigmatization characteristic of Down's syndrome had trasmitted the supernumerary chromosome 21.

The findings presented here suggest a practical application of dermatoglyphics in the search for such hidden mosaicism in the parents of Down's syndrome children; dermatoglyphic analysis could become of great importance in the genetic counselling of such families.

Progress in Dermatoglyphic Research, pages 385-391

PALMAR DERMATOGLYPHICS IN WILMS' TUMOR

V.CURRÓ,P.P.MASTROIACOVO,M.CASTELLO°,C.ROMAGNOLI,
R.MASTRANGELO,G.SEGNI
°Dep. of Pediatrics II°,State Univ. of Rome
Dep. of Pediatrics,Catholic Univ. of Rome
Largo A. Gemelli, 8, 00168 Rome

INTRODUCTION

Dermatoglyphics are cutaneous manifestations of development (Okajima M.,1975), and reflect the influence of environmental and hereditary factors during the first trimester of gestation (Holt S.B.,1968). They are of greatest importance in the study of syndromes resulting from chromosomal abnormalities, such as Down's syndrome, where they can have diagnostic value (Reed T.E.,1970). Dermatoglyphic anomalies are sometimes associated with significant malformations, and these malformations are, in turn, sometimes associated with tumors (Pendergrass T.W.,1976). Aniridia and hemihypertrophy, for example, may be found in patients with Wilms' tumor (Miller R.W.,1964).

The study of dermatoglyphic anomalies when coexistent infantile tumors could help one to better understand the prenatal origin of those tumors, and to determine whether tumorgenesis can be linked to those processes which result in malformation (Cohen A.J.,1979).

MATERIALS AND METHODS

Palmar dermatoglyphics of 30 unrelated children, aged 6 months - 12 years: 13 males and 17 females, affected by Wilms' tumor were examined.

The diagnosis was always confirmed by histological report.

For each patient were registered his own, parents' and his maternal grand-mother place of birth, and made his pedigree. All the subject studied were natives of the Lazio region as well as the 44 control children: 22 males and 22 females.

Fingertips and palmar dermatoglyphics were analized and the prints were recorded on paper, using black finger-print ink (Galton F.,1892;Cummins H.,1929). In younger patients, up to two years, we adopted a method using adhesive tape, we rolled on their hand, previously coloured with cosmetic pencil.

The following dermatoglyphics parameters have been analyzed according to international literature (Penrose,1968):

a) fingerprint patterns;

b) pattern intensity index (PII);

c) total finger ridge count (TRC);

d) hypothenar, thenar/first interdigital patterns and patterns in the interdigital areas of palm;

e) sum (right + left) maximal atd angles;

f) a-b ridge count;

g) Cummins' index.

RESULTS

The results were analyzed, separating males from females (Ohler E.A.,1942), for χ^2 and Student t test by means of an Olivetti 101 computer.

Quantitative Data

a) the mean TRC in Nephroblastoma patients of both sex was significantly lower than the mean TRC in control patients Tab.1:

TRC	N°	MEAN	SD
WILMS' TUMOR			
F	16	123.93	66.57*
CONTROLS			
F	21	176.29	67.68*
WILMS' TUMOR			
M	13	143.53	88.72**
CONTROLS			
M	22	204.22	69.29**

$*p < 0.05$; $**p < 0.05$

b) the mean PII in Nephroblastoma male patients was significantly lower than the mean PII in control patients Tab.2:

PII	N°	MEAN	SD
WILMS' TUMOR			
M	13	11	3.78*
CONTROLS			
M	22	14.13	3.00*

$*p < 0.02$

c) the maximal atd angle in Nephroblastoma female patients was higher than the maximal atd angle in control patients Tab.3:

atd	N°	MEAN	SD
WILMS' TUMOR			
F	17	100.47	19.39*
CONTROLS			
F	22	89.00	11.46*

$*p < 0.01$

d) the mean Cummins' index in Nephroblastoma patients of both sex was lower than the mean Cummins' index in control patients Tab.4:

CUMMINS' INDEX	N°	MEAN	SD
WILMS' TUMOR			
F	17	17.47	3.03*
CONTROLS			
F	21	26.04	2.86*
WILMS' TUMOR			
M	13	17.84	2.76**
CONTROLS			
M	22	28.13	7.04**

$*p < 0.001$; $**p < 0.001$

Qualitative Data

The incidence of radial loops(RL) and whorls (W) in tumor-affected males has decreased compared with controls, while the incidence of arches (A) has increased Tab.5:

FINGERPRINT PATTERNS	N°	RL%	A%	W%	UL%
WILMS' TUMOR					
M	13	1.7*	13.1°	23.1^{+}	62.4^
CONTROLS					
M	22	7.2*	0.0°	41.8^{+}	50.4^

$*p < 0.05$; $°p < 0.0005$; $^{+}p < 0.025$; ^ns

All the other parameters examined didn't show, statistically, remarkable differences between tumor-affected individuals and controls.

DISCUSSION

Dermatoglyphics are quantificable manifestations of early development which remain immutable during the life of an individual (Cummins H.,Midlo C.,1961;Dallapiccola B.,1968).

If studies were to document that children with, for example, Nephroblastoma had distinctive dermatoglyphic features, this documentation could suggest a correlation between the development of fetal characteristics during the first trimester of gestation and tumorigenesis.

During the last several years various authors have considered the relationship between dermatoglyphics and neoplasias (Purvis-Smith S.G., 1973; Singh D., 1979). Many studies have focused on Lymphocytic Leukemia, often with conflicting results. Wertelecki (1969) determined that male leukemics had a higher frequency of both digital whorls and Sydney palmar flexion creases than normals. Verbov (1970), on the other hand while finding a higher frequency of digital whorls among leukemics, found no significant increase in the incidence of Sydney or simian lines. Colombo (1973) supported Wertelecki's finding of a higher frequency of Sydney lines among male leukemics.

Various authors report cases of Retinoblastoma in which the Penrose angle is larger than normal and in which a high number of normally infrequent figures, such as ulnar loop and whorl, are found in the hypothenar area (Vidal O.R., 1969. François (1969) however, reported no statistical difference in dermatoglyphics between patients with retinoblastoma and controls.

The results of our work with patients suffering from Wilms' tumor suggest that there are dermatoglyphic differences between these patients and normals. Male patients showed a higher frequency of finger arches and a lower Cummins' index and a higher atd angle. The greater frequency of finger arches among male patients correlates with a lower PII and TRC.

These results are not coesistant with those of Gutjahr (1975) who studied a group of thirty children with Wilms' tumor. He found a normal dislocation of the axial triradius, a non-transverse course for the A line, no differences in fingertip patterns or TRC, a low a-b ridge count, and an increase in the number of distally opened loops in the third interdigital area.

It is difficult to reconcile the differing results of

the various studies. One could consider them to be artefact arising from the choice of controls, but is perhaps more reasonable to ascribe these differences to the aspecificity of dermatoglyphic anomalies in general, and to accept, therefore, a lack of value in most variation of dermatoglyphic patterns among children with embryonic tumors.

Yet despite inconsistencies among the results of workers who have sought correlations between certain dermatoglyphic patterns and neoplasia, it is perhaps unwise to discard the idea that given prenatal processes may be at once responsible for structure and tumorigenesis (Miller R.W., 1968; 1975). The occasional association of Beckwith's syndrome lends support to this idea.

REFERENCES

Cohen AJ (1979). Hereditary renal- cell carcinoma associated with a chromosomal translocation. N Engl J Med 301:592.

Colombo A, Gasparoni MC, Biscotti G, Severi F (1973). Dermatoglifi e leucemia linfatica acuta nell'infanzia. Min Ped 25:353.

Cummins H (1929). Revised methods for interpreting and formulating palmar dermatoglyphics. Am J Phys Anthropol 12:415.

Cummins H, Midlo C (1961). "Finger prints, palms and soles." New York: Dover Publications Inc.

Dallapiccola B (1968). "I Dermatoglifi della Mano." Milano - Vicenza: Zambon.

François J, Matton Van Leuven M (1969). Les dermatoglyphes dans le retinoblastome. J Genet Hum 17:367.

Galton F (1892). "Finger Prints." London: Macmillan.

Gutjahr P, Wolffram T, Emmrich P (1975). Dermatoglyphische untersuchungen bei kindern mit embryonalen tumoren. Z Kinderheilk 120:101.

Holt SB (1968). "The Genetics of Dermal Ridges." Springfield: Charles Thomas.

Miller RW, Fraumeni JF, Manning MD (1964). Association of Wilms' tumor with aniridia, hemihypertrophy, and other

congenital malformations. New Engl J Med 270:922.
Miller RW.(1968). Relation between cancer and congenital defects. An epidemiologic evaluation. J Nat Cancer Inst 40:1079;
Miller RW (1975). Wilms' tumor: evidence against Knudson's hypothesis (?). Childhood Cancer Etiology Newsletter 15.
Ohler EA, Cummins H (1942). Sexual differences in breadths of epidermal ridges on finger tips and palms. Amer J Phys Anthrop 29:341.
Okajima M (1975). Development of dermal ridges in the fetus. Med Gen 12:243.
Pendergrass TW (1976). Congenital anomalies in children with Wilms' tumor. Cancer 37:403.
Penrose LS (1968). Memorandum on dermatoglyphic nomenclature. Birth Defects Original Series 4:1.
Purvis-Smith SG, Menser MA (1973). Dermatoglyphics in children with acute leukaemia. Brit Med J 4:646.
Reed TE, Borgaonkar DS, Conneally PM, Yu P, Nance WE, Christian JC (1970). Dermatoglyphic nomogram for the diagnosis of Down's syndrome. J Ped 77:1024.
Singh D (1979). Dermatoglyphic study in breast carcinoma. Indian J Pathol Microbiol 22:27.
Verbov J (1970). Dermatoglyphs in leukaemia. J Med Genet 7:125.
Vidal OR, Damel A, Funes JG (1969). Dermatoglyphics in retinoblastoma. J Gen Hum 17:99.
Wertelecki W, Plato CC, Fraumeni JF, Niswander JD (1969). Dermatoglyphics in leukaemia. Lancet 10:806.

Progress in Dermatoglyphic Research, pages 393-420

DIAGNOSTIC SIGNIFICANCE OF DERMATOGLYPHICS IN CERTAIN BIRTH DEFECTS

*Samia A. Temtamy M. D., Ph. D.

Head of Human Genetics Department (HGD)
National Research Centre (NRC)
Dokki, Cairo, Egypt.

Awatif El-Mazni M. D.
Professor of Pediatrics
Children's Hospital Cairo University (CHCU)

Fawzia H. Hussien M. D., Ph. D.
HGD, NRC.

Mouchira Abdel Salam M. D.
HGD, NRC

Amal A. Moussa. M. B., B. Ch.
CHCU

Mouchira E.Zaki, B. Sc.
HGD, NRC

Lilly K. El Meniawi, M. D.
HGD, NRC

*Reprint address.

Birth defects have been defined as abnormal variants originating during prenatal life (Benirschke et al. 1979). They can be caused by various factors, genetic causes, environmental agents or a combination of both. Genetic causes are either due to gene defects or to chromosomal aberrations. The epidermal ridge formation in the hand is not only affected by general factors that alter development but also by local influences of the underlying differentiating digits.

In the diagnosis of birth defects, the importance of dermatoglyphics in some autosomal abnormalities is well established. It is the purpose here to summarise the authors' experience regarding the value of dermatoglyphics in the diagnosis of three categories of birth defects : 1) hand malformation, 2) primary azoospermia with the Klinerfelter pattern of testicular biopsy, and 3) congenitalheart diseases.

DERMATOGLYPHICS IN HAND MALFORMATIONS

Dermatoglyphic patterns are sensitive indicators of the process of differentiation (Cummins 1926). The direction of the dermal ridges has been explained on the basis of response to growth factors operating during the fetal period of ridge differentiation between the sixth week and the fourth month of intrauterine life (Cummins 1923, Penrose, 1968, Mulvihill and Smith , 1969, Alter and Schulenberg). Okajima (1975) demonstrated dermatoglyphic features in fetuses from the 14th week of gestation. Since dermatoglyphics reflect enents of differentiation of the limbs, they are expected to be altered in the different types of hand malformations whenever the abnormality affects limb growth at an early stage of development (Penrose and Ohara 1973). On a similar basis, we studied dermatoglyphics in the different types of hand malformations (Temtamy,1966). Numerous investigators studied different qualitative and quantitative aspects of dermatoglyphics in hand malformations (Cummins 1923, Penrose 1965; Holt, 1968; Mulvihill and Smith 1969; Schaumann and Alter, 1976). Popich and Smith (1970) studied flexion creases in normal and malformed hands. It is the purpose here to discuss the diagnostic and developmental significance of some dermatoglyphic changes in hand malformations, Certain palmar qualitative changes pertinent to the diagnosis of the type of hand malformation will be emphasized. This is particularly evident in four categories of hand malformations. According to the classification of Temtamy and Mckusick (1978) the categories are : 1) absence deformities, 2) syndactyly, 3) polydactyly, and 4) hand malformation associated with congenital ring constrictions. Dermatoglyphics in absence deformities. In one type of absence deformity, ectrodactyly which is a terminal transverse defect characterized by distal absence of digits, palmar dermatoglyphics (Fig. 1) showed transverse orientation of the ridges, presence of digital triradii at the bases of the vestigial digits or nubbins, the most radial of them

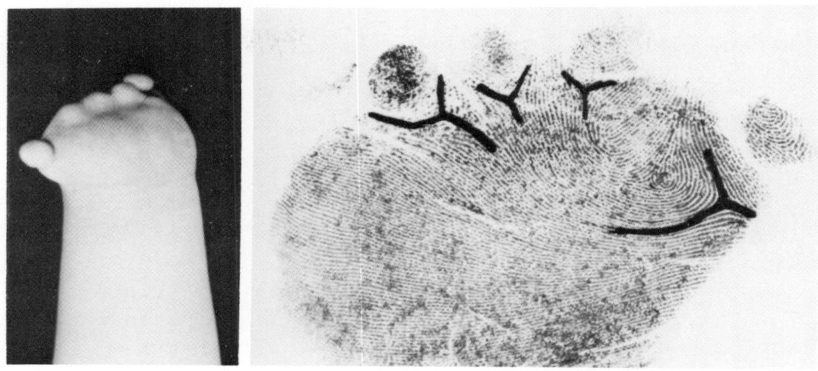

Fig. 1. A) Photograph and B) dermatoglyphics of a left hand with ectrodactyly and vestigial nubbins of digits. Note digital triadii and transverse alignment of palmar ridges.

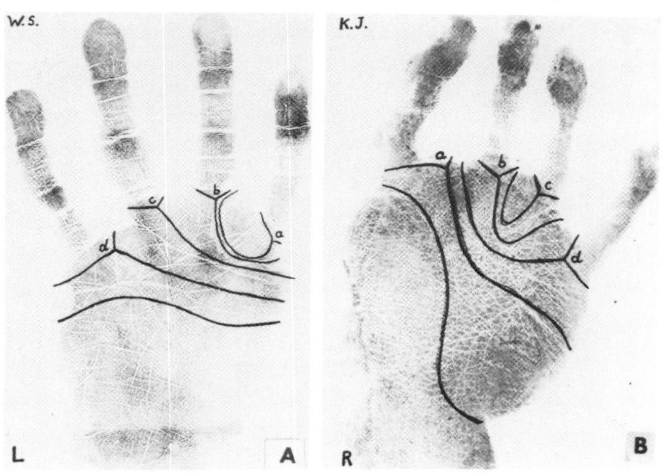

Fig. 2. Dermatoglyphics in hands with absent thumb. In A(left hand) patient had congenital heart, note transverse alignment of dermal ridges and abnormal direction of digital lines. In B(right hand) note oblique alignment of dermal ridges and normal direction of digital lines.

representing a thumb. The hand creases and the axial triradius were absent. In radial dysplasias characterized by various degrees of aplasia or hypoplasia of the thumb or radial digital rays, a consistent finding was absence of the axial triradius in case of absence of the thumb. A correlation was noted between the degree of development of the thumb with its first metacarpal and the presence and level of the axial triradius. The level of the axial triradius was high in cases of a hypoplastic functional thumb. Its position was more distal and radial in cases of non opposable thumb. Abnormal thumb development was usually associated with a complex hypothenar or midpalmar pattern. In some hands with absent thumb, the palmar ridges were transverse and in others they were oblique (Fig. 2). We noted that patients whose hands had absent thumbs, a transverse orientation of palmar ridges and an abnormal termination of digital lines, had associated congenital heart disease. In another type of absence deformaty, split-hand, characterized by absence of axial digital rays, an axial triradius existed when the thumb was present (Fig. 3). Our findings indicate that the transverse alignment of ridges represents the early or initial dermatoglyphic palmar pattern. These results are in agreement with the suggestions of Penrose (1968) and of Mulvihill and Smith (1969) that ridges are aligned transversely at right angle to the compression forces of the lines of growth stress. Ridges start to curve, take an oblique course or a more complex configuration secondary to the existence of a pad or other surface distortion prior to final ridge formation (Mulvihill and Smith 1969). Our observation of transversely aligned dermal ridges in terminal transverse defects and in certain types of radial defects may suggest that such hand malformations have their onset earlier than others which show an oblique course of the ridges and exhibit palmar patterns. These patterns are secondary to the presence of palmar pads. This also agrees with a conclusion by Hale (1952) that ridge direction is conditioned by differential growth of the part covered. Similar changes in palmar dermatoglyphics were noted by other investigators in cases of radial dysplasia as isolated anomalies or as a part of syndromes either genetically determined or due to thalidomide embryopathy or of undetermined causes (Pfeiffer and ZuBerge 1964; Gall et al. 1966; Mulvihill and Smith 1969; Holt 1972 and Arias et al. 1980). Our observation of digital triradii in the hand with terminal trnaverse defects and vestigial nubbins of ditits, the presence of a digital triradius at the base of the vestigial thumb

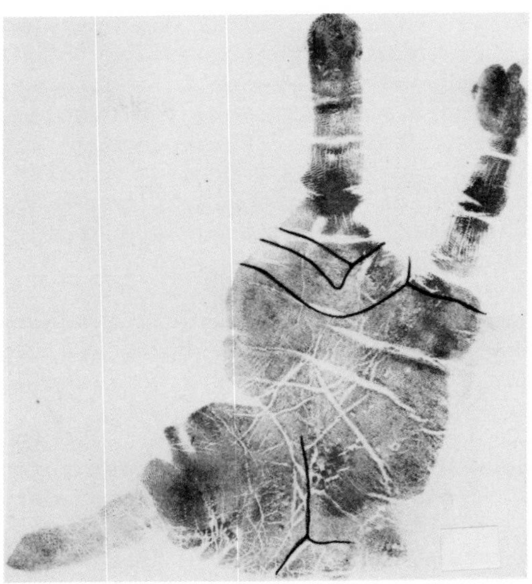

Fig. 3. Dermatoglyphics in split-hand. Note presence of axial triradius.

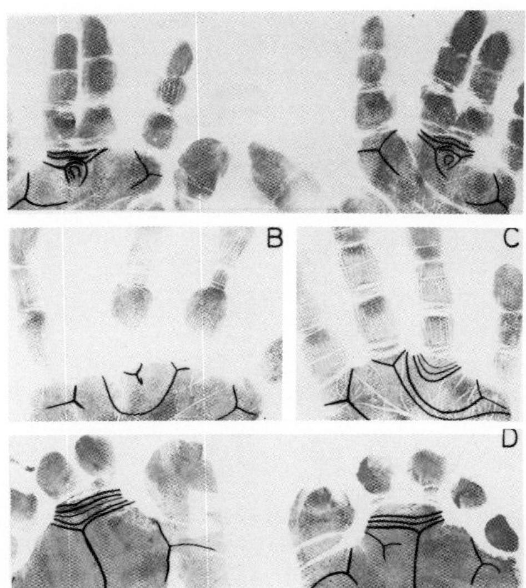

Fig. 4. Dermatoglyphics in zygodactyly A) approximation of b & c digital triradii, B) abortive C line, C) absnet c triradius and D) fused digital triradii.

and the absence of an axial triradius suggests that the axial triradius is the triradius of the thumb and that it attains its normal position by migration due to the normal development of the thumb and the first metacarpal and aquisition of thumb opposability. This is further documented by the relationship between the axial triradius and the different degrees of thumb hypoplasia and opposability and the presence of a normally placed axial triradius in split-hand deformity when the thumb is present.

Two categories of hand malformations syndactyly and polydactyly provide further evidence to the relationship between development of the digital triradii and the eruption of digits.

In syndactyly whether due to soft tissue or bony fusion of digits, the most consistent finding in the palmar area proximal to the webbed digits is the presence of transverely aligned ridged skin and an interdigital triradius at the base of syndactylous digits. This digital triradius replaces two or more digital triradii that are normally present. In zygodactyly or type I syndactyly which is characterized by webbing of the middle and ring fingers, dermatoglyphics (Fig. 4) show that the b & c digital triradii are missing and replaced by a single interdigital triradius which is the result of fusion of the two triradii. This finding indicates eruption of the syndactylous digits as one mass and failure of their cleavage. Another dermatoglyphic expression of zygodactyly is approximation of the b & c digital triradii and a minor expression is absence of the c triradius or presence of an abortive C line. Temtamy and Mckusick (1978) proved that dermatoglyphic changes can increase the penetrance of syndactyly but not 100 %. Similar dermatoglyphic changes in syndactyly were previously reported (Cummins and Sicomo 1923).

Polydactyly or presence of extradigits is associated with presence of an extra digital triradius at the base of the supernumerary digit (Fig. 5). The extra triradius may be the only permanent evidence and an unmistakable sign of an extradigit such as a pedunculated postminimus that has been surgically removed or has fallen spontaneously (Cummins 1932). The presence of an extra digital triradius occurs if the extradigit originally pocesses a triradius. This is an important finding that has been helpful in the diagnosis of preaxial polydactly whether it is due to an extra thumb or

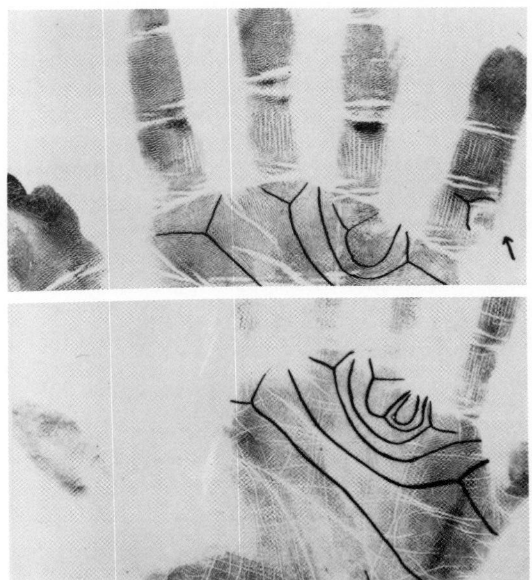

Fig. 5. Dermatoglyphics in postaxial polydactyly: arrow points to triradius of a pedunculated postminimus, lower part shows extradigital triradius and extraline.

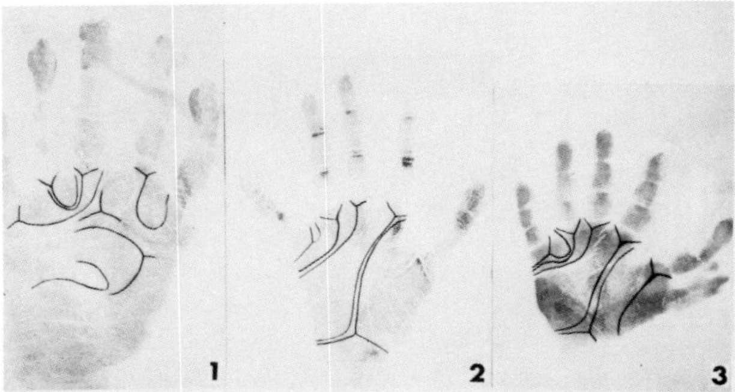

Fig. 6. Dermatoglyphics in three types of preaxial triphalangeal digits 1) triphalangeal nonopposable thumb, an expression of radial dysplasia in the Holt-Oram syndrome, 2) triphalangeal opposable thumb, 3) polydatyly of the index figer.

an extra index finger. Since the thumb does not pocess a digital triradius, polydactyly of a thumb even if it is triphangeal is not associated with an extradigital triradius (Fig. 6). In polydactyly of the index finger we observed an extra "a" triradius and line in an affected father and daughter (Temtamy 1966). Subsequently, Atasu (1976) reported a family with similar involvement in at least 4 generations and also illustrated the dermatoglyphic changes. Dermatoglyphic changes may be a useful clue to the time of digital malformations. In digital anomalies associated with congenital ring constrictions, we observed dermatoglyphic changes in the form of disorganized, dissociated or hypoplastic dermal ridges in the affected fingers, palms or soles whether associated with ring constrictions or not. Abel (1938) discovered similar dermatoglyphic changes and attributed them to the effect of variation in tension and pressure within the epidermis during the period of ridge differentiation. Cummins (1926) due to his observation of such changes concluded that the malformation is determined during or before the 11th week of fetal life. We can also conclude that since hand malformations associated with congenital ring constrictions are in the form of absence deformity and syndactly and can be mistaken with them dermatoglyphic changes can be an aid to differentiate between such etiologically different anomalies. From the above mentioned observations it is possible to conclude that dermatoglyphics provide a reflection of underlying erros of early differentiation of the hand, are useful in diagnosis, and may in some instances replace x-ray examination for the precise indentfication of the type of digital anomaly.

DERMATOGLYPHICS IN PRIMARY AZOOSPERMIA

As part of a clinical, genetic and pathological investigation of 82 patients with primary azoosperima and the Klinefelter pattern of testicular biopsy (Temtamy et al. 1980), dermatoglyphics were studied in 44 cases. The main aim was to investigate the value of dermatoglyphics in the diagnosis of different types of primary azoospermia and to find out whether cases without detectable chromosomal aberrations have dermatoglyphic abnormalities. According to results of Barr body studies, cases were classified into sex chromatin positive or Klinefelter disease and sex chromatin negative or Klinefelter syndrome (Klinefelter 1973). Detailed results of clinical, genetic and cytogenetic studies of these cases have been previously published (Temtamy et al. 1980). The 44 cases were classified into 28 sex chromatin negative and 16 sex chromatin positive. Dermatoglyphics in each of these groups were statistically compared to each other and to those in 50 normal fertile males and 50 female controls. Dermatoglyphic findings in this control group were similar to the results of Temtamy et al. (1976)in 2628 normal males and 517 normal females. Among the 28 sex chromatin negative cases 2 cases proved to have chromosomal mosaicism. One patient was 46, XY/47, XYY and the other was 46, XY/45, XO. Dermatoglyphic parameters studied were : 1) finger print pattern, 2) mean pattern intensity index of fingers (PII), 3) total ridge count (TRC), 4) a-b ridge count, 5) mean "atd" angle, 6) frequency of distal deviation according to the method of Walker (1957) modified, by Penrose (1968), 7) frequency of ulnar triradii, 8) mean pattern intensity index of the palm, 9) mean main line index, 10) frequency of interdigital and hypothenar patterns, 11) extratradii in the 2nd and 4th palmar areas (I_2 & I_4).

Statistical analysis for the whole study was made by Chi square or Fisher's exact significance tests for frequencies and by T-test for means. The level of $P < 0.05$ was considered significant, $P < 0.01$ highly significant and $P < 0.001$ very highly significant. In the text differences were stated as increased or decreased only when they were statistically significant. Results are shown in tables 1 to 4.

Regarding finger print pattern distribution (table 1) and increase of arches($P < 0.01$)was noted in sex chromatin positive cases when compared to all other groups except to female controls. Similar results were noted by previous investigators (Penrose 1963; Forbes 1964; Ushida et al. 1964; Alter 1965; Hunter 1968; Cushman and Soltan 1969; Wisniewski and Gawronska 1971; and Kadowaki 1977). The table shows an increase of arches in sex chromatin negative cases, also compared to male ($P < 0.05$) but not to female controls. An increase of ulnar loops and a decrease of whorls was found comparing patients with both male and female controls. A decrease of ulnar loops was found in sex chromatin positive patients compared to sex chromatin negative patients ($P < 0.05$). Important findings in sex chrmatin -ve group were the increase in arches and in ulnar loops. An increase of arches is characteristic of extra X (Alter 1965) or of extra Y chromosomes (Uchida et al.1964). An increase in ulnar loops is characteristic of single X cases or their equivalents (Holt 1964). The abnormal finger print patterns in the sex

Table 1. Finger Prints in Primary Azoospermia (Frequency of Patterns, PII & TRC).

Dermatoglyphic parameter	Primary azoospermia		Control	
	Sex chromatin -ve(N=28)	Sex Chromatin +ve(N=16)	Male (N=50)	Female (N=50)
Arch	5	10	1.6	5.8
Radial Loop	1.07	0.62	2	1
Ulnar Loop	62.85	50.62	50.4	52
Whorl	31.07	38.75	45.8	41.2
Mean PII	12.46	13.18	14.52	13.62
± SD	± 3.44	± 3.35	± 3.35	± 3.92
Mean TRC	127.67	109.75	141.02	123.49
± SD	±37.01	±44.42	±37.88	±49.99

chromatin negative groups which does not fit any single abnormality of sex chromosome complement suggests etiologic heterogeneity of this group. An evidence is that two cases of the sex chromatin negative group proved by chromosomal study to have abnormal sex chromosome mosaisism (XY/XYY & XY/XO). Their individual dermatoglyphic patterns showed abnormalities suggestive of their chromosome complement. The patient with XO/XY had increased whorls and that with XY/XYY had increased arches. Statistical analysis of dermatoglyphics after exclusion of the findings in these 2 cases from the sex chromatin negative group did not alter the significance of the previous findings.

Regarding the mean PII of fingers our results showed that in patients both sex chromatin positive and negative, there was a lower PII of fingers compared to male controls with no significant differences. We were not able to find comparable literature for mean PII in primary azoospermia.

Regarding TRC the present investigation showed a decreased mean TRC in sex chromatin positive patients ($P < 0.01$) when compared to male controls which is in agreement with previous investigations (Holt 1964; Penrose 1967; Hunter 1968). We observed a reduced value of mean TRC in sex chromatin negative cases compared to male controls. By comparing the mean TRC in sex chromatin positive and negative patients no significant difference was noticed ($P > 0.05$). These findings may also suggest the heterogeneity of our cases with the probalitity of mosaicism for extra sex chromosomes as proved in one of the sex chromatin -ve cases who showed mosaicism for an extra Y chromosome and decrease in TRC. Penrose (1967) noted that the presence of an additional X chromosome diminishes the TRC nearly three times as much as does the presence of an additional Y chromosome.

Analysis of Palm prints (table 2) showed an increase of hypothenar patterns in chromatin positive cases when compared to male controls ($P < 0.01$) but not to female controls. This is similar to previous investigators (Cushman and Soltan 1969) who also found a significant decrease in thenar/first interdigital patterns in XXY patients. Such a difference although noted was not significant in the present study.

Table 2. Palm Prints in Primary Azoospermia (Frequency of Interdigidital and Hypothenar Patterns).

Dermatoglyphic parameter	Primary Azoospermia		Control	
	Sex Chromatin -ve (N=28)	Sex Chromatin +ve (N=16)	Male (N=50)	Female (N=50)
Th/I_1	7.1	3	7	6
I_2	3.5	6	5	3
I_3	33.9	62.5	45	43
I_4	48.2	50	47	54
H_y	17.8	53.12	25	35

Regarding frequency of 2nd and 4th interdigital patterns we found no significant differences between sex chromatin positive cases and controls but we observed an increased frequency of 3rd interdigital patterns similar to previous investigators (Kadowaki 1977). In sex chromatin negative cases we found a decrease in hypothenar patterns between cases and female controls ($P < 0.05$) but not to male controls. There was a general tendency for a decreased interdigital pattern frequency between sex chromatin negative cases and controls. Palmar pattern configurations revealed an increase in frequencies of third interdigital and hypothenar patterns in sex chormatin positive compared to sex chromatin negative patients ($P < 0.01$).

Study of the a-b ridge count (table 3) showed that sex chromatin positive patients had a slightly lower mean value compared to both male and female controls. This is similar to previous observations (Komatz and Yoshida 1976 a). Other investigators noted significant reduction when compared to both male and female controls (Hunter 1968; Kadowaki 1977). We noted an increase of a-b ridge count in sex chromatin negative patients compared to both male and female controls ($P < 0.05$) especially to sex chromatin positive patients ($P < 0.01$). Holt (1964) reported that XO patients have an increased mean a-b ridge count. Our finding of one case of XO/XY in the sex chromatin negative group may suggest the presence of undetected mosaicism in other cases of this group thus causing the observed increase in the mean a-b ridge count.

Table 3. Palm Prints in Primary Azoospermia (a-b Ridge Count & Axial Triradius).

Dermatoglyphic parameter	Primary Azoospermia		Control	
	Sex Chroma-tin -ve (N=28)	Sex Chroma-tin +ve (N=16)	Male (N=50)	Female (N=50)
a-b Ridge count. Mean ± SD	82.75 ±12.08	74.75 ± 9.08	78.02 ±11.24	77.08 ± 9.32
Mean atd angle ± SD	87 ±16.3	89.06 ±18.5	87.38 ±14.83	88.66 ±17.26
Perc. Freq. of Distal deviation	28.1	53.2	27	37
Perc. Freq. of Ulnar triradii	14.2	40.62	14	25

Comparison of atd angle measurements (table 3) showed absence of significant differences between sex chromatin positive and sex chromatin negative patients and both male and female controls. Forbes (1964), Holt (1968), Komatz & Yoshida (1976 b) observed no difference in atd angle between XXY patients and both male & female controls. On the other hand, Hunter (1968) found a proximal displacement of the axial triradius in (12) XXY patients evidenced by a more acute "atd" angle. Measurement of distal deviation (table 3) showed that there was an increase in the frequency of distal axial triradii in sex chromatin positive patients when compared to male controls and not to females ($P < 0.01$). Our findings are in agreement with those of previous investigators (Cushman and Soltan 1969; Schaumann and Alter 1976; Komatz and Yoshida 1976 b). The same authors also noted that while the position of the axial triradii by distal deviation showed a significant increase in the frequency of distal axial triradius, this was not evident by atd angle measurements. These findings confirm that "atd" angle is not an accurate method for determining the position of the axial triradius. Study of sex chromatin negative cases showed no significant differences in either atd angle or frequency of distal deviation when compared to male and female controls.

An increase was found in the frequency of distal triradii in sex chromatin positive compared to sex chromatin negative patients ($P < 0.05$). Palmar ulnar triradii were found frequently associated with hypothenar patterns. As shown in table (3) there was an increase in XXY patients when compared to male controls ($P < 0.01$). Our findings are similar to those of Cushman and Soltan (1969) and Schaumann & Alter (1976) while Ushida et al. (1964) reported a normal frequency of palmar ulnar triradii in XXY patients.

We did not notice any significant differences in the frequency of palmar ulnar triradii between sex chromatin negative cases and controls. But we found a significant increase in frequency of palmar ulnar triradii in sex chromatin positive compared to sex chromatin negative patients.

As shown in table (4) sex chromatin positive patients had an increase in the frequency of accessory triradii in I_4 ($P < 0.01$) compared to both male and female controls and sex chromatin -ve but no significant alterations in I_2.

Table 4. Palm Prints in Primary Azoospermia (Extra Triradii, PII and Main Line Index).

Dermatoglyphic parameter	Primary Azoospermia		Control	
	Sex Chromatin -ve(N=28)	Sex Chromatin +ve(N=16)	Male (N=50)	Female (N=50)
Extra triradii				
I_2	3.5	6	5	2
I_4	12.5	40	9	8
Mean PII $\pm$ SD	10.46 $\pm$ 0.74	11.37 $\pm$1.15	10.92 $\pm$ 1.51	10.72 $\pm$ 1.14
Mean main line Index $\pm$ SD	16.71 $\pm$ 3.08	17.11 $\pm$ 3.59	17.76 $\pm$ 3.62	17.56 $\pm$ 2.85

Our results agree with those of Cushman and Soltan (1969), who on the other hand noted an increase in accessory triradii in I_2. We did not find any significant difference between sex chromatin negative patients and controls in the frequency of accessory triradii neither in the second nor in the fourth interdigital area. These findings suggest that the increase in the frequency of accessory triradii may be related to the presence of an extra X chromosome.

We also observed an increase in PII of palm in sex chromatin positive patients when compared to female ($P < 0.05$) but not to male controls. This increase in PII could be due to the significant increase of accessory triradii in I_4, palmar ulnar triradii and distal axial triradii. On the other hand, there was no significant difference in the mean value of PII of palm between sex chromatin negative cases and controls. Comparison between the 2 groups of azoospermia patients showed a significant increase of mean PII of palm in sex chromatin positive patients compared to the sex chromatin negative group ($P < 0.01$). We were unable to find comparable literature on this dermatoglyphic parameter in primary azoospermia patients.

Analysis of the main line index (table 4) showed no significant difference in the mean value neither between the sex chromatin positive nor sex chromatin negative patients and controls. Yoshida (1977) noted similar results in patients with KF syndrome.

We did not observe any abnormalities of flexion creases in cases of primary azoospermia neither in the sex chromatin positive nor the sex chromatin negative cases. This is in agreement with the results of Cushman and Soltan (1969) and Schaumann and Alter (1976).

From the present study, it is possible to conclude that certain dermatoglyphic changes were observed in both sex chromatin positive and sex chromatin negative patients with primary azoospermia. Differences between sex chromatin positive patients and male controls were significant regarding finger print patterns, mean TRC, frequency of hypothenar patterns palmar ulnar triradii, distal axial triradii accessory triradii in I_4 and PII of palm. No demonstrable differences were found in PII of fingers, mean a-b ridge count, mean "atd" and main line index. In the sex chromatin negative group the study showed that they had abnormal dermatoglyphic patterns. Significant differences between patients, male and female controls were found in finger print pattern distribution, PII of fingers, frequency of hypothenar patterns and mean a-b ridge count. While changes in the sex chromatin positive groups are similar to those of previous investigators and are due to the extra X chromosome, changes in the sex chromatin negative group cannot be explained as the effect of a single specific sex chromosome complement, thus suggesting that the sex chromatin negative group is heterogeneous. This was documented by our finding of two cases mosaic for sex chromosome abnormalities.

Since blood was the only tissue studied for chromosomal complement, mosaicism in other tissues cannot be excluded. Therefore dermatoglyphic studies proved to be a useful adjunct to chromosomal studies. Moreover, dermatoglyphics may even be more sensitive indicators of underlying developmental differences between the sex chromatin negative azoospermia patients and the controls. In such cases where no chromosomal abnormalities were found, genetic changes, environmental prenatal causes,mosaicisim and minor chromosomal abnormalities that could not be revealed by available cytogenetic techniques may be etiological.

DERMATOGLYPHICS IN CONGENITAL HEART DISEASE (CHD)

Previous reports in the literature have suggested that the frequencies of certain dermatoglyphic configurations in patients with CHD differs from those of normal individuals or patients with aquired heart disease. The earliest reports were made by Hale et al. (1961) and Rowe and Uchida (1961). The finger and palm prints were used to compare patients with controls. Later, some authors treated CHD as a group (Saller and Glowatzki 1967; Alter and Schulenberg 1970). Others analysed dermatoglyphics for CHD and for specific defects (Cascos 1964; Kontras and Bodenbender 1965; Weninger et al. 1966; Reyes 1968; Saksena and Kumar 1968; Emerit et al. 1968; Laurenti 1969; Paci et al. 1969; David 1969; Preus et al. 1970 and Magotra and Chakrabarti 1976).

The present investigation included 200 patients with CHD not associated with apparent congenital malformations. Table (5) shows classification of the cases according to sex and type of CHD. In 133 patients, diagnosis was confirmed by cardiac surgery or by catheterization. The rest were diagnosed by full clinical, electrocardiographic and radiologic evaluation.

Table 5. Classification of Cases According to Type of CHD and to Sex.

Type of CHD	Sex and Number		
	Males	Females	Total
Tetralogy of Fallot (F_4)	17	9	26
Pulmonary stenosis (PS)	7	10	17
Aortic stenosis (AS)	3	3	6
Coarctation of the aorta (AC)	5	2	7
Patent ductus arteriosus (PDA)	8	15	23
Interatrial septal defect(ASD)	11	7	18
Interventricular septal defect(VSD)	3	5	8
Multiple CHD (MD)	1	6	7
Miscelaneous	11	10	21
Cases diagnosed clinically	33	34	67
Total	99	101	200

170 prints of controls matched for age and sex were collected representing different Egyptian Provinces. None

of the patients or controls were relatives.

Quantitative and qualitative data for finger and palm prints used comprised the 11 parameters included in the azoospermia study. Additional methods used in the analysis were : 1) in evaluation of the axial triradius, methods of measuring lateral deviation of the axial triradius by the mean of the adt angle and the frequency of different types of deviations by Cascos (1965) and the new method of David (1971) which corrects the atd angle for any lateral deviation, 2) the distal palm configuration described by Holt (1968) according to D line exit which classifies the palm into types α, β, γ, δ and ϵ, 3) main line variations, 4) main line terminations A,B,C and D , and 5) the topographic approach of Hanna and Schmidt (1976) for quantitative evaluation of the total degree of transversality of the palm creases.

Statistical tests similar to the azoospermia study were used. Comparisons were carried out between patients and controls, both sexes, each sex separately, summed hands, each hand, each digit and between patients with specific cardiac defects and controls.

Analysis of the results summerized in table (6) showed that FPP (Finger print pattern distribution) in CHD as a whole exhibited a decrease in ulnar loops and an increase in whorls in both sexes mainly due to diminished UL on 4th & 5th digits and increase in W on the 5th digit of the right hand. Analysis by sex revealed that the differences were significant in females. Our findings agree with those of Cascos (1964) and Paci et al. (1969) regarding the group as a whole. The results of Saller and Glowatzki (1967) and Alter and Schulenberg (1970) did not reveal significant differences in either sex. Analysis of each digit separately comparing males with females revealed a decrease in UL and an increase in W on the 5th digit of the right hand in males, and of the right hand particularly the 4th digit in females. In F_4 we observed an increase in UL on the left hand especially its first digit in males and a decrease in UL and an increase in W in females. Combining both sexes, no differences were noted between cases and controls. The latter finding agrees with the results of Preus et al. (1970). An increase in W was also observed by previous investigators (Cascos 1964); Kontras and Bodenbender 1965; Paci et al.(1969) and Magotra and Chakrabarti(1976). In PS in the whole group we observed a decrease in UL and an increase in W. Analysis of each sex separately showed no differences in males and a decrease of UL and an increase in W particularly on the right hand in females. We did not observe any significant changes in AS which agrees with the results of Emerit et al. (1968). In PDA we noted an increase in arches in the whole group which agrees with the findings of Paci et al. (1969) and Preus et al. (1970). Analysis by sex showed no significant differences in males but an increase in arches in females in both hands and mainly in the right hand. In ASD we noted a significant increase in arches in the whole group. Analysis by sex revealed an increase in arches and in radial loops (RL)and a decrease in UL in females, mainly due to increased arches on the left third digit and a decrease in UL on digit 5 of both hands and an increase in RL on digit 2 on the left hand. In VSD we noted a decrease in UL and an increase in W in the whole group which agrees with the results of Paci et al. (1969). This was mainly due to a decrease in UL on digit 5 right and left and an increase in W on digit 5 right and digit 5 and 3 left in males. In females a decrease in W was noted on digit 2 left and an increase of W on digit 4 left. In AC, there was a decrease in UL and an increase in W. Analysis of each sex separately showed that changes were significant in females. Cascos (1964) observed a similar increase in W.

In total finger ridge count (FRC) we observed no significant differences between patients and controls even after separation by sex. Analysis of digits seperately and combined also showed no significant differences. In specific types of CHD we observed no differences except in ASD in females where we noted a decreased FRC on the left third and fifth digits. Similarly, Burguet and Collard (1968) and Alter and Schulenberg (1970) who analysed the group of CHD as a whole observed no significant differences in TFRC (Total finger ridge count).

Study of finger pattern intensity index(FPII) in the group as a whole showed no significant differences between patients and controls and in both sexes separately. Analysis of specific types of CHD revealed in F_4 females a higher PII on both hands particularly on the right. Also there was a significant increase in PII in AC in females and in VSD in males in both hands summed and separate.

Analysis of patterns in interdigital areas showed no

significant differences between patients and controls when both sexes were combined. Our findings are in agreement with those of other investigators (Alter and Schulenberg 1970; Preus et al. 1970; Magotra and Chakrabarti 1976). Patterns in Th/I_1 showed a significant increase only in females with PDA. Analysis of frequency of patterns in I_2, I_3 and I_4 showed no significant differences in the group as a shole. In males, in CHD as a whole, and in those with F_4 and ASD we noted a decrease in loops in I_3 particularly on the right hand and in PDA on the summed hands. In females with ASD we noted an increase W on I_4 in both hands and in AS increased W on the left I_4 and increased loops on summed I_2.

In the Hy area we did not observe any significant differences between patients and controls. Similar findings were noted by previous investigators (Ciccarelli et al., 1968; Alter and Schulenberg 1970; Preus et al. 1970; Magotra and Chakrabarti 1976). In the specific types of CHD no significant changes in frequency of Hy patterns were observed except in patients with AS, where we noted an increased frequency in both males and females similar to the observation of Preus et al. (1970). We also noted an increase of bilateral Hy patterns in females with F_4 and in males with VSD.

"a-b" ridge count showed no differences between patients and controls which agrees with the findings of Alter and Schulenberg (1970). A significant decrease of a-b ridge count was found in females with CHD mainly on the left hand and in females with AC on the right and summed hands.

Study of Palm pattern intensity index(PPII) showed an increase in the right hand of females with PS and males with VSD on the left hand.

Evaluation of the position of the axial triradius by various methods showed that by measurement of distal deviation of "t" we noted an increase in the frequency of t', t'', t''' in the whole group of CHD. In males, an increase was noted in t'', t''' on the summed hands. In females, the increase was in t' particularly on the left hand. In F_4 an increase of t''' and t' was noted in males and females, respectively. In females with PS and AC, and in males with AS, we noted an increase in t' on the summed. In males with VSD an increase in t''' on each hand was noted. In females with multiple

CHD a decrease in t' was noted on the left hand. Using the mean atd angle and matching the patients and controls for age and sex we found a significantly wider atd angle on the right hand in males aged 7-12 years as a whole and in the group of F_4. There was a decrease in the mean atd angle on the right hand in males with PDA in the age group above 18 years. Chance alone may explain these findings since previous investigators who performed similar matching noted similar results (Friend and Neel 1962; Hook et al. 1974) while others (Reyes 1968; Burguet and Collard 1968; Burguet et al. 1970; Alter and Schulenberg 1970; Magotra and Chakrabarti 1976) who found significant increase of wide atd angle, did not match their patients for neither sex nor age. Applying the new David's formula for correction of the atd angle, no significant difference was found in the group of CHD as a whole. However, in F_4 we noted an increase in the mean atd angle on the right and left and summed hands in males aged 7-12 years and in the left and summed hands in females above 18 years. No previous investigators used David's formula to evaluate the atd angle. Evaluation of the lateral deviation of the axial triradius using the mean adt angle showed an increase in the left adt angle in the right and summed hands in females aged 1-6 years and a decrease in males 7-12 years on the right hand in CHD as a whole, and in F_4. In females with PDA aged 13-18 years an increase was noted. An increase in the mean adt angle indicates ulnar deviation while a decrease indicates radial deviation. Determination of different types of deviation according to the method of Cascos (1965) and matching for sex, we found no significant differences in the group of CHD when both sexes were analysed. The only exception was in ASD which showed an increase in the frequency of middle 't' in comparison with the controls. Cascos (1965) observed a more radial axial triradius in CHD patients especially in those with F_4. Matching the patients and controls for sex in our study showed a decrease in the frequency of the radial 't' on the summed hands. Females with F_4 showed an increase in ulnar 't' on the summed hands, those with PS a highly significant ulnar 't' on the right hand, those with multiple CHD a decrease of radial 't' and an increase of middle 't' on summed hands. Males with ASD had an increase of middle 't' on the right hand while those with VSD had a decrease in the frequency of middle 't' on the summed hands. Study of the frequency of multiplicity of the axial triradius (MAT) by all methods of analysis revealed insignificant differences between patients and controls which conforms with the results of other investigators (Christensen and Nelson 1963; Emerit et al. 1968; Preus et al. 1970; Laurenti 1969 and Sharets 1974). However, in F_4 in females, there was a significant increase in multiple axial triraduii and in females with PS an increase was noted in the right hand only. Males with AS, AC and VSD showed an increase in MAT.

Study of the main lines of the palm showed that in the main line variation, the CHD group as a whole showed a decrease of γ variation particularly in females. Males with F_4 had a decrease of bilateral γ variation. Females with PS had an increase in α on the right hand and β on the left hand. In AC there was an increase of β variation in the left hand in males and in both hands in females. In ASD there was an increase of α variation in the left hand in males and bilateral β variation in females.

Study of main line terminations showed non-significant differences between patients as a whole and controls. The most common termination for main line A was in area 3. In males with F_4 and females with PS there was an increase in 5 exit on the left hand, in females with AS an increase in 5' exit on the right hand and in males with VSD an increase in 1' exit on the left hand, indicating a longitudinal course. Regarding main line D we noted a decrease in exit 7 on the right hand in females, males with AC had increased exit 9 on the left hand and in males with PDA on the right hand. Males with ASD had a decrease in exit 11 on the right hand. For the main line B exit, we noted a decrease in the frequency of 5" exit on the left hand in males. In PS, males had an increase of bilateral 5' exit and females an increase of 5" exit on the left hand. Males with AS had an increase of 9 exit on the right hand and 6 exit on the left hand. Females with PDA showed a decrease of 5 exit on the left hand. Males with ASD had a decrease of 7 exit on the right hand. Females with VSD had an increase of 5' exit on the right hand. Regarding the main line C we found no differences between male patients and controls but a decrease in abrupt ending of main line C on the right hand in females. In F_4 we noted a decrease in exit 5 on the left hand in males and a decrease of abrupt ending on the right hand in females. Males with PS had an increase of exit 5 on the left hand. Males with AS had an increase in exit 11 on the right hand. Males with PDA had an increase in exit 7 on the right hand.

Females with multiple CHD had an increase in exit 7 on the left hand.

Regarding the main line index, there was no significant difference between patients and controls except in females with PS and AS where there was an increase in the main line index on the right hand. Study of the total degree of transversality of the creases showed no significant differences between cases and controls except for an increase in males with CHD as a whole and in males with F_4.

Study of the transverse creases of the palm revealed no significant differences between patients and controls regarding Sydney line. The frequency of simian creases showed no differences except for an increase in males with VSD. Previous investigators noted no differences in simian creases in the whole group of CHD (Burguet and Collard 1968; Emerit et al. 1968; Alter and Schulenberg 1970; Preus et al. 1970).

It is worth pointing out that in the present study,up to our knowledge, certain parameters were investigated unpreceeded by others in CHD e.g. PII of fingers and palms, frequency of main line variation, frequency of main lines B and C exits, main line index, frequency of Sydney line, degree of transversality of palm creases, and the corrected atd angle by David's method, analysis of each hand and each digit seperately and separation by sex in all parameters and by age in some parameters. In our discusion we mentioned points of agreement only with previous investigators. In most cases disagreement between our findings and those of other authors could be due to small sample size and failure to specify exclusion of other congenital abnormalities.

It is possible to conclude from the present study of CHD that analysis of each hand separately revealed changes in one hand and not in the other, analysis of each sex separately yielded new findings and that matching patients and controls for age and sex is of utmost importance for accuracy of the results. As shown in table (6) certain types of CHD in the different sexes showed changes more than others examples are F_4 in both sexes, PS in females, VSD in males. The study of dermatoglyphics in CHD in general showed that the presence of any pattern in an individual is not necessarily pathognomonic , but can share in the battery of investigations to ascertain the diagnosis. Certain dermatoglyphic parameters

Table 6. Significant Dermatoglyphic Changes in Patients with Congenital Heart Disease.

Dermatoglyphic parameter	CHD		F_4		PS		AS		PDA		ASD		VSD		AC		Freq. signif. NP = 16
	M	F	M	F	M	F	M	F	M	F	M	F	M	F	M	F	
FPP (Both hands)		+	+	+		+				+		+	+	+		+	9
FRC												+					1
FPII				+									+			+	3
Th/I_1										+							1
I_2, I_3 & I_4	+		+					+	+		+	+					6
H_y				+			+						+				3
a-b ridge count		+														+	2
PPII						+							+				2
Distal deviation	+	+	+	+		+	+						+			+	8
atd angle	+		+						+								3
David's method			+	+													2
Mean adt	+	+	+							+							4
Cascos method		+		+		+					+		+				5
MAT				+		+	+						+		+		5
Main line variation		+	+			+					+	+			+	+	7
Main line A			+			+		+					+				4
Main line D		+							+		+				+		4
Main line C		+	+	+	+		+		+								6
Main line B	+			+	+	+	+			+	+			+		+	9
Main line index						+		+									2
Crease transvers.	+		+														2
Syndey line																	0
Simian crease													+				1
Freq.Signif.NP=23	6	8	10	9	2	9	5	3	4	4	5	4	9	2	3	6	

\+ = Significant T = Total M = Male F = Female NP = Number of parameters may be more important than others not only in the group of CHD as a whole but also in the specific types. Noteworthy examples as shown in table (6) are finger print pattern distribution, distal deviation of the axial triradius, main line variations, exits of main lines B and C and frequency of patterns in I_2, I_3 and I_4.

In conclusion, we agree with Reed (1981) that dermatoglyphic studies should be an integral part of the physical examination of every patient with a birth defect.

Acknoweldgement : Thanks are due to Prof. Dr. A. S. Ibraheem Prof. of Statistics, The National Cancer Institute , Cairo University for directing and revising the statistical analysis of data in CHD.

Abel W (1938). Kritische Studien uber die Entwicklung der Papillarmuster auf den Fingerbeeren. Z Menschl Vererb. -u Konstit-Lehre 2 : 497.

Ater M (1965). Is hyperploidy of sex chromosomes associated with reduced total finger ridge count? Am J Hum genet 17 : 473.

Alter M and Schulenberg GR (1970). Dematoglyphics in CHD. Circulation XII : 49.

Arias S, Penchaszadeh VB, Pinto-Cisternas J, and Larrauri S (1980). The IVIC syndrome: A new autosomal dominant complex pleiortropic syndrome with radial ray hypoplasia hearing impairment, external ophthalmoplegia and thrombocytopenia. Am J Med Genet 6 : 25.

Atasu M (1976). Hereditary index finger polydactyly. Phenotypic radiological dermatoglyphic and genetic findings in a large family. J Med Genet 13 : 469.

Benirschke K, Lowry RB, Opitz JM, Schwarzacher HG and Spranger JW (1979). Developmental terms-some proposals: First Report of an International Working Group. Am J Med Genet 3 : 297.

Birnholz JC (1972). Dermatoglyphics in CHD. Am J Roentgenol Radium Nucl Med 116 : 539.

Burguet W, and Collard P (1968). Dermatoglyphics in Congenital heart disease. Lancet 2 : 106.

Burguet W, Collard P and Janovic M (1970). Study of extracardiac malformation anomalies of dermatoglyphics in group of patients with CHD. Acta Cardiol (Brux) 25 : 291.

Cascos AS (1964). Finger-print patterns in CHD. Brit Heart J 26 : 624.

Cascos AS (1965). Palmarprint pattern in CHD. Brit Heart J 26 : 428.

Cascos AS (1968). Dermatoglyphics in CHD. Acta Pediat Scand 27 : 9.

Cascos AS and Hermida LF (1969). Dermatoglyphics in Eisenmenger reactions.Acta Cardiol (Brux) 24 : 382.

Ceccarelli M, Giorgi PL and Paci A (1966). Further study of dermatoglyphics in CHD. a-b ridge count.Minerva Pediat 21 : 867.

Christensen FK and Nelson RM (1963). Similar congenital heart disease in siblings. J Thorac Cadiovasc Surgery 45 : 597.

Cummins H, and Sicomo J (1923). Plantar epidermal configuration in low grade syndactylism (Zygodactyly) of the second and third toes.Anat Rec 25 : 355.

Cummins H (1923). The configuration of epidermal ridges in a human acephalic monster. Anat Rec 26 : 1.

Cummins H (1926). Epidermal ridge configuration in developmental defects with particular reference to ontogenetic factors which condition ridge direction. Amer J Anat 38 : 39.

Cummins HS (1932). Spontaneous amputation of human supernumerary digits pedunculated postminimi. Am J Anat 51 : 381.

Cushman CJ and Soltan HC (1969). Dermatoglyphics in Klinefelter's syndrome (47,XXY). Human Hered 19 : 641.

David TJ (1969). Finger print in CHD. Bristol Medicochir J 48 : 167.

David TJ (1971). The palmar axial triradius a new method of location. Hum Hered 21 : 624.

Emerit I, Vernant P and Corona P (1968). Les dermatoglyphes des malades proteurs d'une cardiopathie congenitale. Acta genet Med Gemellol 17 : 523.

Forbes AP (1964). Finger prints and palm prints (dermatoglyphics) and Palmar-flexion creases in gonadal dysgenesis, pseudohypoparathyroidism and Klinefelter's syndrome. N Engl J Med 270 : 1268.

Fried K, and Neel JV (1962). Palmar dermatoglyphics in CHD. Abstract of Am Soc Hum Genet.

Gall JC JR, Stern AM, Cohen MM, Adams MS and Davidson PT (1966). Holt-Oram syndrome: Clinical and genetic study of a large family. Am J Hum Genet 18 : 187.

Hale AR (1952). Morphogenesis of volar skin in the human fetus Amer J Anat 91 : 147.

Hale AR, Phillips JH, and Burch GE (1961). Feature of palmar dermatoglyphics in CHD. A report of the variant frequently associated with CHD. 176 : 41.

Hanna D and Schmidt R (1976). Topographic approach for analysis of palm crease variant. J Med Gen 13 : 310.
Holt SB (1964). The role of dermatoglyphics in medical biology. Med World London 101 : 112.
Holt SB (1968). "The Genetics of Dermal Ridges". Springfield, III. Charles C thomas.
Holt SB (1972). The effect of absence of thumb on palmar dermatoglyphics. J Med Genet 9 : 448.
Hunter H (1968). Finger and palm prints in chromatin positive males. J Med Genet 5 : 112.
Kadowaki SH (1977). Dermatoglyphics of Klinfelter's syndrome. J Med Genetics 14 : 187
Klinefelter HF Jr (1973). Background of the recognition of Klinefelter syndrome as a distinct pathologic entity. Am J Obstet gynecol 116 : 436.
Komatz Y and Yoshida O (1976 a). The palmar a-b ridge counts in patients with KF syndrome (47, XXY) among Japanese. Hum Biology 48 , 581 : 84.
Komatz Y, and Yoshida O (1976 b). Position of axial triradius in 51 cases of 47, XXY Klinefelter syndrome. Jap J Hum Genet 21 : 123.
Kontras SB, and Bodenbender JQ (1965). Dermatoglyphic survey of CHD. (Abstr.) Midwest Soc Pediat Res (Quoted from Cascos 1968).
Laurenti R (1969). "Etudo dos dermatoglifos am partadores de cardiopatias congenitas" (Thesis) Sao Paulo.
Magotra ML and Chakrabarti MC (1976). Dermatoglyphics in CHD. Indian Pediatr 13 : 225.
Mulvihill JJ and Smith D (1969). The genesis of dermatoglyphics. J Pediatr 75 : 579.
Okajima M (1975). Development of dermal ridges in the fetus. J Med Genet 12 : 243.
Paci A, Giorgi PL, Ceccarelli M and Baldini Q (1969). Digital dermatoglyptics and CHD. Minerva Pediatr 21 : 658.
Penrose LS (1963). Finger-prints, palms and chromosomes. Nature 197 : 933.
Penrose LS (1965). Dermatoglyphic topoloy. Nature 205 : 544.
Penrose LS (1967). Finger print patterns and the sex chromosomes. Lancet 1 : 298.
Penrose LS (1968). Memorandum on dermatoglyphic nomenclature. Birth Defects: Orig Art Ser 4 The National Foundation the March of Dimes. New York.
Penrose LS and Ohara PT (1973). The development of the epidermal ridges. J Med Genet 10 : 201.
Pfeiffer RA and ZuBerge S (1964). Untersuchungen Zur Frage der Hautleisten und Furchen bei Extremitatenmissbildungen. Z. Menschl Vererb Konstit.-Lehre 37 : 677.

Popich GH and Smith DW (1970). The genesis and significance of digital and palmar hand creases. Preliminary report. J Pediat 77 : 1017.

Preus M, Fraser FC, and Levy EP (1970). Dermatoglyphics in congenital heart malformations. Hum Hered 20 : 388.

Reed T (1981). Review Dermatoglyphics in Medicine-Problems and use in abnormalities. Am J Med Genet 8 : 411.

Reyes L (1968). Abnormal dermatoglyphics in CHD. Chicago Pediatric Society 27 : 86.

Row RD, and Uchida JA (1961). Dermatoglyphic heterogenity in Mongols with CHD. Am J Med Genet 31 : 726.

Saksena PN, and Kumar N (1968). Evaluation of dermatoglyphics in CHD. and Turner's syndrome. Indian Pediatr 5 : 315.

Saller VK, and Glowatzki G (1967). CHD and Dermatoglyphics Med Klin 62 : 1458.

Schaumann B, and Alter M (1976). "Dermatoglyphics in Medical Disorders". Springer-Verlag.

Sharets Yu D (1974). Characteristics of the palmar axial tradius in patients with CHD and their next of kin. Bull Exp Biol. and Med 77 : 567.

Temtamy SA (1966). "Genetic Factors in Hand Malformations" Ph. D. Thesis. Johns Hopkins University.

Temtamy S and Mckusick VA (1969). Synopsis of hand malformations with particular emphasis on genetic factors. Birth Defects OAS 3 : 125.

Temtamy SA , El-Darawy ZI, El-Zawahry M, Mobarak ZM and El-Laithy SA (1976). Dermatoglyphic studies in Egyptians. Abstracts of papers presented at the Vth International Congress of Human Genetics Mexico Cit. Mexico, October 10-15.

Temtamy S A and Mckusick VA (1978). "The Genetics of Hand Malformations". Alan R Liss Inc. New York.

Temtamy SA, Ibrahim AA, Salam AM, Boulos SY, El-Miniawy L, Hussien FH and Mahmoud KZ (1980). Genetic studies in Azoospermia patients with the Klinefelter pattern of Testicular Biopsy. Andrologia 12 : 345.

Uchida IA, Miller JR and Soltan HC (1964). Dermatologyphics associated with XXYY chromosomes. Am J Hum Genet 16 : 284.

Walker NF (1957). The use of dermal configuration in the diagnosis of mongolism. J Pediatr 50 : 19.

Weninger M, Kaindi F, Rothenbuchner G, and Scober B (1966). Hautleistenuntersuchungen bei angeborenen M: Abbildunger der Herzens und der grosse gefasse. Weiner Klin Wschr, 23 : 905.

Wisnieski L, and Awronska H (1971). Dermotoscopic and Cytogenetic studies in the parents of children with congenital anomalies and in persons with Down's and KF Syndromes.Genet Pol 12 : 621.

Yoshida D (1977). Terminations of palmar main lines and main line indices in 47, XXY KF'S syndrome. J Hum Gent 22 : 281.

Progress in Dermatoglyphic Research, pages 421-425

A STUDY OF DERMATOGLYPHICS AND MYOCARDIAL INFARCTION

M.P. Mi and Florence C.C. Mi

Department of Genetics
University of Hawaii
Honolulu, Hawaii 96822

Cardiovascular disorders are the most important causes of morbidity and mortality in all industrialized nations. In the United States these disorders account for approximately one-half of all deaths each year, the majority being due to ischemic heart disease or coronary heart disease (CHD). Myocardial infarction (M.I.) is the catastrophic, often fatal form of CHD, usually resulting from precipitous reduction or arrest of a significant portion of the coronary flow and is known to be responsible for approximately two-thirds of CHD deaths.

Many risk factors have been reported for CHD (Levy and Feinleib, 1980). These include hypertension, cigarette smoking, hyperlipidemia, physical inactivity, stress, diabetes, and obesity. Some of these factors also demonstrate familial aggregation.

Previous studies in two samples of Japanese males in Hawaii have shown that patients with M.I. had a higher frequency of whorl pattern types and a higher ridge count on fingers than controls (Rashad and Mi, 1975; Rashad et al., 1978). As this observed association suggests a possible involvement of antenatal factors in the etiology of myocardial infarction, the use of dermatoglyphic characteristics in identifying individuals at high risk would be of great importance from a preventive medicine standpoint. Therefore, there is an urgent need to explore further the association and to test the validity of the original findings.

In Hawaii many racial groups are represented (Lind, 1967; Nordyke, 1977). These are mainly Caucasian, Chinese, Filipino, Hawaiian, and Japanese. Significant racial variations in digital dermatoglyphic traits are presented in two other reports (Mi et al., 1981a,b). Based on our previous analysis four dermatoglyphic clusters can be identified. The first cluster consists of the Hawaiian people who have the highest frequency of whorl pattern types and the highest ridge counts. The Caucasian group is at the other extreme, being low in whorls and ridge counts. For most dermatoglyphic traits the Chinese, Filipino and Part-Hawaiian who are not significantly different from the population mean fall into one single cluster. The Japanese group is intermediate between the Caucasian and the population mean.

There is no information available about the incidence of myocardial infarction among racial groups in Hawaii. Table 1 gives mortality rates for heart disease (ICD 410) in Hawaii for the 10-year period from 1966 to 1975. These rates were computed based on death statistics from the Hawaii State Department of Health and the 1970 Census data, and were adjusted for age based on Segii World Population. The Caucasian and Hawaiian groups, which are significantly different from each other in most digital dermatoglyphic traits, have similar higher rates as compared with other groups. This apparently contradicts the implication based on the observed results among Japanese males that high ridge count and high frequency of whorl patterns are associated with high risk for myocardial infarction. For this reason, it would be equally important to test the association in other racial groups.

TABLE 1. AGE-ADJUSTED MORTALITY RATES* FOR HEART DISEASE

Racial Group	Male	Female
Caucasian	3.25 4.06	1.43 1.96
Japanese	1.45 1.91	0.95 1.30
Chinese	1.42 2.43	0.07 1.48
Hawaiian	3.11 4.51	2.09 3.22
Filipino	1.98 2.78	0.70 1.69
All races	2.34 2.68	1.31 1.58

* Upper and lower 95% confidence intervals per 1,000 population

It is well established that many dermatoglyphic traits are under genetic control. All heritability estimates for the total ridge count are in the high range of over 0.7 (Holt, 1952, 1956, 1957; Vogelius Anderson, 1963; Bonne et al., 1971; Matsuda, 1973; Mi and Rashad, 1975). By comparing estimates derived from the regression coefficients of offspring on father, mother and midparent and full-sib correlation, there is sufficient evidence that most of genetic variance, if not all, is additive. This mode of inheritance provides a unique opportunity to test whether the high ridge count associated with M.I. patients has a genetic basis. The alternative hypothesis is that some environmental influences occur during the prenatal life.

We are conducting a study in Hawaii to confirm the association between total ridge count and M.I. in several racial groups and to test that M.I. patients with higher ridge counts have a genetic basis. Our current efforts are in data collection. Data are being collected from two sources. One source is the fingerprint file of approximately 435,000 residents for the population registration in Hawaii during 1942 to 1943. By computerized linkage it is possible to locate records in the fingerprint file of individuals with confirmed diagnosis of M.I. and their spouses and first-degree relatives. The second source is the recruitment of M.I. patients and their relatives through the cooperation of three major clinics in Honolulu.

To date, fingerprint records representing more than 150 families have been collected. There are three basic types of familial data for analysis. The first type consists of families with one or both parents affected. The regression coefficient of offspring on mid-parent value will be tested for heterogeneity as compared to the same coefficient derived from control families. Families involving one or more M.I. patients and their normal siblings provide the second type of data. If parental information is available, each offspring can be expressed as a deviation from the mid-parent value. The within sibship variance estimated from families with M.I. patients will be compared with that derived from the control families. When parental information is not available, full-sib correlation will be derived for comparison. As yet, the number of families collected is too small to allow for discrimination between the genetic and the intrauterine environmental hypotheses.

ACKNOWLEDGEMENT

This work was supported in part by U.S. PHS Grant HL-23386 from the National Heart, Lung and Blood Institute.

REFERENCES

Bonne B, Ashbel S, Tal A (1971). The Habbanite isolate. II. Digital and palmar dermatoglyphics. Hum. Hered. 21:473-192.

Holt SB (1952). Genetics of dermal ridges: Inheritance of total finger ridge-count. Ann. Eugen., London 17:140-161.

Holt SB (1956). Genetics of dermal ridges: Parent-child correlations for total finger-ridge count. Ann. Hum. Genet. 20:270-281.

Holt SB (1957). Genetics of dermal ridges: Sib pair correlations for total finger-ridge count. Ann. Hum. Genet. 21:352-362.

Levy RI, Feinleib M (1980). Risk factors for coronary artery disease and their management. In Braunwald (ed): "Heart Diseases." Philadelphia: W.B. Saunders, p 1246-2578.

Lind AW (1967). "Hawaii's People." Honolulu: The University Press of Hawaii, 121p.

Matsuda, E (1973). Genetic studies on total finger ridge-count among Japanese. Jap. J. Human Genet. 17:293-318.

Mi MP, Budy AM, Rashad MN (1981a). A population study of finger dermal patterns and ridge counts.

Mi MP, Budy AM, Rashad MN (1981b). Ridge count of finger dermal patterns.

Mi MP, Rashad MN (1975). Genetic parameters of dermal patterns and ridge counts. Hum. Hered. 25:249-257.

Nordyke EC (1977). "The Peopling of Hawaii." Honolulu: The University Press of Hawaii, 221p.

Rashad MN, Mi MP (1975). Dermatoglyphic traits in patients with cardiovascular disorders. Amer. J. Phy. Anthrop. 42:281-283.

Rashad MN, Mi MP, Rhoads G (1978). Dermatoglyphic studies of myocardial infarction patients. Hum. Hered. 28:1-6.

Vogelius Anderson CH (1963). On the genetics of certain dermatoglyphic traits. Proc. II Intern. Congr. Human Genet. 3:1509-1516.

Progress in Dermatoglyphic Research, pages 427-433

DERMATOGLYPHICS IN VITILIGO

M. Oyhenart-Perera, R. Kolski, G. Salvat

Dpt. Genética. Facultad de Humanidades y Ciencias

Montevideo - Uruguay

The present communication tackles the description of the digital and palmar dermatoglyphics in vitiligo patients. Vitiligo is a cutaneous disease characterized by the appearance of hypocromic areas. These areas, of a quite symmetrical arrangement, progress generally, although they may stop and even regress. In regards to its etiology, the significance of Cu (Genov et al. 1972, Newbold 1973) and the possibility of immunological factors (Carter and Jegasothy, 1976) has been underlined. Several authors believe in the existance of a hereditary component in the disease (Gorl 1934, Gates, 1948, Cauwenberghe 1958, Lerner 1959, Vogel and Dorn, 1966, Silvers and Glickman 1970, Bader et al. 1975, Thumon et al. 1975, Goncalvez 1976, Mayenburg 1976, Oyhenart-Perera and Kolski 1980), with the features -according to the almost absolute majority- an autosomic dominant mechanism of variable expressivity and penetrance.

The hereditary nature of this disease, the common embryological origin of the skin and dermatoglyphics, and the great variation on the age when the visible signs of vitiligo (hypocromic areas) appear, stimulates the execution of this study in search of signs that would help to diagnose it.

Material and Methods

We took the files from patients diagnosed to have vitiligo from the Dermatological Clinics of the Central Military Hospital and The Pasteur Hospital (Ministerio de

Salud Pública, Montevideo, Uruguay), and the patients recived an appointment by mail. Had they not come to it, they would have received another and last one. Thanks to this procedure we were able to interview 43 caucasoid patients of both sexes (19 males and 24 females).

The patients were informed about the object of the interview. They were questioned in order to obtain data in relation to their case history as vitiligo patients, their relatives case history, etc. -material covered in another communication (Oyhenart-Perera and Kolski 1980)-, and finger and palm prints were taken of them.

The methodology and symbology used here follow the usual criteria (Cummins and Midlo 1961, Penrose 1968). The control for digital dermatoglyphics were taken from studies on normal samples of our population (Kolski and Scazzocchio 1961, Oyhenart-Perera 1977). For the palmar control of values we used a sample of both sexes, caucasoid, equivalent in number to the one covered here. This sample was selected at random among the palmar prints of normal individuals from the files of the Genetics Department of the Facultad de Humanidades y Ciencias in Montevideo. We adjusted the results to proofs of statistical significance -according to the circumstances, x^2 or t of Student-, considering the level of significance under .05

Results and Conclusions

In the study of digital dermatoglyphs we tackle two aspects: The frequency of designs per hand and sex that we compare to the sample on the Kolski and Scazzocchio's study (1961), table 1; and the total quantitative value (T.R.C.) per sex that we evalute with data from Oyhenart-Perera (1977), table 2.

On males, the comparison with the control came out highly significant in regards to the alternatives of right hand and both hands: The difference existent in the left hand did not achieve statistic significance (x^2 = 4.21). These differences are due to a pronounced increase in the number of arches (A) in detriment of the whorls (W) frequency. It is important to emphasize that in the preceding study on this theme of Sahasrabuddhe et al. (1973), a decrease in the frequency of W in males and an increase of A in the middle finger were found in a sample of 25 males and 25 females vitiligo patients.

Among women, the comparisons among the three alternatives gave highly significant differences, due to the substantial increase in the frequency of W and a consequent disminution on the remaining figures. This remark is common to all the alternatives. Comparing these results with the study mentioned above (Sahasrabuddhe et al. 1973) we find a difference, since those authors underline an increase in the A frequency.

As far as the T.R.C. is concerned, the tendency to decrease in males and to increase in females stands out. That is coherent with the qualitative remarks produced: Increase in A among the former and increase in W among the latter.

TABLE 1 - Finger Prints

SEX	HAND	SAMPLE	W	U	R	A
M	R	V	28.9	55.5	3.3	12.2
		C	37.5	52.3	5.3	4.9
	L	V	20.0	66.3	3.1	10.5
		C	29.7	61.0	3.5	5.8
	R+L	V	24.3	61.1	3.2	11.3
		C	33.6	56.7	4.4	5.3
F	R	V	46.4	50.4	1.6	1.6
		C	30.1	60.4	3.1	6.4
	L	V	45.8	49.2	2.5	2.5
		C	28.7	58.4	4.3	8.6
	R+L	V	46.1	49.8	2.0	2.0
		C	29.4	59.4	3.7	7.5

TABLE 2 - T.R.C. Values

SEX	VITILIGO PATIENTS	CONTROL
M	124.72 $\pm$ 63.98	136.17 $\pm$ 49.58
F	153.29 $\pm$ 45.42	128.18 $\pm$ 47.38

In the study on palms we tackle two characteristics: The frequency in the presence or absence of designs in the five palmar areas jointly per hand and sex -table 3-, and the a-b ridge count equally per hand and sex -table 4-. On these two studies the control -which appears in the respective tables- suited the sample selected for this work.

The differences found in the presence of figures in the palmar areas did not reach a level of statistic sigficance. In males and in females, respectively to the order outlined on talbe 3, we obtained $x^2 = 0.094$; $x^2 = 0.366$; $x^2 = 0.046$; $x^2 = 0.276$; $x^2 = 0.154$; $x^2 = 0.424$. Sahasrabuddhe et al. (1973) indicated a minor frequency of designs in the thenar area, and l (T/l) in women. Although we did not study areas separately, we noticed a general tendency towards a decrease of figures in this sex. The opposite happens to males, in which appears an increase on the number of figures, except in the right hand.

Conserning the a-b ridge count, the differences among the sample of vitiligo patients and control sample are minimal, and we do not find any special tendency worth pointing out.

We summarized then, according to the present study -on the appearance of particular features in the digital and palmar dermatoglyphics in vitiligo patients- not necessarily coincident in both sexes. The tendencies noticed could be enumerated as follows:

1.- A pronounced increase in the number of A in the digital dermatoglyphics in males and a decrease of the number of W -reaching statistic significance the differences of right hand and both hands. Among women there is a relevant increase on the number of W, with a decrease in the number of the other designs. The differences reach a level of statistic significance on both hands jointly as well as separately.

2.- The T.R.C. has a tendency to decrease in males and to increase in females.

3.- The designs of female palms tend to decrease; and to increase in male's, though without such a pronounced tendency.

Among these mentioned tendencies, the increase of A and the decrease of W in the digital designs among males stand out. This observation coincides with the cited work of Sahasrebuddhe et al. (1973).

TABLE 3 - Palmar Patterns

SEX	HAND	SAMPLE	PRESENCE	ABSENCE
M	R	V	36.6	63.3
		C	38.8	61.1
	L	V	43.3	56.6
		C	38.8	61.1
	R+L	V	40.0	60.0
		C	38.8	61.1
F	R	V	34.4	65.6
		C	37.6	62.4
	L	V	35.2	64.8
		C	37.6	62.4
	R+L	V	34.8	65.2
		C	37.6	62.4

TABLE - a-b Ridge Count

SEX	HAND	VITILIGO PATIENTS	CONTROL
M	R	37.55 ± 6.52	37.44 ± 4.68
	L	38.17 ± 5.97	39.44 ± 3.89
	R+L	75.72 ± 12.17	76.89 ± 6.81
F	R	42.44 ± 4.74	41.32 ± 5.49
	L	42.12 ± 4.48	42.72 ± 5.84
	R+L	84.96 ± 8.24	84.04 ± 10.67

References

Bader PL, Diegel A, Epinette WW, Nance WE (1975). Vitiligo and dysgammaglobulinemia. A case report and family study. Clin Genet 7:62.

Carter MD, Jegasothy BV (1976). Alopecia areata. Arch Dermatol 112:1397.

Cauwenberghe D (1958). Vitiligo dans 3 générations. Arch belges de Dermatol 14:115.

Cummins H, Midlo Ch (1961). "Finger Prints, Palms and Soles: An Introduction to Dermatoglyphics." N. York: Dover Publications, Inc.

Gates RR (1948). "Human Genetics." N. York: McMillan Co., Vol. I, p 295.

Genov D, Bozhkov B, Zlatkov NB (1972). Copper pathochemistry in vitiligo. Clin Chim Acta 37:207.

Goncalves A (1976). Vitiligo familiar averiguado em quatro generacoes. An bras Dermatol 51:109.

Gorl L (1934). Vitiligo, alopecia areata. Dermatologische Wochenschrift 98:58.

Kolski R, Scazzocchio C (1961). Estudio de la frecuencia de caracteres dermopapilares en nuestra población. Rev Fac Hum Cienc (Montevideo) 22:221

Lerner AB (1959). Vitiligo. Jour Inv Dermatol 32:285.

Mayenburg J, Vogt HJ, Ziegelmayer G (1976). Vitiligo bei einem Eineiigenzwillingspaar. Hautarzt Deutchland 27:426.

Newbold PCH (1973). The skin in genetically-controlled metabolic disorders. Jour Med. Genet 10:101.

Oyhenart-Perera MF (1977). Contribución al estudio de los dermatoglifos digitales de la población de Montevideo (Uruguay). I Caracteres cuantitativos. Rev Biol Uruguay 5:47

Oyhenart-Perera MF, Kolski R (1980). Vitiligo: Contribución al conocimiento de su herencia. Actas dermo-sifiliográficas 71:383.

Penrose LS (1968). Memorandum on Dermatoglyphic Nomenclature. Birth Defects Original Article Series, June.

Sahasrabuddhe RG, Agrawal SP, Singh G (1973). Dermatoglyphic patterns in patients of vitiligo. IDA News Bulletin 2:16.

Silvers SH, Glickman FS (1970). Familial vitiligo. Cutis (N. York) 618:875.

Thumon TF, Jackson J, Fowler CG (1975). Deafness and vitiligo. Birth Defects Conference, Kansas City, Missouri.

Vogel F, Dorn H (1966). Vitiligo. In Becker PE (ed.): "Genética Humana." Barcelona: Toray.

Progress in Dermatoglyphic Research, pages 435–449

THE DERMATOGLYPHICS OF JEWISH XXY KLINEFELTER'S AND X TURNER'S PATIENTS.

M. BAT-MIRIAM KATZNELSON, Ph.D.

Dept. of Human Genetics, Tel-Aviv University
Medical School
Institute of Genetics, The Sheba Medical Center,
Tel-Hashomer, Israel

In a study of finger print patterns, Sachs and Bat-Miriam (1957) found that normal Jewish males had on the average more whorls and fewer loops than normal European males. These findings held true for each of the nine major Jewish communities as well as for one Arab community. Subsequent analysis (Katznelson and Ashbel, 1973) have shown that the average total ridge counts of Jews, both males and females, are significantly higher than those of European, namely that in terms of the total ridge count this Jewish excess of whorls more than compensates for the deficiency of loops.

Dermatoglyphic studies of patients with sex chromosomal aneuploidy which were done predominantly among populations of non-Jewish origin have shown that these conditions greatly affect the total ridge count. For example, patients with the 47,XXY karyotype have total ridge counts which are about 25% lower than those of normal males, while the counts of patients with the 45,X karyotype are some 15% higher (Holt and Lindsten, 1964; Penrose, 1967).

It has not been possible to tell whether these quantitative effects of an additional or a missing chromosome were absolute or rather relative.

It was thought that while the same effects of aneuploidy could be expected within Jewish populations, the differences between the respective normal controls might contribute to an understanding of the nature of the effects themselves.

Consequently a dermatoglyphic study of various Jewish aneuploids was undertaken.

The present paper summarizes the findings among 119 Jewish patients with Klinefelter's syndrome and 51 Turner's syndrome.

MATERIAL AND METHODS

The patients with sex chromosome aneuploidy were all Jewish, though from various populations. They were referred to us by the male fertility clinic of our hospital, the sterility clinic and the rest by pediatricians and general practitioners. Each patient went through a thourough medical examination in addition to sex chromatin evaluation of buccal smears and leucocyte culture for determining the karyotype.

200 controls were chosen (100 males and females).

The Faurot Inkless method and the Hollister Foot Printer were used. The prints were analyzed with the aid of a magnifying glass and a disseeting microscope. Dermatoglyphic patterns were formulated according to the rules set out be the Memorandum on Dermatoglyphic Nomenclature (Penrose, 1968) and the useful classification originated by Penrose and Loesch(1969, 1970).

RESULTS

Digital Patterns(Table 1)

The most significant difference between XXY patients and controls is found regarding the frequency of arches. The XXY patients show a significant increase of arches as compared with the male controls (X^2 = 15,68; $p < .001$).

Table 1: DIGITAL PATTERNS FREQUENCY IN JEWS WITH SEX CHROMOSOME ABERRATIONS AND CONTROL

Sex Chromosome Complement	X (N = 51)	XX (N=100)	XY (N=100)	XXY (N=119)
Patterns				
Whorl	32.45	32.20	39.33	43.55
Ulnar Loop	63.21	55.80	52.30	46.41
Radial Loop	3.21	4.90	5.20	2.80
Arches	1.13	7.10	3.20	7.25

There is an opposite tendency regarding the distribution of both radial and ulnar loops: When compared to both male and female controls the XXY patients show a significant decrease in these patterns. There is no difference in the frequency of whorls when compared with male control, even though there is a slight increase. However, when the same comparison is done with female controls there is a highly significant difference regarding all patterns but the arches (Table 4).

The X group showed an excess of ulnar loops and a deficit in arches, radial loops and whorls. The differences of whorls, ulnar loops and arches are statistically significant when compared to male controls. When compared to female controls significant differences exist only for ulnar loops and arches. The findings with **X females** regarding the digital patterns are the opposite of those found for XXY patients.

These results do not agree with previous studies in which there was shown an excess of whorls in the X females (Holt, 1968), but agree with Saldana-Garcia (1979).

Total Ridge Count (Table 2)

The average mean obtained for the XXY Klinefelter's (135 $\pm$ 50.41) is significantly lower than the mean for the male controls ($t = 2.67$; $p < .005$). It does not differ from female controls.

It was postulated by Penrose (1968) that finger pattern size, as measured by the total ridge count is influenced by the sex chromosome complement. Our results indicate that an excess of sex chromosome both reduces the complexity of the digital patterns (by an increase of arches) and consequently reduces the total ridge count. However, it is of interest to notice that in contrast to all previous reports of digital patterns of Klinefelter's from other populations (Alter, 1965), the Jewish Klinefelter's manifest a significant increase in whorls. This increase, however, does not elevate the mean total ridge count, as expected. The high total ridge count obtained for the X females (169.31 $\pm$ 31.86) exceeds significantly that of both male and female controls (Table 4).

As stated by Penrose (1967) a deficit in the amount of X chromosome tends to produce in X females the reverse effect upon the total ridge count than an excess of it. This explains the results of the high total ridge count

Table 2: Frequencies of Palmar Patterns of Jews with Sex Chromosome Aberrations and Controls

Sex Chromosome Complement:

Parameters	X (N=51)		XX (N=100)		XY (N=100)		XXY (N=119)	
	Mean	S.D.	Mean	S.D.	Mean	S.D.	Mean	S.D.
TRC	169.31	± 38.66	138.21	± 49.09	152.	± 39.93	135.24	± 51.03
a-b	86.26	± 16.27	81.43	± 11.15	82.9	± 12.23	75.76	± 11.59
maximal atd	101.46	± 21.03	88.22	± 14.83	89.5	± 18.0	86.36	± 14.23
Ridge width	492.30	± 51.24	507.03	± 47.26	558.	± 46.11	594.73	± 47.0
M.L.I.	16.03	± 3.88	17.60	± 4.02	17.47	± 3.64		
Pattern intensity	1.71		1.96		1.86		1.72	

obtained for the X females without an excess of whorls. However, these loops are undoubtedly large and thus contribute to the big mean of the total ridge count obtained for this group of patients (Table 1).

a-b Ridge Count (Table 2)

The mean a-b ridge count (75.76 ± 11.59) count for the XXY patients is significantly ($p < .001$) lower than for both male and female controls (Table 4). This observation confirms the results obtained by others for British patients and their controls (Holt, 1968; Penrose and Loesch, 1970; Saldana-Garcia, 1979).

The mean a-b ridge count, 86.26 ± 16.27 for X females is significantly higher than both male and female controls. Holt (1968) stated that a reduction of X chromosome material is associated with marked increase in the distance between a-b palmar triradii.

Ridge Width

It was postulated by Penrose (Penrose and Loesch,1970) that the ridge width tends to increase with the number of sex chromosomes. Thus the mean for ridge width of the XXY patients, 594.94 ± 53.33 (Table 2) exceeds significantly that of both male and female controls (Table 4).
Males on the average have a higher value for ridge width, and as it is positively related to body size and stature it reflects on the greater height that males have, on the average, than females. Thus the high mean of the ridge width obtained for the XXY may be a reflection of their increased height.

With the X females the results are quite the opposite. The ridge width for these females is lower than both male and female controls (492.30 ± 51.24). This was observed too by Penrose and others (Penrose and Loesch, 1970; Saldana-Garcia, 1979). Since ridge width is positively related to body size the very low mean of the ridge width for Turner's syndrome (X) is clearly associated with their unusually short stature (Penrose and Loesch, 1970).

Maximal atd Angle

No significant difference was found between the values of the XXY patients and both male and female controls (Table 4).

There is an elevation of the maximal atd angle in Turner's patients X (101.46° ± 21.03) and it differs significantly from both male and female controls (Table 4). This observation is well correlated with the high incidence of the various t triradii (Table 4) found in the X females; it differs significantly from both male and female controls.

Palms (Table 3)

The palmar configurations did not show gross deviations from normals. The existing differences between the two groups with sex chromosomal aberrations and corresponding control groups were mainly of quantitative nature.

Table 3: FREQUENCIES OF PALMAR CHARACTERS OF JEWS WITH SEX CHROMOSOME ABERRATIONS AND CONTROLS

Sex Chromosome Complement:	X	XX	XY	XXY
Loops:				
I	4.41	8.5	10	6.92
I^R	8.82	6.0	11	7.14
II	5.88	8.5	10.5	5.46
II	1.47	0.0	0.0	0.0
III	47.06	51.5	50.5	44.95
III	1.47	0.0	0.0	0.0
III^T	2.94	9.5	15.5	9.24
IV	35.29	56.5	55.5	61.34
$\widehat{IV}$	1.47	4	3	1.26
V	26.47	12	12.5	9.66
$\hat{V}$	36.76	27.5	25	29.31
V^R	1.47	2	2	7.14
Triradii				
e,f	11.76	13.5	20	13.8
t	61.76	67.5	76.5	64.71
t'	35.29	36.5	29.5	29.41
t"	20.59	7.5	8	8.82
t^b-t^o	41.18	29.5	22.5	29.41
t^u	1.47	1	2	5.0
z'	10.29	2	0	7.14
z"	7.35	3.5	2.5	7.56

According to Saldana-Garcia (1977) "the patterns in the thenar / first interdigital area (area I) decrease in frequency with increasing number of sex chromosomes, showing the greatest incidence in Turner's and the lowest in Klinefelter's X > XX > XY > XXY". However, the Jews do not conform at all to this observation. The order of incidence of patterns in the area I is XY > XX > XXY > X. Penrose (Penrose and Loesch, 1970) also found that the two groups with sex chromosome aberration have the lowest incidence of patterns in area I.

In area II there was a deficit of loops for both XXY and X patients. There was a definite deficit in the III^{T} of the X females. The XXY Klinefelter's resemble the normal female control. In Turner's there was a deficit of loops in region IV, and an excess of them in area V with corresponding excess of t" and t^{b}, whereas XXY did not show a real difference from the normal controls.

Interdigital triradii indicating a zygodactylous tendency like fusion of a and b triradii (z triradius) was not observed in any group. The z' triradius (fused triradii bc) and z" triradius (fused cd) occurred with high frequency in both groups with sex chromosomes anomalies than in both control groups. This finding is in line with the general observation that zygodactyly tends to occur with greater intensity with sex chromosome errors than on the hands of normals.

Pattern Intensity

Pattern intensity is measured by total number of loops is low when the number of sex chromosomes is altered (Table 2). This observation does not follow the conclusion by others (Penrose and Loesch, 1970; Saldana-Gracia, 1979) that the pattern intensity is low only when the number of sex chromosomes increases.

No statistical difference was found regarding the main line index (A and D). Komatz and Yoshida (1977) reported the same findings for a group of 65 cases of Japanese Klinefelter's syndrome.

Table 4: STATISTICAL DIFFERENCES BETWEEN JEWISH XXY, X PATIENTS AND CONTROLS

	XXY vs.		X vs.	
Parameters	XX	XY	XX	XY
W	****	-	-	****
UL	****	*	**	****
RL	**	****	-	-
A	-	****	****	*
TRC	-	***	**	*
a-b	****	****	**	*
Ridge width	****	***	-	****
atd	-	-	****	****
d	*	-	*	-
e,f	-	*	-	-
III^T	-	*	-	-
IV	-	-	*	*
$V, \hat{V}, V^R$	-	-	**	****
t'				**
t	-	*	****	-
$t^u - t^b$	***	***	-	*
t"	-	-	*	***
z'	-	*	*	-
z"	**	***	-	-
z' - z"			*	**

* $p < .02-.05$

** $p < .01$

*** $p < .005$

**** $p < .001$

Table 5: COMPARISONS OF DERMATOGLYPHIC PARAMETERS BETWEEN JEWISH AND BRITISH X AND XXY PATIENTS

	X		XXY	
	Jewish	British	Jewish	British
W	32.45	26.90	43.55	26.9
UL	63.21	65.80	46.49	62.8
RL	3.21	3.5	2.80	5.8
A	1.13	2.9	7.25	4.4
TRC	169.31 ± 38.66	169.3 ± 41.6	135.24 ± 50.41	117.8 ± 41.9
a-b	86.26 ± 16.27	95.7 ± 11.9	75.76 ± 11.59	80.3 ± 11.5
Maximal atd	101.46 ± 21.03	105.2 ± 23.4	86.33 ± 14.23	84.8 ± 12.9
Ridge width	492.30 ± 51.24	486. ± 51.24	594.73 ± 47	587. ± 50.
MLI	16.03 ± 3.89		17.38 ± 3.41	

DISCUSSION

The analysis of dermatoglyphic parameters of Jewish and British normal population differ significantly in a number of digital and palmar traits (Katznelson Bat-Miriam and Ashbel, 1973), the trends being identical in both males and females. The most ethnic difference is in the presence of the abortive C (III^T) in the Jewish sample with a frequency of 12.5% as opposed to its complete absence in the British.

When comparing the differences between Klinefelter's patients and normal males and females in each population the pattern of deviation seems to be different. The Jewish patients (Table 3) differ more markedly from males than from females (8 significant differences).

Table 6: STATISTICAL DIFFERENCES BETWEEN BRITISH XXY AND X PATIENTS AND CONTROLS

	XXY vs.		X vs.	
Parameters	XX	XY	XX	XY
W	-	-	-	-
UL	-	-	-	-
RL	-	-	-	-
A	-	-	-	***
TRC	-	**	***	-
a-b	-	***	***	***
Ridge width	***	**	***	***
atd	-	-	***	***
V, $\hat{V}$, V^R	*	***	*	*
t'	-	-	***	**
t"	-	-	***	***
z'	-	*	-	*
z"	-	**	-	**

* $p < .01$
** $p < .005$
*** $p < .001$

The British (Table 6) with sex chromosomes anomalies differ more markedly from males (6 significant differences) than from females (2 significant differences). However, the significant deviations involve different parameters in the two populations. Superficially it may seem that these findings would indicate perhaps that the extra X chromosome acts differently in the two populations. But when individual parameters are compared the tend of deviations of the Klinefelter patients seem to be the same in the two populations. The mean total ridge count (Fig. 1) for the XXY patients is the lowest count in each population; but the values for ridge width (Fig. 2) are the highest for the Klinefelter's patients.

When comparing Turner's patients with normal males and females in each population (Table 3) they differ significantly in the same trend from the X patients (13 and 12 significant differences). The British Turner's manifest the same trend, though the actual number of the significant parameters is lower (9 parameters when compared to males and 7 significant parameters when compared to females).

The value for total ridge count (fig. 1) is the highest for Turner's in both populations, while the mean for ridge width is the lowest (Fig. 2) in the two populations. Most parameters studied showed the same phenomenon; namely that the aneupoid patients, irrespective of their ethnic origin, show the same direction of deviation.

These significant findings raise the question whether an extra X-chromosome or its absence, exerts a different type of dermatoglyphic deviation in two populations, or whether it is rather a difference between the two basic respective normal populations which is responsible for these findings. This latter possibility seems more likely both because of theoretical considerations and because the two populations have been known to differ in frequencies of dermatoglyphic traits.

It seems plausible to conclude that the differences between the two groups of patients originated primarily from differences in the respective normal populations, on which these deviations were superimposed in essentially the same direction.

The possibility of an additional, specific influence of either an extra X-chromosome or its absence in specific populations cannot be totally discarded, and should be further investigated on a larger scale.

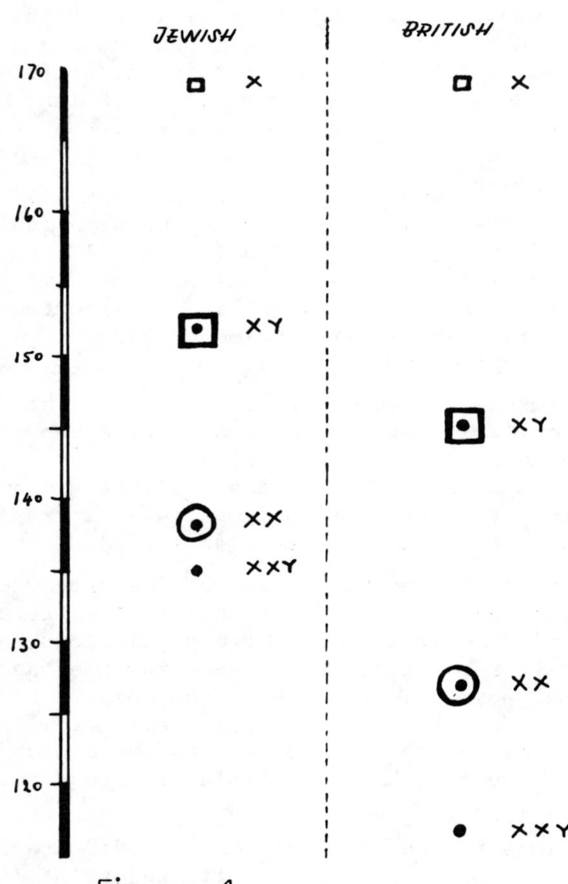
TOTAL RIDGE COUNT
IN
JEWISH & BRITISH
JEWISH
BRITISH
170
160
150
140
130
120
X
XY
XX
XXY
X
XY
XX
XXY

Figure 1.

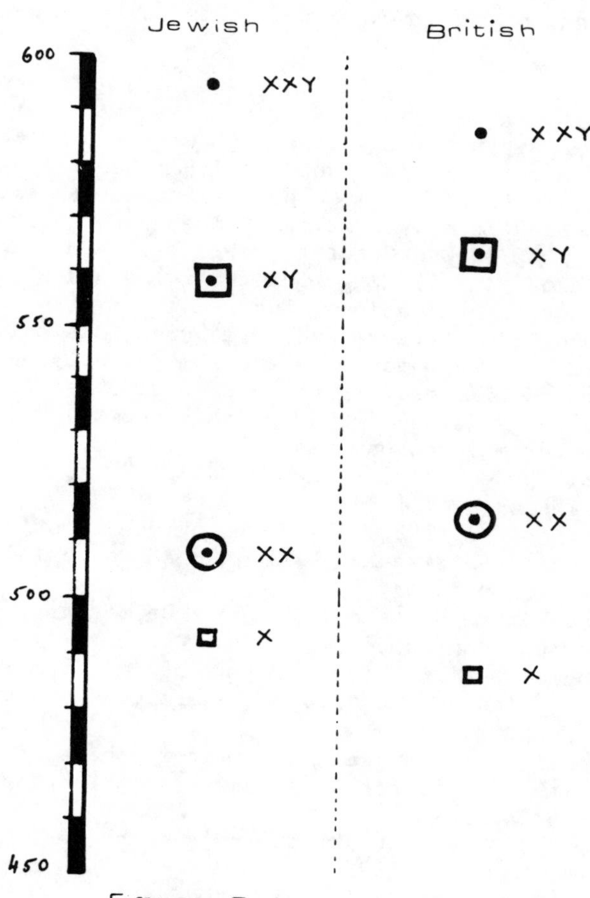
RIDGE WIDTH
in
JEWISH & BRITISH.
Jewish
British
600
550
500
450
XXY
XY
XX
X
XXY
XY
XX
X

Figure 2.

This study has once again demonstrated how essential it is to obtain detailed analysis of normal population for evaluating the significance of dermatoglyphic findings in patients derived from that population.

ACKNOWLEDGMENT

The authoress is deeply indebted to Mrs. R. Grossman whose co-operation and optimism made this publication possible.

REFERENCES

Alter M (1965) Is hyperploidy of sex chromosomes associated with reduced total ridge count? Am J Hum Genet 17:473.

Borgaonkar DS, Mules E (1970) Comments of patients with sex chromosome aneuploidy: Dermatoglyphics, parental ages, Xg^{a} blood group. J Med Genet 1:345.

Cummins H, Midlo C (1961)"Fingerprints, Palms and Soles". New York: Dover Publications, Inc.

Forbes AP (1964) Fingerprints and palm prints and palmar flexion creases in gonadal dysgenesis, pseudohypoparathyroidism and Klinefelter synd. New Engl J Med 270:1268.

Holt SB, Lindsten J (1964) Dermatoglyphic anomalies in Turner's syndrome. Ann Hum Genet 28:87.

Holt SB (1968)"The Genetics of Dermal Ridges". Springfield Illinois: Thomas.

Hreczko TA, Sigmon BA (1980) The dermatoglyphics of a Toronto sample of children with XXY, XXYY and XXX aneuploidies. Am J Phys Anthrop 52:33

Katznelson Bat-Miriam M, Ashbel S (1973) Dermatoglyphics of Jews. Z Morph Anthrop 65:14.

Komatz J, Yoshida O (1977) Terminations of palmar main lines and main line indices in 47,XXY Klinefelters syndrome. Jap J Hum Genet 22:28.

Komatz Y, Yoshida O (1978) Palmar dermatoglyphics of the patients with Klinefelter's syndrome (47,XXY). Jap J Hum Genet 23:245

Penrose LS (1967) Finger-print pattern and the sex chromosomes. Lancet 1:298.

Penrose LS, Loesch D (1967) A study of dermal ridge width in the second (palmar) interdigital area with special refernce to aneuploid states. J Ment Defic Res 11:36.

Penrose LS (1968)"Memorandum on Dermatoglyphic Nomenclature" Birth Defects Original Article Series 4. New York: The National Foundation.

Penrose LS, Loesch D (1970) Topological classification of palmar dermatoglyphics. J Ment Defic Res 14:111.
Saldana-Garcia P (1977) A dermatoglyphic study of the thenar/first interdigital area of the palm in females and males with sex chromosomal abnormalities. J Ment Defic Res 21:127.
Saldana-Garcia P (1979) Dermatoglyphics in sex chromosome anomalies. J Ment Defic Res 23:91.

Progress in Dermatoglyphic Research, pages 451-458

DERMATOGLYPHIC FINDINGS IN FAMILIES WITH X-LINKED HYPOHIDROTIC(OR ANHIDROTIC)ECTODERMAL DYSPLASIA(HED)

Alexander Rodewald[§],Prof PhD,and Karin Zahn-Messow,MD[+]

Institute of Human Genetics,University of the land Saar,D-6650 Homburg,and[+]Department of Pediatrics, University of Munich,Federal Republic of Germany

Hereditary hypohidrotic(or anhidrotic)ectodermal dysplasia(HED)is a rare disease characterized by a diminished ability to sweat and by nondevelopment or underdevelopment of certain ectodermal structures,namely,the skin(there may be partial or complete absence of sweat glands,or of sweat pores on the papillary ridges)and its appendages(hypotrichosis),and the teeth(hypodontia,abnormal teeth tending to be conical in shape).Other features include,in the affected males,characteristic facies with prominence of the forehead and depressed nasal bridge,protruding thick lips, and large deformed ears(Lapiere and Dodinval,1967;Messow et al.,1977).Inheritance of the condition is determined by an X-linked recessive gene and the heterozygote carrier mothers of these patients may show some manifestations,such as hypodontia and hypohidrosis.The carrier status cannot be readily recognized clinically.Frias and Smith(1968) and Passarge and Fries(1973)considered that counting the sweat pores on the finger tips is an important means of detecting heterozygote carrier females. Nacata et al.(1980)found that heterozygous female carriers had significantly smaller teeth than did normal controls and a 10-fold increase in the frequency of congenitally absent teeth.Fuenmayor et al. (1981)reported a family with three affected males, in wich in two sisters this severe affection occurs in association with a pericentric inversion of chro-

§ Senior and corresponding author

mosome 9. Concerning this aspect, they concluded that the clinical manifestations of ectodermal dysplasia in the carrier females with the pericentric inversion of chromosome 9 has occurred as a consequence of a non-random (preferential) inactivation of the paternal X chromosome caused by the inversion 9.

Unusual dermatoglyphics in male patients with HED and in carrier mothers were reported by Lapière and Dodinval (1967) and by Verbov (1970). In this comunication we report new dermatoglyphic findings for a family with HED and gather previously published data. The clinical findings for the family members described here are reported elsewhere (Messow et al., 1977).

MATERIALS AND METHODS

Fingertip, palm and sole prints were obtained from a male patient with HED, and from his mother and grandmother (both carriers; Fig. 1). The control group consisted of 552 unrelated healthy individuals (270 females and 282 males) living in Southern Germany.

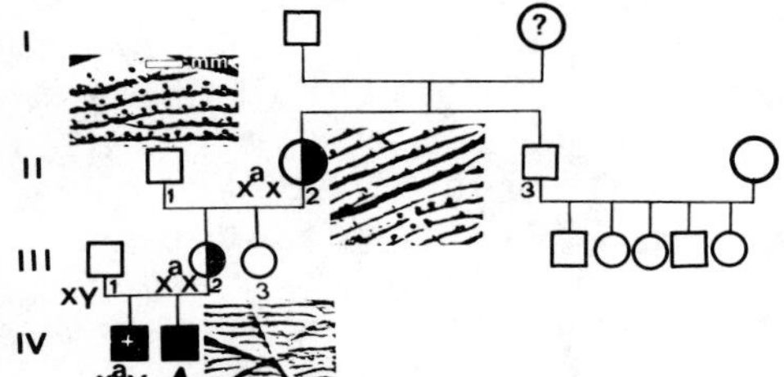

Fig. 1. Pedigree of the family with HED. Notes the absence of visible sweat pores on the ridges in the affected male and the patchy distribution of areas lacking sweat pores in the carrier mothers, and grandmother. x^a=pathol. X-chromosome

Rolled prints were taken using Kleenprint ink and paper and were analyzed according to the methods advocated by Cummins and Midlo (1961) and Penrose (1968). For statistical analysis, the X^2 test and Student's t-test were used, with P=0.5 taken as the limit of significance.

RESULTS

Dermatoglyphic analysis of the palms and soles in the males with HED was often difficult because of the distortion, dysplasia and flattening of the dermal ridges, as a result of the ectodermal defect.

Table 1. Dermatoglyphic findings[a]

Digital patterns

	Left 5	4	3	2	1	Right 1	2	3	4	5	TFRC
Patient	U	U	A	A	U	U	A	U	U	U	73
Mother	U	U	A	A	A	U	A	U	U	U	70
Grandmot.	U	U	A	W	R	U	A	A	A	U	65

Palmar patterns

			S.l.	H.c.
Patient (IV/2)	R:	11 .9.7 .5′–t.t″–L^u.V.V.L^d.V	+	+
	L:	11 .9.7 .5′–t.t″–L^u.O.V.L^d.V	+	+
Mother (III/2)	R:	11 .9.7 .5.–t.t″–L^u.O.V.L^d.O	–	–
	L:	11 .9.7 .5.–t. –A^u.O.O.L^d.V	+	–
Grandmot. (II/2)	R:	11–7.9.5″.4.–t′.t^b–L^c.O.V.L^d.L^d	(+)	–
	L:	9–7.9.5″.4.–t^b –A^r.V.O.L^d.L^d	+	–

Toe patterns

	Left 5	4	3	2	1	Right 1	2	3	4	5
Patient	A	A	A	L^f	A	L^t	L^f	L^f	A	A
Mother	A	A	L^f	L^f	A	L^f	L^f	L^f	A	A
Grandmother	A	A	W^d	L^t	W^d	L^f	L^t	W^d	A	A

	a-bRC	b-cRC	c-dRC	atd angle (right/left)	
Patient	36/40	18/17	31/29	76/79(°)	48/50(%)
Mother	31/31	18/21	30/28	46/35	40/17
Grandmot.	32/33	31/31	34/30	52/-	35/-

Plantar patterns

			p	p′	p″	e	f	hal. cre.	ab-Trir.
Patient (IV/2)	R:	A^f.O .L^d.O.O.	–	–	–	–	+	+	–
	L:	A^f.O .L^d.O.O.	–	–	–	–	+	+	–
Mother (III/2)	R:	l^d.L^p.L^d.O.L^t.	+	–	–	–	+	–	+
	L:	l^d.V .L^d.O.L^t.	+	–	–	–	+	–	+
Grandmo. (II/2)	R:	W^s.O .W^s.O.L^t.	+	–	–	+	+	–	+
	L:	l^d.V .W^d.O.L^t.	+	–	–	–	+	–	+

[a]Nomenclature from Penrose (1968) S.l.=Sydney line
H.c.=Hypothenar cre.

In all the affected individuals, many of the fingertip patterns were distorted, showing numerous "white lines", and some of them were undecipherable. A high incidence of arches on the fingertips was observed in the one patient of Lapière and Dodinval (1967; 7 arches) and in our patient (3 arches). Lapière and Dodinval (1967) reported in the same patient a bilateral simian crease; our patient has a bilateral Sydney line and a hypothenar crease on the palms, and a hallucal crease on the soles (Tables 1 and 2).

The percentage frequencies of the palmar pattern types in patients with HED, their mothers and sisters,

TABLE 2. Fingertip and palmar patterns in members of families with HED (Nomencl. from Penrose, 1968)

Family No.	Patients with HED	TFRC	No. of arches on fingertips	d' Trir. L	d' Trir. R	atd angle° (%) L	atd angle° (%) R	t' trir. L	t' trir. R	Hyp. pat. L	Hyp. pat. R	T line L	T line R	CREASES transv. L	transv. R	hypot. L	hypot. R	halluc. L	halluc. R	Dyspl./Hypopl.	Ridge flatt.	AUTHOR
1.	our ♂	73	3	–	–	79 (50)	76 (48)	+	+	L^u	L^u	13	13	+	+	+	+	+	+	(+)/+	+	Rodewald
2.	III/7 ♂	.	7	.	.	63	68	+	+	–	L^u	11	11	+	+	.	.	.	.	+/+	+	Lapière and Lodinval
3	III/13 ♂	.	.	+	+	80	70	+	+	–	W	11	13	–	–	.	.	.	.	+/+	+	
4.	(A) ♂	.	.	.	.	65	58	+	+	–	–	.	.	.	.	.	.	.	.	+/+	+	Verbov
5.	(B) ♂	.	.	.	.	?	100	?	+	–	–	.	.	.	.	.	.	.	.	+/+	+	
6.	(C) ♂	.	.	.	.	69	61	+	+	–	L^u	.	.	.	.	.	.	.	.	+/+	+	
7.	(D) ♂	.	.	.	.	49	48	–	–	–	–	.	.	.	.	.	.	.	.	+/+	+	
8.	(E) ♂	.	.	.	.	60	60	+	+	L^u	L^u	.	.	.	.	.	.	.	.	+/+	+	
	Mothers of patients																					
1.	our case	70	4	–	–	35 (17)	46 (40)	–	+	–	L^u	13	13	Sl	–	–	–	–	–	–/+	+	Rodewald
2.	II/11	.	.	.	.	.	38	.	–	–	L^u	.	.	.	.	.	.	.	.	–/+	+	Lapière and Lodinval
3.	II/7	.	.	.	.	.	63	.	+	–	W	.	.	.	.	.	.	.	.	–/+	+	
4.	(A)	.	.	.	.	76	66	+	+	L^u	–	.	.	.	.	.	.	.	.	–/+	+	Verbov
5.	(B)	.	.	.	.	80	80	+	+	L^u	L^u	.	.	.	.	.	.	.	.	–/+	+	
6.	(C)	.	.	.	.	60	41	+	–	L^u/L^r	L^r	.	.	.	.	.	.	.	.	–/+	+	
7.	(D)	.	.	.	.	42	60	–	+	–	–	.	.	.	.	.	.	.	.	–/+	+	
8.	(E)	.	.	.	.	40	41	–	–	L^u	L^u	.	.	.	.	.	.	.	.	–/+	+	
1.	Our grandmother	65	4	+	+	–	52 (35)	–	–	A^r	L^c	13	13	Sl	–	–	–	–	–	–/+	+	Rodewald
	Sisters of patients																					
2.	III/8	.	.	.	.	.	50	–	–	L^u	L^u	.	.	.	.	.	.	.	.	–/–	.	Lapière and Lodinval
4.	(A)	.	.	.	.	44	44	–	–	–	L^r	.	.	.	.	.	.	.	.	–/–	.	Verbov
5.	(B)	.	.	.	.	80	45	–	+	L^u	–	.	.	.	.	.	.	.	.	–/–	.	
6.	(C)	.	.	.	.	41	41	–	–	–	L^r	.	.	.	.	.	.	.	.	–/–	.	
7.	(D1)	.	.	.	.	40	40	–	–	–	–	.	.	.	.	.	.	.	.	–/–	.	
	(D2)	.	.	.	.	42	58	–	+	–	–	.	.	.	.	.	.	.	.	–/–	.	
8.	(E)	.	.	.	.	43	45	–	–	–	–	.	.	.	.	.	.	.	.	–/–	+	

Sl. = Sydney line ; L^u = ulnar loop ; L^r = radial loop; A^r = radial arch; W = whorl ; L^c = carpal loop; . = no data; + = present; – = absent *and control individuals differed significantly in some respects(Table 2 and 3). The males with HED had significantly higher frequencies of t'' triradii and of hypothenar patterns(especially of ulnar loops)on the palms than the controls did.The carrier mothers of the patients also had more t''triradii and ulnar loops on the hypothenar than the controls.A high maximal atd angle has been a common finding in affected male individuals and in their mothers(Table3).*

Table 3.Percentages of t''triradii,hypothenar patterns and the means of atd angle in the analyzed groups

	L^u hypoth.		t''trirad.		mean atd angle	
HED pat.	pres.	abs.	pres.	abs.	left	right
N=16palms	37.5	62.5	81.3	18.7	66.4±10.9	67.6±15.6
Mothers N=16palms	50.0	50.0	50.0	50.0	55.5±19.4	54.4±15.1
Sisters N=14palms	21.4	78.6	14.3	85.7	48.3±15.6	46.9± 6.1
Controls N=1104 pa.	9.1	90.9	8.5	91.5	♂=44.0±9.3 ♀=43.3±8.2	45.0± 8.6 45.2± 8.6

L^u on hypothenar				
X^2	HED	Mo.	Si.	Co.
HED				++
Mo.				++
Si.				
Co.	++	++		

t'' triradii				
X^2	HED	Mo.	Si.	Co.
HED			++	++
Mo.				++
Si.	++			
Co.	++	++		

X^2: ++ $P < 0.01$

Mean of the atd angle(right/left)

't'	HED	Moth.	Sist.	Contr.
HED			++/++	++/++
Mo.				++/++
Si.	++/++			
Co.	++/++	++/++		

't': $\alpha < 0.01$; $f > 120$

The carrier grandmother of our patient has 4 arches on the fingertips,an abortive form of simian crease, a t' triradius and a carpal loop on the hypothenar of the right palm,a Sydney line on the left palm,and slight hypoplasia of the dermal ridges.

The digital and palmar imprints of the affected males with HED clearly demonstrated a complete or almost complete absence of visible sweat pores on the dermal ridges. Our male patient with HED had no visible sweat pores on his fingertips,palms,or soles.

The mean pore counts in our patient's mother and grandmother(mean,$\bar{x}$,number of sweat pores per cm of dermal ridge,determined in 10 measurements,5 on the fingertips and 5 on the left hypothenar area) were 16.0 and 17.4,respectively(ranges 7-20 and 8-25,respectively).These mean values are in agreement with those found by Frias and Smith(1968),Passarge and Fries(1973),and Verbov(1970),and are markedly lower than those for 5 normal adult females($\bar{x}$=24.6 sweat pores per cm dermal ridge;range 19-31).Like Passarge and Fries(1973),we found that the sweat pores of the carrier mother and grandmother were distributed patchily,with some areas having a normal number and others entirely lacking sweat pores,but none with an intermediate pattern.The sisters of the male patients with HED reported by Lapière and Dodinval(1967) and by Verbov(1970) had hypoplasia and flattening of the dermal ridges(in 3 cases out of 7),distal dislocation of t triradius(in 3 cases out of 7),and in 2 cases ulnar loops on the hypothenar areas on the palms.

DISCUSSION

This study seems to be the first convincing demonstration of a typical pattern combination in male patients with HED and in the heterozygote female carriers of the HED gene. This for HED characteristical pattern combination include:high frequencies of arches on the fingertips,of t'' triradii,of ulnar loops on the hypothenar areas,of simian creases or Sydney lines on the palms, and wide atd angles.Significant differences from the distributions of all these patterns were found in affected males and female carriers of the gene compared to the control healthy individuals.The analyzis of the number and the distribution of the sweat pores in our two female carriers confirmed the all-or-none mosaic distribution of sweat pores found by Passarge and Fries (1973).This is a good example in man of the effects of the random inactivation of one X-chromosome in an X-linked integumentary genetic marker,that is comparable to those in the mouse(Lyon,1962).

The patchy distribution of areas lacking sweat pores is a finding significant for the detection of heterozygous status for the HED gene,and is valuable for genetic counselling.Distortion,dysplasia,and structural disturbance combined with flattening of the dermal ridges was a common finding in the affected males.The carrier females showed also ridge flattening and ridge hypoplasia(Lapière and Dodinval, 1967;Passarge and Fries,1973;Verbov,1970).

The significance of this characteristic combination of high atd angle values,t'' triradii,and ulnar loops on the hypothenars in the affected males and in female carriers of the HED gene is not clear, but is not surprising,because these patterns are strongly correlated.It is possible that,both for HED male patients and for carrier females,the effect of environmental and/or genetic factors in utero at the time of epidermal ridge formation,on the basis of the Lyon's hypothesis of X-inactivation,could account for this interesting dermatoglyphic findings. Further data are needed,especially concerning the combination of patterns on the soles in HED patients and in carrier females,and special attention should be given to the structure of the dermal ridge,the number and localization of the sweat pores, and the patterning of the sole areas.

REFERENCES

Cummins H, Midlo C(1961).Finger prints,palms and soles.New York,Dover Publications.

Familusi JB, Jaiyesimi F, Ojo CO, Attach ED(1975). Hereditary anhidrotic ectodermal dysplasia.Arch Dis Chilh 50:642.

Frias JL, Smith DW(1968).Diminished sweat pores in hypohidrotic ectodermal dysplasia:a new method for assessment.J Ped 72:606.

Fuenmayor HM, Roldan-Paris L, Bermudez H(1981).Ectodermal dysplasia in females and inversion of chromosome 9. J Med Gen 18:214.

Lapière S, Dodinval P(1967).Dysplasie ectodermique anidrotique chez trois frères et leur cousin germain.Ann Dermat Syphilig 94:477.

Lyon M(1962).Sex chromatin and gene action in the mammalian X-chromosome.Am J Hum Genet 14:135.

Messow K, Götz A, Murken JD, Rodewald A, Riegel K (1977).Ektodermale Dysplasie vom anhydrotischen Typ.-Identifizierung heterocygoter Merkmalsträgerinnen.Z Geburts u Perinat 181:129.

Nakata M, Koshiba H, Eto K, Nance WE(1980).A genetic study of anodontia in X-linked hypohidrotic ectodermal dysplasia.Am J Hum Genet 32:908.

Passarge E, Fries E(1973).X chromosome inactivation in X-linked hypohidrotic ectodermal dysplasia. Nature New Biology 245/141:58.

Penrose LS(1968).Memorandum on dermatoglyphic nomenclature.Birth Defects Orig Article Series 4/No 3.

Verbov J(1970).Hypohidrotic(or anhidrotic)ectodermal dysplasia-an appraisal of diagnostic methods. Br J Dermat 83:341.

AKNOWLEDGMENTS

We wish to thank Prof.Dr.J.-D.Murken MD(Kinderklinik,University of Munich) for his critical reviewing of the manuscript and for comments in this study.

SUMMARY

Data from finger,palmar,and plantar prints of 8 males with X-linked hypohidrotic ectodermal dysplasia(HED),8 carrier mothers, 7 sisters,and 1 carrier grandmother are compared with data from 552 controls. The patients with HED and the carrier females had higher incidencis of arches on the fingertips,of t'' triradii, of hypothenar patterns(especially ulnar loops), and of a transversal direction of the main lines on the palms than the control individuals did. The affected males were also characterized by severe hypoplasia and/or dysplasia of the dermal ridges("ridge flattening"); the carrier females also showed ridge flattening and hypoplasia.

KEY WORDS: anhidrotic ectodermal dysplasia, X-linked,dermatoglyphics, female carriers.

Requests for reprints to Professor Dr. A Rodewald,Institute of Human Genetics,University of the land Saar,D-6650 Homburg,Universitätskliniken Bau 68,Federal Republic of Western Germany.

Subject Index

PROGRESS IN CLINICAL AND BIOLOGICAL RESEARCH

Vol 1: **Erythrocyte Structure and Function,** George J. Brewer, *Editor*

Vol 2: **Preventability of Perinatal Injury,** Karlis Adamsons and Howard A. Fox, *Editors*

Vol 3: **Infections of the Fetus and the Newborn Infant,** Saul Krugman and Anne A. Gershon, *Editors*

Vol 4: **Conflicts in Childhood Cancer: An Evaluation of Current Management,** Lucius F. Sinks and John O. Godden, *Editors*

Vol 5: **Trace Components of Plasma: Isolation and Clinical Significance,** G.A. Jamieson and T.J. Greenwalt, *Editors*

Vol 6: **Prostatic Disease,** H. Marberger, H. Haschek, H.K.A. Schirmer, J.A.C. Colston, and E. Witkin, *Editors*

Vol 7: **Blood Pressure, Edema and Proteinuria in Pregnancy,** Emanuel A. Friedman, *Editor*

Vol 8: **Cell Surface Receptors,** Garth L. Nicolson, Michael A. Raftery, Martin Rodbell, and C. Fred Fox, *Editors*

Vol 9: **Membranes and Neoplasia: New Approaches and Strategies,** Vincent T. Marchesi, *Editor*

Vol 10: **Diabetes and Other Endocrine Disorders During Pregnancy and in the Newborn,** Maria I. New and Robert H. Fiser, *Editors*

Vol 11: **Clinical Uses of Frozen-Thawed Red Blood Cells,** John A. Griep, *Editor*

Vol 12: **Breast Cancer,** Albert C.W. Montague, Geary L. Stonesifer, Jr., and Edward F. Lewison, *Editors*

Vol 13: **The Granulocyte: Function and Clinical Utilization,** Tibor J. Greenwalt and G.A. Jamieson, *Editors*

Vol 14: **Zinc Metabolism: Current Aspects in Health and Disease,** George J. Brewer and Ananda S. Prasad, *Editors*

Vol 15: **Cellular Neurobiology,** Zach Hall, Regis Kelly, and C. Fred Fox, *Editors*

Vol 16: **HLA and Malignancy,** Gerald P. Murphy, *Editor*

Vol 17: **Cell Shape and Surface Architecture,** Jean Paul Revel, Ulf Henning, and C. Fred Fox, *Editors*

Vol 18: **Tay-Sachs Disease: Screening and Prevention,** Michael M. Kaback, *Editor*

Vol 19: **Blood Substitutes and Plasma Expanders,** G.A. Jamieson and T.J. Greenwalt, *Editors*

Vol 20: **Erythrocyte Membranes: Recent Clinical and Experimental Advances,** Walter C. Kruckeberg, John W. Eaton, and George J. Brewer, *Editors*

Vol 21: **The Red Cell,** George J. Brewer, *Editor*

Vol 22: **Molecular Aspects of Membrane Transport,** Dale Oxender and C. Fred Fox, *Editors*

Vol 23: **Cell Surface Carbohydrates and Biological Recognition,** Vincent T. Marchesi, Victor Ginsburg, Phillips W. Robbins, and C. Fred Fox, *Editors*

Vol 24: **Twin Research, Proceedings of the Second International Congress on Twin Studies,** Walter E. Nance, *Editor*
Published in 3 Volumes:
Part A: **Psychology and Methodology**
Part B: **Biology and Epidemiology**
Part C: **Clinical Studies**

Vol 25: **Recent Advances in Clinical Oncology,** Tapan A. Hazra and Michael C. Beachley, *Editors*

Vol 26: **Origin and Natural History of Cell Lines,** Claudio Barigozzi, *Editor*

Vol 27: **Membrane Mechanisms of Drugs of Abuse,** Charles W. Sharp and Leo G. Abood, *Editors*

Vol 28: **The Blood Platelet in Transfusion Therapy,** G.A. Jamieson and Tibor J. Greenwalt, *Editors*

Vol 29: **Biomedical Applications of the Horseshoe Crab (Limulidae),** Elias Cohen, *Editor-in-Chief*

Vol 30: **Normal and Abnormal Red Cell Membranes,** Samuel E. Lux, Vincent T. Marchesi, and C. Fred Fox, *Editors*

Vol 31: **Transmembrane Signaling,** Mark Bitensky, R. John Collier, Donald F. Steiner, and C. Fred Fox, *Editors*

Vol 32: **Genetic Analysis of Common Diseases: Applications to Predictive Factors in Coronary Disease,** Charles F. Sing and Mark Skolnick, *Editors*

Vol 33: **Prostate Cancer and Hormone Receptors,** Gerald P. Murphy and Avery A. Sandberg, *Editors*

Vol 34: **The Management of Genetic Disorders,** Constantine J. Papadatos and Christos S. Bartsocas, *Editors*

Vol 35: **Antibiotics and Hospitals,** Carlo Grassi and Giuseppe Ostino, *Editors*

Vol 36: **Drug and Chemical Risks to the Fetus and Newborn,** Richard H. Schwarz and Sumner J. Yaffe, *Editors*

Vol 37: **Models for Prostate Cancer,** Gerald P. Murphy, *Editor*

Vol 38: **Ethics, Humanism, and Medicine,** Marc D. Basson, *Editor*

Vol 39: **Neurochemistry and Clinical Neurology,** Leontino Battistin, George Hashim, and Abel Lajtha, *Editors*

Vol 40: **Biological Recognition and Assembly,** David S. Eisenberg, James A. Lake, and C. Fred Fox, *Editors*

Vol 41: **Tumor Cell Surfaces and Malignancy,** Richard O. Hynes and C. Fred Fox, *Editors*

Vol 42: **Membranes, Receptors, and the Immune Response: 80 Years After Ehrlich's Side Chain Theory,** Edward P. Cohen and Heinz Köhler, *Editors*

Vol 43: **Immunobiology of the Erythrocyte,** S. Gerald Sandler, Jacob Nusbacher, and Moses S. Schanfield, *Editors*

Vol 44: **Perinatal Medicine Today,** Bruce K. Young, *Editor*

Vol 45: **Mammalian Genetics and Cancer: The Jackson Laboratory Fiftieth Anniversary Symposium,** Elizabeth S. Russell, *Editor*

Vol 46: **Etiology of Cleft Lip and Cleft Palate,** Michael Melnick, David Bixler, and Edward D. Shields, *Editors*

Vol 47: **New Developments With Human and Veterinary Vaccines,** A. Mizrahi, I. Hertman, M.A. Klingberg, and A. Kohn, *Editors*

Vol 48: **Cloning of Human Tumor Stem Cells,** Sydney E. Salmon, *Editor*

Vol 49: **Myelin: Chemistry and Biology,** George A. Hashim, *Editor*